Clinical Neurophysiology in Pediatrics

Clinical Neurophysiology in Pediatrics

A Practical Approach to Neurodiagnostic Testing and Management

EDITOR

Gloria M. Galloway, MD, FAAN

Professor, Department of Neurology
Neuromuscular Division
Ohio State University Medical Center
Columbus, Ohio

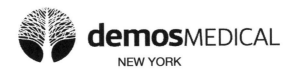

demosMEDICAL

NEW YORK

Visit our website at www.demosmedical.com

ISBN: 9781620700457
e-book: 9781617052118

Acquisitions Editor: Beth Barry
Compositor: Exeter Premedia Services Private Ltd.

Medicine is an ever-changing science. Research and clinical experience are continually expanding our knowledge, in particular our understanding of proper treatment and drug therapy. The authors, editors, and publisher have made every effort to ensure that all information in this book is in accordance with the state of knowledge at the time of production of the book. Nevertheless, the authors, editors, and publisher are not responsible for errors or omissions or for any consequences from application of the information in this book and make no warranty, expressed or implied, with respect to the contents of the publication. Every reader should examine carefully the package inserts accompanying each drug and should carefully check whether the dosage schedules mentioned therein or the contraindications stated by the manufacturer differ from the statements made in this book. Such examination is particularly important with drugs that are either rarely used or have been newly released on the market.

Library of Congress Cataloging-in-Publication Data
Clinical neurophysiology in pediatrics : a practical approach to neurodiagnostic testing and management / [edited by] Gloria M. Galloway.
    p. ; cm.
Includes bibliographical references and index.
ISBN 978-1-62070-045-7 — ISBN 978-1-61705-211-8 (e-book)
I. Galloway, Gloria M., 1960– , editor.
[DNLM: 1. Child. 2. Nervous System Diseases—diagnosis. 3. Diagnostic Techniques, Neurological.
4. Infant. 5. Nervous System Diseases—therapy. 6. Neurophysiology—methods. WS 340]
  RJ486
  618.92'8—dc23
                                      2015014554

Special discounts on bulk quantities of Demos Medical Publishing books are available to corporations, professional associations, pharmaceutical companies, health care organizations, and other qualifying groups. For details, please contact:

Special Sales Department
Demos Medical Publishing, LLC
11 West 42nd Street, 15th Floor
New York, NY 10036
Phone: 800-532-8663 or 212-683-0072
Fax: 212-941-7842
E-mail: specialsales@demosmedical.com

Printed in the United States of America by McNaughton & Gunn.
15 16 17 18 / 5 4 3 2 1

Contents

Contributors

Mark B. Bromberg, MD, PhD Professor, Department of Neurology, University of Utah, Salt Lake City, Utah

Russell J. Butterfield, MD, PhD Assistant Professor, Departments of Neurology and Pediatrics, University of Utah, Salt Lake City, Utah

Mark Eric Dyken, MD Director, Sleep Laboratory, Professor, Department of Neurology, University Iowa Hospitals, Iowa City, Iowa

Ronald G. Emerson, MD Director of Intraoperative Monitoring, Department of Neurology, Hospital for Special Surgery; Professor, Department of Neurology, Weill Cornell Medical Center, New York, New York

Gloria M. Galloway, MD, FAAN Professor, Department of Neurology, Neuromuscular Division, Ohio State University Medical Center, Columbus, Ohio

Aatif M. Husain, MD Professor, Department of Neurology, Duke University Medical Center; Director, Neurodiagnostic Center, Veterans Affairs Medical Center, Durham, North Carolina

Ze Dong Jiang, MD, PhD Professor, Department of Pediatrics, Children's Hospital, Fudan University, Shanghai, China; Senior Researcher, Department of Pediatrics, University of Oxford, Oxford, United Kingdom

Charuta N. Joshi, MBBS, FRCPC Clinical Professor, Pediatric Neurology; Director of Pediatric Epilepsy, Department of Pediatrics, University of Iowa Children's Hospital, Iowa City, Iowa

Nancy L. Kuntz, MD   Associate Professor of Pediatrics and Neurology, Departments of Pediatrics, Neurology, Northwestern Feinberg School of Medicine; Medical Director, Mazza Foundation Neuromuscular Disorders Program, Department of Pediatrics, Ann & Robert H. Lurie Children's Hospital of Chicago, Chicago, Illinois

Jason T. Lerner, MD   Associate Professor, Department of Pediatrics, Division of Pediatric Neurology, David Geffen School of Medicine at UCLA, Los Angeles, California

Deborah C. Lin-Dyken, MD   Clinical Associate Professor of Pediatrics, Division of Pediatric Neurology, Development and Behavior, Carver College of Medicine, University of Iowa, Center for Disability and Development, Iowa City, Iowa

Jaime R. López, MD   Associate Professor, Departments of Neurology and Neurological Sciences and Neurosurgery, Stanford University School of Medicine, Stanford, California

Joyce H. Matsumoto, MD   Health Science Assistant Clinical Professor, Department of Pediatrics, Division of Pediatric Neurology, David Geffen School of Medicine at UCLA, Los Angeles, California

Marc R. Nuwer, MD, PhD   Professor and Vice Chair, Department of Neurology, Reed Neurological Research Center, David Geffen School of Medicine at UCLA; Department Head, Clinical Neurophysiology Department, Ronald Reagan UCLA Medical Center, Los Angeles, California

Theresa Oswald, BS, MS   Instructor in Pediatrics, Department of Pediatrics, Northwestern Feinberg School of Medicine, Chicago, Illinois

Pallavi P. Patwari, MD   Assistant Professor of Clinical Pediatrics, Director of Pediatric Sleep Medicine Program, Interim Chief of the Division of Pediatric Critical Care Medicine, Department of Pediatrics, University of Illinois Hospital and Health Science System, University of Illinois College of Medicine, Chicago, Illinois

Lekha M. Rao, MD   Health Sciences Assistant Clinical Professor, Department of Pediatrics, Division of Pediatric Neurology, David Geffen School of Medicine at UCLA, Los Angeles, California

Zarife Sahenk, MD, PhD, FAAN   Director, Neuromuscular Disease Laboratory, Neuromuscular Division, Center for Gene Therapy, Department of Pediatrics, Nationwide Children's Hospital, Columbus, Ohio

Jorge Vidaurre, MD   Assistant Professor/Director, Pediatric Clinical Neurophysiology Program–EEG Laboratory, Pediatric Neurology Division, Nationwide Children's Hospital–The Ohio State University, Columbus, Ohio

Thoru Yamada, MD, FACNS   Director, Neurophysiology Laboratory, University of Iowa Hospitals, Iowa City, Iowa

Preface

The field of clinical neurophysiology has expanded with the development of new approaches, techniques, and studies over the last two decades. In many cases, new neurophysiologic procedures and interpretations have allowed more accurate diagnosis, aided in diagnosis, and set the gold standard for diagnostic confirmation in numerous neurological disorders. Thus, clinical neurophysiology has grown and increasingly gained respect due to its diagnostic acumen. With this growth has come a wide diversity of subspecialty skills. Each subspecialty lends itself to focused research and, in many cases, clinical certification. In this regard, neurophysiologists skilled in sleep studies, for example, would find themselves unlikely to spend much of their time evaluating complex electromyography (EMG) cases. Pediatric or adult training creates another layer of differentiation so that the interpretation of an electroencephalogram (EEG) in an infant or child differs greatly from that of an adult. A lack of information focused on *pediatric* clinical neurophysiology exists, with most texts written largely with the adult patient in mind. This book uniquely bridges that gap by providing information from a pediatric perspective in various aspects of clinical neurophysiology. Contributors to this book are thought leaders and researchers in their respective fields of clinical neurophysiology. Each has provided discussion in their subspecialty area with a pediatric focus emphasizing diagnostic neurophysiologic techniques. Each chapter emphasizes a different focused area of neurophysiology and brings together the clinical and technical information needed for understanding. Chapters are devoted to pediatric sleep disorders, epilepsy, febrile seizures, and nonepileptic paroxysmal disorders. Other chapters are devoted to pediatric muscular dystrophies, EMG, brachial plexopathies, and peripheral neuropathy. A chapter devoted to intraoperative monitoring is included along with other chapters on evoked potentials and autonomic disorders. In several chapters, multiple authors have contributed, each providing aspects related to their research or area of unique expertise.

This book will serve as an excellent reference for the clinical provider as well as for trainees and technologists in gaining greater knowledge in the various subspecialty areas of clinical neurophysiology.

I want to thank the contributors of this book who, through their passion for the field of clinical neurophysiology, devoted much time to writing and sharing their wealth of information. Additionally, none of the research or clinical data would be possible without the patients who entrusted their care to us. Of course, the time devoted to research and dedication to the field of clinical neurophysiology would not be possible without the encouragement of mentors and the support of our families. My parents' encouragement has been invaluable throughout my life. I dedicate this book to them and to my sons Nadeem and Corey who taught me how deep love can be. Never stop following your dreams, my darlings.

Gloria M. Galloway, MD, FAAN

EEG Monitoring in Neonatal Epilepsies

Lekha M. Rao, MD
Joyce H. Matsumoto, MD
Jason T. Lerner, MD
Marc R. Nuwer, MD, PhD

Electroencephalographers often approach neonatal studies with trepidation. Neonatal studies vary from traditional electroencephalograms (EEGs) in both technical and visual aspects. Half of the full electrode set is used, placed at double distance, and the recording lasts for 60 minutes in order to catch a full sleep-wake cycle. Extra electrodes are also essential for interpreting the recording, such as ocular leads, chin electromyogram (EMG), and cardiac and respiratory monitoring. When interpreting the neonatal EEG, the paper speed is slowed to 15 mm/sec in order to more easily recognize the slower delta frequencies, which dominate in neonatal records. The low-frequency filter is set to 0.5 Hz in order to clearly interpret slow eye movements (1). Sensitivity is often lowered below the standard 7 mv/sec, given that amplitudes are not as high and scalp impedance is lower. Although these differences exist, with experience and knowledge of these EEG differences, interpretation in this age group is readily accomplished.

Much of the trepidation associated with the interpretation of neonatal EEG stems from the fact that "normal" background is somewhat of a moving target. Findings that are acceptable at 30 weeks conceptional age (CA) are grossly abnormal at 36 weeks. Therefore, neonatal EEG is best interpreted by first noting the infant's current CA and then recognizing the characteristics that should be present in the EEG background of a normal neonate. CA is calculated by adding the estimated gestational age at birth to the current chronologic age (in weeks). If not given the correct gestational age, an age range can be estimated based on recognized patterns.

NEONATAL EEG BACKGROUND

Neonatal EEG studies should be systematically evaluated, with interpretation phrased in terms of several key features:

▨ Continuity

▨ Amplitude

▨ Symmetry

▨ Interhemispheric synchrony

▨ Normal named patterns

In extreme prematurity, normal electrographic findings are typically discontinuous, with bursts of continuous cerebral activity separated by intervals of relative quiescence and lower amplitude. This discontinuity improves with age, with the interburst interval becoming progressively shorter and higher in amplitude as the baby approaches full term. By 40 to 44 weeks CA, the EEG background becomes continuous in both wake and sleep (2).

Differentiation between wake and sleep states initially appears around 30 weeks CA. By definition, the infant is awake whenever his/her eyes are open and asleep when eyes are closed. Sleep is further subdivided into active sleep (AS, characterized by irregular respirations, occasional limb movements, and rapid horizontal eye movements) and quiet sleep (QS), characterized by deep, regular respirations and paucity of limb/trunk movement. Electrographically, wakefulness and AS in infants more than 30 weeks CA demonstrate fairly continuous cerebral activity, developing into a characteristic mixed frequency, moderate-amplitude *activité moyenne* pattern.

Because neonatal background abnormalities may become most apparent during deeper sleep stages, a complete assessment of the EEG background requires thorough evaluation of QS. To this end, continuous EEG (cEEG) provides a significant advantage over routine EEG in ensuring that a generous sample of QS is captured for review. As the invariant, nonreactive pattern of burst suppression seen in extremely preterm infants transitions into more defined wake-sleep stages around 30 weeks CA, the final remnants of EEG discontinuity linger in QS. As development proceeds, QS discontinuity gradually resolves, with gradual improvement in the duration and amplitude of the interburst activity. Between 30 and 32 weeks CA, QS activity consists of a *tracé discontinue* pattern in which periods of cerebral activity are separated by nearly isoelectric periods of quiescence with voltage less than 25 μV. With time, the voltage of the interburst intervals gradually increases such that by 35 to 36 weeks CA, QS typically transitions to a *tracé alternant* pattern, in which cerebral activity is consistently maintained above 25 μV but cycles between higher-amplitude bursts and more quiescent periods. The interburst amplitude continues to increase until no periods of relative quiescence are perceived, and a *continuous slow-wave sleep* pattern is fully established around 44 weeks CA (3,4).

Bursts of activity appearing in one hemisphere within 1.5 seconds of the other hemisphere are considered to be synchronous. Prior to 30 weeks CA, cerebral activity occurs nearly simultaneously in both the right and left hemispheres, a phenomenon described as a *hypersynchrony* (5). The reason for early interhemispheric hypersynchrony is unknown, though it has been postulated to be related to prominent thalamic drivers without significant cortical input. Following 30 weeks, occasional asynchronous bursts are seen, which progressively diminish until 100% synchrony is reestablished around 37 weeks CA.

BACKGROUND PATTERNS

A. Excessive sharps

B. Excessive discontinuity

C. Brief ictal/interictal rhythmic/repetitive discharges (BIRDs)

D. Other patterns (depressed/undifferentiated, low voltage)

EEG background findings (Table 1.1) are also frequently employed to assess the functional integrity of the neonatal brain and to aid in the evaluation of neurologic prognosis. At the same time, however, many patterns are nonspecific and of uncertain clinical significance.

TABLE 1.1 EEG Background in Prematurity

CONCEPTIONAL AGE (WEEKS)	MAXIMUM INTERBURST DURATION (SEC)	EEG BACKGROUND FEATURES
24–25	60	No sleep organization or reactivity
27–30	35	Discontinuous in both wake and sleep, some reactivity
31–33	20	Differentiation between active and quiet sleep patterns
		Wake and active sleep: mixed frequency continuous (*activité moyenne*)
		Quiet sleep: interburst intervals amplitude nearly isoelectric, <25 µV (trace discontinue pattern)
34–36	10	Wake and active sleep: mixed frequency continuous (*activité moyenne*)
		Quiet sleep: Interburst intervals increase in amplitude, eventually exceeding 25 µV (trace alternant pattern)
37–40	6	Wake and active sleep: mixed frequency continuous (*activité moyenne*)
		Quiet sleep: Interburst intervals continue to increase in amplitude, increasing continuity (trace alternant) transitioning to continuous slow-wave sleep pattern

Source: Adapted from Refs. 5, 8, 9.

Excessive Sharps

Temporal sharp transients are normally seen during sleep in the term neonate, are often bilateral and asynchronous, and should be surface negative in polarity. If they occur in runs, are unilateral, or appear in wakefulness, they are more likely to be considered abnormal. Sharp waves occurring outside of the temporal or centrotemporal regions would also be considered abnormal. No official criteria exist in which temporal sharps are defined as excessive, and it has been proposed that greater than 13 over the course of a 60-minute recording in a term neonate would be considered excessive [criteria adapted from (6,7)].

Excessive Discontinuity

In the term neonate, periods of attenuation during QS should not exceed 2 to 4 seconds in duration. Interburst intervals longer than this are considered excessively discontinuous. This pattern can be associated with dysmaturity or incorrect gestational dating but can also be a nonspecific marker for neonatal encephalopathy.

Brief Ictal/Interictal Rhythmic/Repetitive Discharges

First described by Shewmon in 1990, this pattern is considered interictal but on the ictal spectrum. It usually occurs in the context of electrographic seizures and is characterized by a run of epileptiform discharges with evolution but lasting less than 10 seconds. Their clinical significance is not yet completely understood, but given their presence in neonates with seizures, they may be associated with neurologic morbidity.

Depressed/Undifferentiated or Low Voltage

A depressed and undifferentiated pattern (Figure 1.1) is most commonly associated with severe underlying neurologic injury to the cortical generators of electrocerebral activity. Low voltage is considered to be background activity persistently less than 10 μV without normal background features. The recording will also show poor reactivity, no alteration in frequencies with external stimulation, and no sleep-wake cycling.

SEIZURE DETECTION

Seizure is the most common neurologic disorder in the neonatal period. There are numerous potential etiologies for neonatal seizures, and timing of presentation as well as electrographic findings can be of potential use in elucidating their etiology. Seizures can be transient due to an acute injury, markers of an underlying genetic or metabolic disorder, or signs of an underlying structural abnormality.

EEG evaluation and confirmation of seizure activity is particularly important in the neonatal population, given the high rate of subclinical or subtly clinical seizures and because newborns may often have unusual movements that can be mistaken for seizure activity. For instance, a systematic video review of 526 electrographic seizures in nine infants revealed that only 34% of seizures were associated with clinical manifestations, and only 27% of these clinical seizures

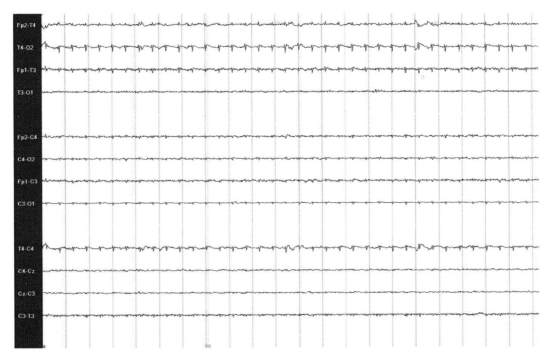

FIGURE 1.1 A 38-week-old baby boy born via emergency Caesarean-section (C-section) for polyhydramnios and nonreassuring fetal heart tracings with severe hypoxic-ischemic encephalopathy. Background shows low voltage (<10 μV) without reactivity.

(9% of overall seizures) were recognized by nursing staff. Of more concern, 73% of "seizures" documented by the neonatal intensive care unit (NICU) nursing staff were not epileptic seizures. Rather, the events marked by NICU nursing were not epileptic in nature. Instead, these movements commonly consisted of likely nonepileptic events such as jitteriness, mouthing, and fisting (10). Therefore neonatal seizure quantification solely by clinical observation is plagued by both high false-positive and high false-negative rates. To ensure an accurate assessment of seizure detection and treatment response, EEG monitoring is essential.

Subclinical Seizures

EEG confirmation of seizure cessation following anticonvulsant treatment is also recommended. Neonates are particularly vulnerable to the phenomenon of electroclinical uncoupling, in which clinical evidence of seizure activity ceases, following the administration of seizure medications, while subclinical electrographic seizure activity continues unabated. Although subclinical seizures are known to occur in critically ill children and adults (11,12), features of chloride homeostasis unique to the immature brain contribute to a high likelihood of electroclinical uncoupling. The potassium-chloride cotransporter (KCC2), which is the predominant type of chloride channel in the adult brain, transport chloride ions outside of neurons and have a hyperpolarizing effect. In contrast, the predominant chloride channel in the immature brain is the sodium-potassium-chloride cotransporter (NKCC1), which transports chloride ions into neurons and has a depolarizing effect. Gamma aminobutyric acid (GABA), a neurotransmitter that activates chloride channels, can therefore have a paradoxically excitatory effect in developing neurons due to the predominance of NKCC1 channels (13). Because the transition from NKCC1 to KCC2 chloride channels occurs in a caudal-to-rostral progression, GABA initially becomes inhibitory in subcortical structures such as the brainstem and basal ganglia while remaining excitatory in the cortex. Commonly used medications such as phenobarbital, which exert their effects through GABA agonist activity, may therefore suppress brainstem motor output, while allowing electrographic seizure activity to continue in the cortex.

The high risk of subclinical seizures has been well documented in the NICU population (14–17). For instance, cEEG monitoring of neonates randomized to initial treatment with either phenobarbital or phenytoin demonstrated that while 24 of 50 infants responded completely to the first seizure medication administered, 15 of the remaining 26 neonates (58%) demonstrated electroclinical uncoupling, with suppression of clinical seizure activity during all or the majority of posttreatment electrographic seizures (18).

Neonatal Seizure Semiology

Seizure semiology in the newborn is variable but can be grouped into the following categories: clonic, tonic, and myoclonic (Table 1.2). These are focal, repetitive, and cannot be suppressed by the examiner. Due to incomplete myelination, infants cannot generate generalized tonic-clonic seizures, but they can have multifocal seizures that can appear generalized to the untrained or inexperienced examiner. Infants can also have generalized epileptic spasms that are hypothesized to be more subcortically driven.

Because infants often have repetitive movements which can be difficult to interpret, EEG is often relied upon to distinguish stereotyped or rhythmic movements as epileptic or nonepileptic. Oral automatisms, bicycling, roving eye movements, and other nonrhythmic but repetitive movements are often seen in critically ill infants. Without clear electrographic correlate, these had been previously termed *clinical only* seizures, but are now more commonly presumed to be

TABLE 1.2 Neonatal Seizure Types

MOVEMENT TYPE	LOCALIZATION/CLINICAL	ELECTROGRAPHIC CORRELATE
Clonic	Focal rhythmic jerking of an extremity	Yes
	Nonsuppressible	
Tonic	Focal sustained extension or flexion of an extremity	Yes
	Not able to overcome with external manipulation	
	Sustained extension of the whole body	Not usually
Myoclonic	Single jerk or multiple nonrhythmic jerks of an extremity	Usually
Spasms	Focal or generalized	Yes
	Flexor, extensor, or mixed flexor-extensor	

nonepileptic in nature. These movements tend to occur more often in encephalopathic infants and are also associated with poor prognosis (19).

Role of Amplitude-Integrated EEG

The use of amplitude-integrated EEG (aiEEG) is now growing in the NICU, because it offers an opportunity for continuous monitoring of cerebral activity in a manner that can be interpreted at the bedside by the neonatologist rather than requiring a certified electroencephalographer. With the growing use of therapeutic hypothermia for hypoxic-ischemic encephalopathy (HIE) in the NICU, aiEEG has become more widely used concurrently in monitoring for seizures and change in background activity.

aiEEG differs from conventional EEG in that it involves the use of only four electrodes and relies on the trending of voltage and comparison between the two hemispheres. The timescale is also broader, with the evaluation of 8 to 12 hours of data on one screen, as opposed to 20 to 30 seconds per screen of a conventional EEG.

Background activity on conventional EEG can be assessed using continuity, amplitude, and symmetry, all of which can also be assessed on aiEEG in a different manner. Interburst interval cannot be precisely interpreted with this method, but voltage over time is averaged in order to give a range of activity, which can then be interpreted. This is tightly linked to amplitude, where the peak-to-peak interval of minimum and maximum voltage ranges is represented as bandwidth. If the minimum voltages are consistently less than 5 µV and maximum less than 10 µV, this is considered a low-voltage, suppressed background. Normal activity is considered to be a minimum voltage of greater than 5 µV and maximum voltage greater than 10 µV.

Seizures are detected on aiEEG as a relative increase in overall amplitude over a given period of time. These can be detected by relative increases of the peak-to-peak amplitude with narrow bandwidth. Some indication of localization can be inferred if this occurs only in one hemisphere. Overall seizure burden can also be inferred, based on the number of peaks of increased voltage peaks. (20)

However, a limitation of condensing this data and relying on voltage alone is that aiEEG can be ripe with artifact. When the baby is handled and high-amplitude electrode artifact is generated, this will appear as an amplitude spike on aiEEG. Similarly, when continuous external artifacts such as EKG rhythm occur in the setting of a low-voltage, suppressed background, this can be misrepresented as a normal voltage range on aiEEG.

aiEEG has been shown in studies to be sensitive, but not very specific for the identification of an abnormal background and seizures (21). Regardless, given the ease of use, the widespread availability, and the ability for bedside interpretation, aiEEG has now become part of the standard of care during therapeutic hypothermia for HIE of the newborn (22–24). Studies have shown that the use of aiEEG may even be beneficial in that neonates are being treated for seizures only with electrographic confirmation, rather than purely on a clinical basis (25).

TRANSIENT OR "BENIGN" NEONATAL SEIZURES

Hypoxic-Ischemic Encephalopathy

HIE is the leading cause of seizures in the neonatal period, with an incidence of 2 to 5 per 1,000 live births. Seizures have been found in up to 80% of this population, but this may be an underestimation, given that continuous EEG monitoring is not routinely used. aiEEG is often used in the NICU to fulfill the need for continuous electrographic monitoring.

Therapeutic hypothermia has also become the standard of care in the treatment of infants with HIE and has been shown to improve neurodevelopmental background. Evaluation of background activity can be useful for prognostication in infants with HIE. Persistently abnormal background activity without evidence of improvement over time is more likely to be associated with a worse neurodevelopmental outcome. A normal background or improvement in background is less likely to be associated with poor neurodevelopmental outcome.

Recent studies have shown a high incidence of seizures in infants undergoing therapeutic hypothermia for HIE, up to 40% to 60%, with 35% to 75% of these being subclinical (26,27) (Figure 1.2). The burden of seizures is highest in the first 24 to 48 hours, with a natural decline after 72 hours (28). It is presumed that a higher burden of seizures is associated with worse neurodevelopmental outcome; however, this is a topic of much debate, as infants with more severe HIE are also likely to have more refractory seizures. Additionally despite advances in antiepileptic drug development, relatively few advances have been made in the treatment of seizures due to HIE, and many treatments also have potential unwanted side effects in the developing brain (29,30).

Benign Familial Neonatal Convulsions

Benign familial neonatal convulsions are often seen around the fifth day of life, giving them the frequently used descriptive term of "fifth day fits." Most are associated with a mutation in the *KCNQ2* gene coding for a voltage-gated potassium channel, which has autosomal transmission, but other potassium channels as well as the sodium channel, such as *SCN2A* mutation, have also been implicated (31). There is often a family history of neonatal seizures, and the electrographic background is frequently normal but can show excessive discontinuity and excessive sharp transients. These were initially termed benign because there was thought to be no long-term consequence, although recent studies have shown that this is not always the case. *KCNQ2* mutations have also been associated with Ohtahara syndrome, and the phenotype can be variable, with seizures persisting well beyond the neonatal period (32,33).

Stroke

Perinatal stroke is also a common cause of neurologic morbidity in the newborn period. The majority are arterial ischemic, although at least 30% can be venous in nature (34). Seizures are a common presentation of neonatal arterial ischemic stroke; up to 72% present with seizures (35). In a neonate with persistently unilateral seizures, arterial ischemic stroke should be strongly considered as an etiology and neuroimaging should be undertaken.

Hypoglycemia and Other Reversible Causes

Neonatal hypoglycemia is a frequent complication of infants of mothers with gestational diabetes, but can also be seen in well neonates with poor feeding. The occipital lobes are particularly at risk because of the high metabolic demand of the visual cortex. Persistent focal seizures can be seen emanating from either posterior quadrant. Imaging can show diffusion restriction in the areas affected, partly due to frequent seizures and increased local metabolism and partly due to watershed ischemia. These areas can later undergo laminar necrosis and develop the appearance of ulegyria.

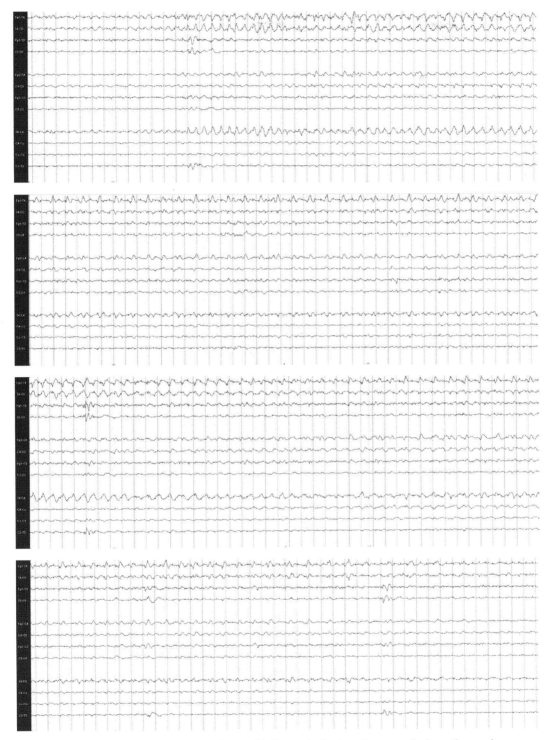

FIGURE 1.2 A 41+1-week-old baby boy with hypoxic-ischemic encephalopathy and meconium aspiration syndrome on selective hypothermia therapy, with seizures starting on the first day of life. This recording shows a seizure starting at T4.

Other electrolyte and metabolic disturbances can also precipitate seizures in the neonatal period, similar to adults. Hypomagnesemia, hypocalcemia, hyponatremia, and hyperbilirubinemia can also lead to neonatal seizures. In these instances, correction of the underlying etiology is necessary to effectively treat the seizures (34).

CATASTROPHIC EPILEPTIC ENCEPHALOPATHIES

There are several conditions presenting in the neonatal period which have been termed "catastrophic," in that they are associated with frequent seizures and severe interictal background abnormalities which, without prompt remedy, almost inevitably result in poor neurodevelopmental outcome (Table 1.3).

Ohtahara Syndrome

Ohtahara syndrome, also known as early infantile epileptic encephalopathy with suppression-burst presents in early infancy. Initial symptoms are seen within the first 3 months, frequently within the first 2 weeks. Clinically this presents with brief (less than 10 seconds) tonic spasms (generalized or focal), which occur independently or in clusters. Other seizure types including focal seizures, hemiconvulsions, or tonic-clonic seizures are seen in approximately 33%. Most cases are related to a variety of structural brain lesions, although metabolic and genetic disorders have been reported. Mutations associated include syntaxin binding protein 1 (STXBP1), Aristaless-related homeobox (ARX), sodium channel SCN2A, and KCNQ2 (36–39).

The typical EEG pattern is a consistent (wake and sleep) "suppression-burst" pattern with periods of diffuse amplitude suppression alternating with bursts of high amplitude spike and polyspike discharges.

Diagnosis of Ohtahara syndrome is based on the clinical picture and EEG findings. The prognosis is poor, with many affected children dying in infancy. Survivors have developmental impairment and many have chronic seizures or evolve into Lennox-Gastaut or West syndrome. Anti-seizure medications are used; however, there is no specific evidence-based therapy known. Surgery has been performed for cases with clear focal lesions (40).

TABLE 1.3 Neonatal Epilepsy Syndromes

EPILEPSY SYNDROME	INTERICTAL EEG BACKGROUND	SEIZURE TYPES
Ohtahara syndrome	Burst-suppression (wake and sleep)	Tonic spasms Focal Tonic-clonic
Early myoclonic epilepsy of infancy	Burst-suppression (more prominent in sleep)	Multifocal myoclonic
Malignant migrating partial seizures of infancy	Multifocal sharps	Focal, arising from multiple regions
Pyridoxine-dependent epilepsy	Continuous spike-wave Burst suppression	Infantile spasms Multifocal myoclonic Focal Tonic

Early Myoclonic Epilepsy of Infancy

Early myoclonic epilepsy of infancy (EMEI) was described shortly after Ohtahara syndrome and there are a number of similarities between them. EMEI also begins within the first 3 years, although it can present as early as a few hours after birth. Clinically this begins with focal myoclonus that can shift between different body parts often in an asynchronous and random pattern. A wide range of focal seizures (anything from tonic posturing to autonomic signs) is very common and tonic spasms are also seen. There is a range of underlying disorders associated with EMEI including structural lesions and metabolic and genetic abnormalities. In contrast to Ohtahara syndrome, diffuse cortical atrophy, rather than focal structural lesions, is typically seen. A variety of metabolic abnormalities have been associated, in particular, non-ketotic hyperglycinemia (41). Mutation of the v-erb-a erythroblastic leukemia viral oncogene homologue 4 (ErbB4), which is associated with cortical migration, is also related (42).

The typical EEG pattern of EMEI is similar to the suppression-burst pattern seen in Ohtahara syndrome; however, in EMEI the suppression-burst pattern is not continuous and occurs more prominently (or exclusively) in sleep. The myoclonic seizures are not generally associated with changes on the EEG.

EMEI is also diagnosed clinically and treated with antiseizure medications. Additionally treatment of the underlying metabolic disorder may be helpful. The prognosis of EMEI is also very poor, with 50% of patients dying by 3 years and the survivors having severe developmental impairment (40).

Malignant Migrating Partial Seizures of Infancy

Malignant migrating partial seizures of infancy (MMPSIs) present in the first 6 months of life with multifocal, bilateral, independent seizures. Seizures are very difficult to control and are associated with progressive developmental impairment and a decrease in the head circumference. The underlying etiology is unknown; however, it is likely genetic. Mutations have been found in a number of genes including *SCN1A*, phospholipase C beta 1 (*PLCB1*), *KCNT1*, and *TBC1D24*.

The ictal EEG shows focal seizures initiating from different locations in both hemispheres that "migrate" from one area to another (Figure 1.3).

MMPSI is diagnosed by clinical presentation along with the typical EEG pattern and has a poor prognosis. Status epilepticus is common and may be related to patients dying in the first 2 years of life (43).

OTHER EPILEPSY SYNDROMES PRESENTING IN NEONATES

Hemimegalencephaly (HME) is a severe developmental brain anomaly characterized by the overgrowth of one hemisphere. This is associated with epilepsy, psychomotor retardation, and contralateral motor defect. Seizure types include focal motor seizures, asymmetric tonic or clonic seizures, and epileptic spasms. HME is one of the causes of Ohtahara syndrome (Figure 1.4) and West syndrome and is associated with a variety of genetic abnormalities and neurocutaneous syndromes; however; it may be an isolated syndrome.

Patients with West syndrome associated with HME may have a unique EEG background called hemihypsarrhythmia (high amplitude, poorly organized with multifocal spikes over the affected side only) (Figure 1.4).

(*text continues on page 16*)

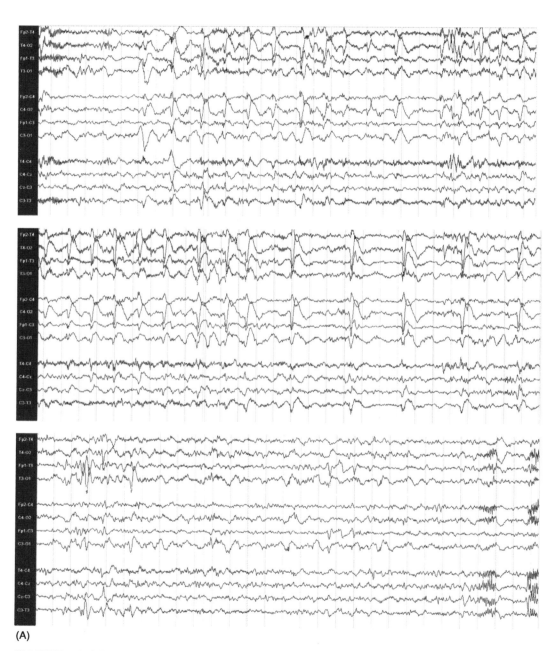

(A)

FIGURE 1.3 (A) A 40+1-week-old baby boy with seizures starting on the first day of life, consisting of clonic movements of any extremity. This shows a seizure over the right posterior quadrant. (*continued*)

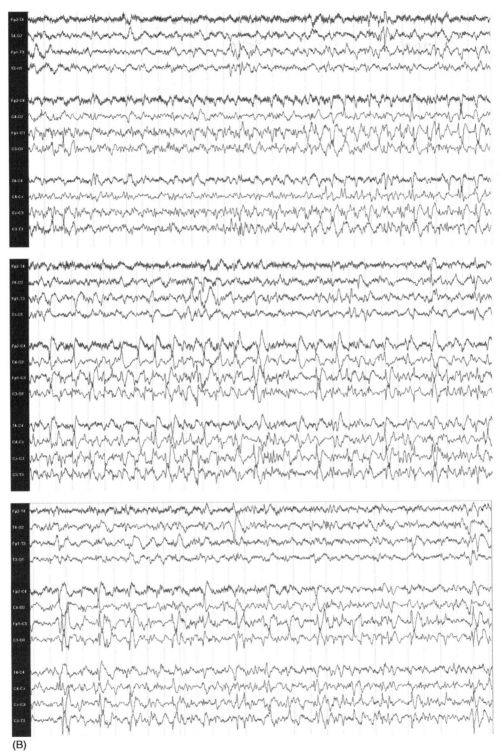

(B)

FIGURE 1.3 (*continued*) (B) Seizures arose from all electrodes, often with a new seizure emerging amidst the existing seizure at a noncontiguous electrode. This demonstrates seizures occurring independently at C3 and C4, as evidenced by nonsynchronous frequencies. (*continued*)

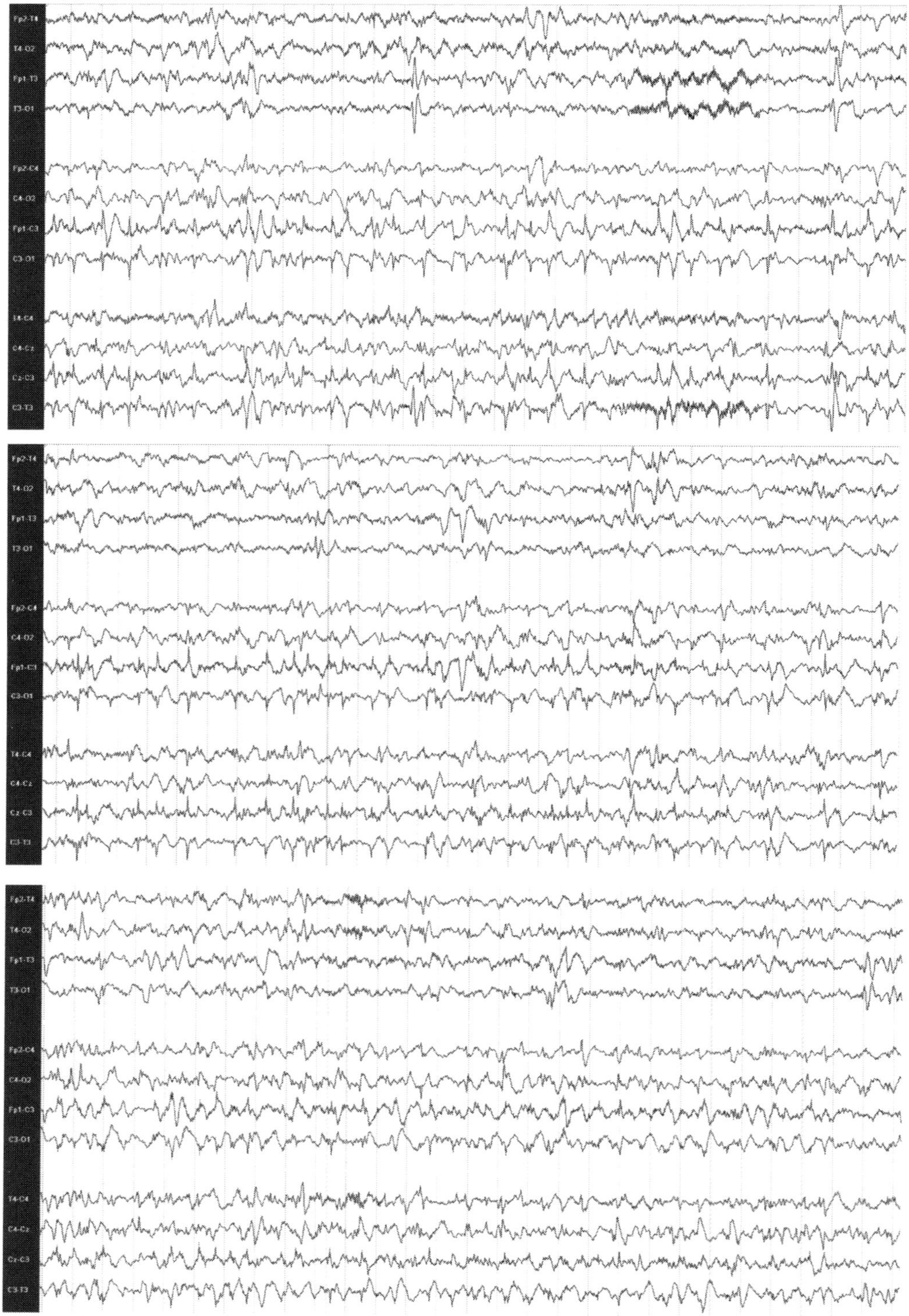

(B) (*continued*)

FIGURE 1.3 (*continued*)

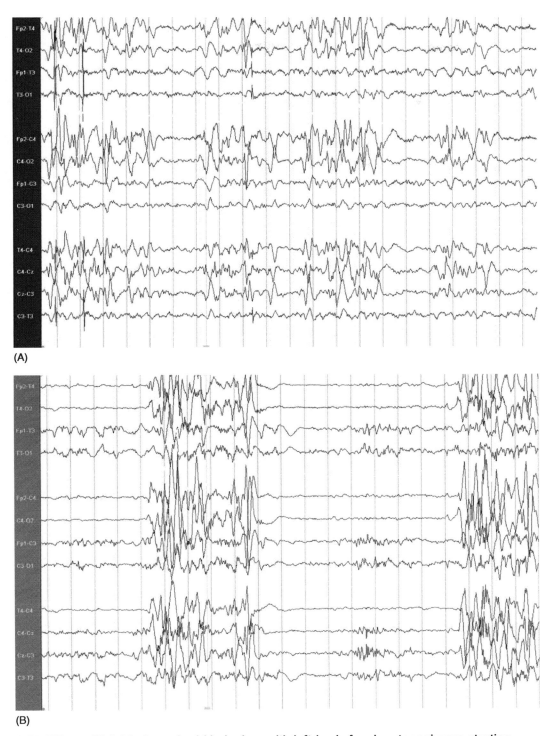

(A)

(B)

FIGURE 1.4 (A) A 38+6-week-old baby boy with left-body focal motor seizures starting day of life 1, found to have right hemimegalencephaly. This background in wakefulness demonstrates epileptiform discharges over the right hemisphere. (B) In sleep, the background is discontinuous with excessive discontinuity more prominent over the right hemisphere. (*continued*)

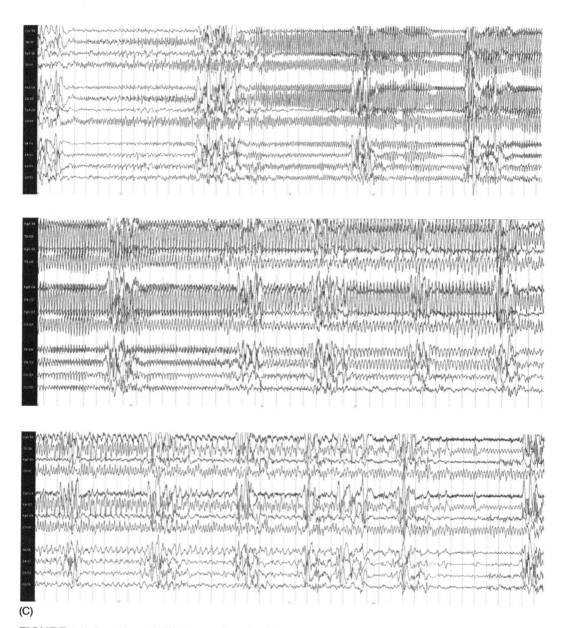

(C)

FIGURE 1.4 (*continued*) (C) The patient had focal left-body tonic seizures, as demonstrated here with a buildup of sharply contoured alpha over the occipital region, which then spreads anteriorly and builds in amplitude. (*continued*)

Diagnosis of HME is based on imaging including asymmetry of the hemispheres and ventricles, loss of gray-white differentiation, neuronal heterotopia, thick cortex, and abnormalities in the gyri, basal ganglia, and internal capsule. The clinical course and prognosis is dependent on seizure control, the severity of the affected side, the ability of the contralateral side to compensate, and early surgery (44).

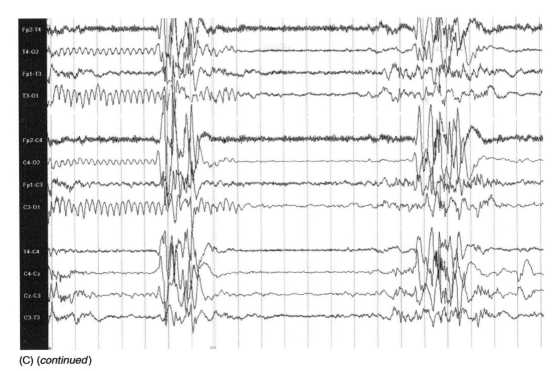

(C) (*continued*)

FIGURE 1.4 (*continued*)

METABOLIC EPILEPSIES

Pyridoxine-dependent epilepsy was first described by Hunt and colleagues in 1954. This syndrome is unique in that it is severe but treatable, and thus early recognition is of tantamount importance. This syndrome has an estimated birth incidence between 1:400,000 and 1:750,000. Seizures can be prenatal in onset and can include multiple seizure types, including infantile spasms and focal, multifocal myoclonic, and tonic seizures. There can also be an associated encephalopathy, which may manifest as tremulousness, irritability, or hypothermia. The baseline EEG will show a continuous spike-wave or burst-suppression pattern. Diagnosis is established by giving an intravenous dose of 100-mg pyridoxine during EEG monitoring, which will often lead to the resolution of epileptiform activity and improvement of the background (Figure 1.5). The response is often seen rapidly, although delayed responses have also been reported. Relapses can occur after a median of 9 days if pyridoxine therapy is withheld, and therefore patients need to remain on lifelong therapy (45).

Folinic acid–responsive seizures are another treatable cause of neonatal seizures. EEG background features and seizure types can be similar to pyridoxine-dependent seizures, and concurrent pyridoxine dependency can occur within individuals. Seizures respond to 2.5- to 5-mg folinic acid given twice daily, and daily doses should be added for patients with an incomplete response to pyridoxine treatment.

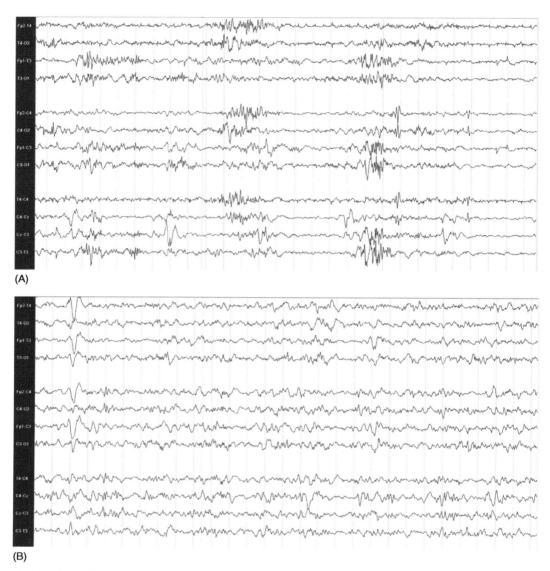

FIGURE 1.5 (A) A 40+5–week-old baby boy who presented with "jitteriness" and episodes of flexor spasms 3 hours after birth. Initial background was discontinuous and asynchronous. (B) After pyridoxine administration, the background normalized, becoming synchronous and continuous.

REFERENCES

1. American Clinical Neurophysiology Society. Guideline two: minimum technical standards for pediatric electroencephalography; 2006. http://www.acns.org/pdf/guidelines/Guideline-2.pdf. Accessed March 12, 2015.
2. Ellingson RJ, Dutch SJ, McIntire MS. EEG's of prematures: 3–8 year follow-up study. *Dev Psychobiol.* 1974;7(6):529–538.
3. Clancy R, Berggvist AC, Dlugos D. Neonatal encephalography. In: Ebersole JS, Pedley T, eds. *Current Practice of Clinical Electroencephalography.* 3rd ed. Philadelphia, PA: Lippincott Williams & Wilkins; 2003:160–234.

4. Vecchierini MF, Andre M, d'Allest AM. Normal EEG of premature infants born between 24 and 30 weeks gestational age: terminology, definitions and maturation aspects. *Neurophysiol Clin.* 2007;37:311–323.
5. Vecchierini MF, d'Allest AM, Verpillat P. EEG patterns in 10 extreme premature neonates with normal neurological outcome: qualitative and quantitative data. *Brain Dev.* 2003;25:330–337.
6. Tsuchida TN, Hahn CD, Riviello JJ, et al. ACNS standardized EEG terminology and categorization for the description of continuous EEG monitoring in neonates: report of the American Clinical Neurophysiology Society Critical Care Monitoring Committee. *J Clin Neurophysiol.* 2013;30(2):161–173.
7. Mizrahi EM, Hrachovy RA, Kellaway P, et al. Patterns of uncertain diagnostic significance. In: *Atlas of Neonatal Electroencephalography.* 3rd ed. Philadelphia, PA: Lippincott Williams & Wilkins; 2004:93–115.
8. Hahn JS, Monyer H, Tharp BR. Interburst interval measurements in the EEGs of premature infants with normal neurological outcome. *Electroencephalogr Clin Neurophysiol.* 1989;73:410–418.
9. Selton D, Andre M, Hascoët JM. Normal EEG in very premature infants: reference criteria. *Clin Neurophysiol.* 2000;111:2116–2124.
10. Murray DM, Boylan GB, Fitzgerald AP, et al. Persistent lactic acidosis in neonatal hypoxic-ischaemic encephalopathy correlates with EEG grade and electrographic seizure burden. *Arch Dis Child Fetal Neonatal Ed.* 2008;93:183–186.
11. Abend NS, Arndt DH, Carpenter JL, et al. Electrographic seizures in pediatric ICU patients: cohort study of risk factors and mortality. *Neurology.* 2013;81(4):383–391.
12. Glass HC, Wusthoff CJ, Shellhaas RA, et al. Risk factors for EEG seizures in neonates treated with hypothermia: a multicenter cohort study. *Neurology.* 2014;82(14):1239–1244.
13. Staley K, Smith R. A new form of feedback at the $GABA_A$ receptor. *Nat Neurosci.* 2001;4(7):674–676.
14. Nash KB, Bonifacio SL, Glass HC, et al. Video-EEG monitoring in newborns with hypoxic-ischemic encephalopathy treated with hyporthermia. *Neurology.* 2011;76:556–562.
15. Lynch NE, Stevenson NJ, Livingstone V, et al. The temporal evolution of electrographic seizure burden in neonatal hypoxic ischemic encephalopathy. *Epilepsia.* 2012;53(3):549–557.
16. Glass HC, Glidden D, Jeremy RJ, et al. Clinical neonatal seizures are independently associated with outcome in infants at risk for hypoxic-ischemic brain injury. *J Pediatr.* 2009;155(3):318–323.
17. Yap V, Engel M, Takenouchi T, Perlman JM. Seizures are common in term infants undergoing head cooling. *Pediatr Neurol.* 2009;41(5):327–331.
18. Scher MS, Alvin J, Gaus L, et al. Uncoupling of EEG-clinical neonatal seizures after antiepileptic drug use. *Pediatr Neurol.* 2003;28(4):277–280.
19. Mizrahi EM, Kellaway P. Characterization and classification of neonatal seizures. *Neurology.* 1987;37(12):1837–1844.
20. El-Dib M, Chang T, Tsuchida TN, Clancy RR. Amplitude-Integrated Electroencephalography in Neonates. *Pediatr Neurol.* 2009;41(5):315–326.
21. Evans E, Koh S, Lerner JT, et al. Accuracy of amplitude integrated EEG in a neonatal cohort. *Arch Dis Child Fetal Neonatal Ed.* 2010;95(3):F169–F173.
22. Shankaran S, Pappas A, McDonald SA, et al. Predictive value of an early amplitude integrated electroencephalogram and neurologic examination. *Pediatrics,* 2011;128:e112–e120.
23. Sarkar S, Barks JD, Bhagat I, Donn SM. Effects of therapeutic hypothermia on multiorgan dysfunction in asphyxiated newborns: whole-body cooling versus selective head cooling. *J Perinatol.* 2009;29:558–563.
24. Shah PS. Hypothermia: a systematic review and meta-analysis of clinical trials. *Semin Fetal Neonatal Med.* 2010;15(5):238–246.
25. Shellhaas RA, Barks AK. Impact of amplitude-integrated electroencephalograms on clinical care for neonates with seizures. *Pediatr Neurol.* 2012;46:32–35.
26. Glass HC, Kan J, Bonifacio SL, Ferriero DM. Neonatal seizures: treatment practices among term and preterm infants. *Pediatr Neurol.* 2012;46:111–115.
27. Abend NS, Gutierrez-Colina AM, Monk HM, et al. Levetiracetam for treatment of neonatal seizures. *J Child Neurol.* 2011;26(4):465–470.
28. Lynch NE, Stevenson NJ, Livingstone V, et al. The temporal evolution of electrographic seizure burden in neonatal hypoxic ischemic encephalopathy. *Epilepsia.* 2012;53(3):549–557.

29. Bittigau P, Sifringer M, Genz K, et al. Antiepileptic drugs and apoptotic neurodegeneration in the developing brain. *Proc Natl Acad Sci USA*. 2002;99(23):15089–15094.
30. Painter MJ, Scher MS, Stein AD, et al. Phenobarbital compared with phenytoin for the treatment of neonatal seizures. *N Engl J Med*. 1999;341(7):485–489.
31. Zara F, Specchio N, Striano P, et al. Genetic testing in benign familial epilepsies of the first year of life: clinical and diagnostic significance. *Epilepsia*. 2013;54(3):425–436.
32. Weckhuysen S, Mandelstam S, Suls A, et al. *KCNQ2* encephalopathy: emerging phenotype of a neonatal epileptic encephalopathy. *Ann Neurol*. 2012;71:15–25.
33. Kato M, Yamagata T, Kubota M, et al. Clinical spectrum of early onset epileptic encephalopathies cause by *KCNQ2* mutation. *Epilepsia*, 2013;54(7):1282–1287.
34. Ferriero DM. Neonatal brain injury. *N Engl J Med*. 2004;351:1985–1995.
35. Kirton A, Armstrong-Wells J, Chang T, et al. Symptomatic neonatal arterial ischemic stroke: the international pediatric stroke study. *Pediatrics*. 2011;128(6):e1402–e1410.
36. Fullston T, Brueton L, Willis T, et al. Ohtahara syndrome in a family with an ARX protein truncation mutation. *Eur J Hum Genet*. 2010;18(2):157–162.
37. Nakamura K, Kato M, Osaka H, et al. Clinical spectrum of SCN2A mutations expanding to Ohtahara syndrome. *Neurology*. 2013;81(11):992–998.
38. Saitsu H, Kato M, Shimono M, et al. Association of genomic deletions in the STXBP1 gene with Ohtahara syndrome. *Clin Genet*. 2012;81(4):399–402.
39. Saitsu H, Kato M, Koide A, et al. Whole exome sequencing identifies KCNQ2 mutations in Ohtahara syndrome. *Ann Neurol*. 2012;72(2):298–300.
40. Beal JC, Cherian K, Moshe SL. Early-onset epileptic encephalopathies: Ohtahara syndrome and early myoclonic encephalopathy. *Pediatr Neurol*. 2012;47:317–323.
41. Wang PJ, Lee WT, Hwu WL, et al. The controversy regarding diagnostic criteria for early myoclonic encephalopathy. *Brain Dev*. 1998;20(7):530–535.
42. Backx L, Ceulemans B, Vermeesch JR, et al. Early myoclonic encephalopathy caused by a disruption of the neuregulin-1 receptor ErbB4. *Eur J Hum Genet*. 2009;17(3):378–382.
43. DeFilippo MR, Rizzo F, Marchese G, et al. Lack of pathogenic mutations in six patients with MMPSI. *Epilepsy Res*. 2014;108:340–344.
44. Honda R, Kaido T, Sugai K, et al. Long-term developmental outcome after early hemispherectomy for hemimegalencephaly in infants with epileptic encephalopathy. *Epilepsy Behav*. 2013;29:30–35.
45. Pearl PL. New treatment paradigms in neonatal metabolic epilepsies. *J Inherit Metab Dis*. 2009;32:204–213.

Pediatric Febrile Seizures

Charuta N. Joshi, MBBS, FRCPC
Thoru Yamada, MD, FACNS

In this chapter, we discuss the basics of febrile seizures and the controversies pertaining to them and provide insights into the understanding of these seizures from the Consequences of Prolonged Febrile Seizures in Childhood (FEBSTAT) study.

Febrile seizures are generally defined as seizures occurring in the presence of a fever higher than 100.4°F in the absence of central nervous system infection, metabolic disturbance, or a previous history of afebrile seizures (1). These are the most common types of convulsive events in infants and young children under 5 years of age and remain the most common childhood neurological emergency affecting 2% to 5% of children. The typical age of the occurrence is between 3 months and 5 years with a peak incidence at 9 to 20 months. The prevalence is 3% to 7% in children up to 7 years, with the above range due to the variability in definition and inclusion criteria in different settings (2). Febrile seizures are classified as simple or complex (Table 2.1) (3). Febrile status epilepticus is a febrile seizure lasting more than 30 minutes and is an extreme form of a complex febrile seizure. It constitutes 5% of febrile seizures (4) and contributes to 25% to 30% of pediatric status epilepticus (5).

ETIOLOGY

Febrile seizures are thought to be an age-specific phenomenon. These are genetically and environmentally modified (6). Febrile seizures are more common in monozygotic (7) than dizygotic twins (9%–22% versus 11%), and by linkage analysis, several loci have been associated with febrile seizures (FEB 1–FEB 11) (8). Some of these, among other loci, are on chromosome 8q13-q21 (FEB1), 19p (FEB2), 2q23-q24 (FEB3 or SCN1A,), 5q14-q15 (FEB4), 6q22-q24 (FEB5), 18p11 (FEB6), 21q22, 5q31.1-q33.1, 3p24.2-p23, and 19q13.1 (SCN1B). These genes encode for various proteins, which are involved in the electrical activity of

TABLE 2.1 Classification of Febrile Seizures

FEBRILE SEIZURE TYPE	DURATION	TYPE OF SEIZURE	RECURRENCE IN 24 HOURS
Simple	<15 min	Generalized	None
Complex	>15 min	Focal	> once

neurons, such as sodium channels (SCN1A/SCN1B) or the receptors for the transmitter gamma-aminobutyric acid (GABRG2 in the region 5q34). These genes are also frequently affected in other febrile seizure–related epileptic syndromes, such as generalized epilepsy with febrile seizures plus (GEFS+) and severe infantile myoclonic epilepsy (Dravet syndrome) as described later.

As far as environmental influences are concerned, risk factors implicated include increasing temperature, fever mediators, genetic factors, and hyperthermia-induced hyperventilation with alkalosis. Although all rat/mouse models of seizures seize with hyperthermia, the threshold temperature needed to cause the seizure varies, with different strains implicating genetic factors. Febrile seizure susceptibility is modified by genes coding sodium channels, gamma-aminobutyric acid (GABA) A receptors, and interleukins. Fever and hyperthermia (after hot water baths or with anticholinergic medications) are both associated with the release of interleukin 1β in the brain (9), which then increases neuronal excitability via glutamate and GABA (10,11).

Fever induced by human herpes virus 6 (HHV6) infection is highly associated with febrile seizures (12). Hyperthermia-induced hyperventilation and therefore alkalosis seems to provoke neuronal excitability (9), contributing to seizure pathophysiology where latency between fever and seizure is greater than 30 minutes (9).

SHOULD CHILDREN WITH FEBRILE SEIZURES BE VACCINATED? DO VACCINATIONS CAUSE FEBRILE SEIZURES?

Vaccine administration is the second leading cause of febrile seizures. Febrile seizure occurrence in children is a serious concern because it leads to public apprehension of vaccinations (13). Seizures following vaccination are most likely associated with the febrile episode and not with vaccination itself. Vaccination causes febrile seizure onset in approximately one-third of the patients with Dravet syndrome (14). The condition of vaccine-associated encephalopathy is poorly defined. However it is thought to be a clinical state where a previously well infant develops seizures and encephalopathy soon after vaccination. In a seminal paper by Berkowicz et al., out of 14 patients with vaccine-associated encephalopathy, 11 were found to have mutations in their sodium channel and all 14 had a diagnosis of a specific epilepsy syndrome, suggesting that the concept of vaccine-associated encephalopathy may be more a myth than a fact (15). According to a recently published position statement by the Italian league against epilepsy (16), although it is apparent that vaccines for diphtheria-tetanus-pertussis (DTP) and measles-mumps-rubella (MMR) are at a higher risk for febrile seizures, the rate of febrile seizures is similar in children with and without a personal history of previous febrile seizures.

Vaccine-induced febrile seizures are no more frequent than febrile seizures with any other cause of fever. The risk of nonfebrile seizures following vaccine-induced febrile seizures is not higher than in children who have not shown vaccine-induced febrile seizures.

EVALUATION OF FEBRILE SEIZURES

The main role of the physician responding to a child with a febrile seizure is to investigate for the cause of fever and rule out meningitis. The latest American Academy of Pediatrics (AAP) guideline (17) unfortunately focuses only on simple febrile seizures and states that in the evaluation of simple febrile seizures, serum electrolytes, complete blood count, calcium, and phosphorus should not be considered. A CT scan and an electroencephalogram (EEG) are not indicated in the evaluation of simple febrile seizures. A lumbar puncture is indicated in any child who appears ill or has signs of meningismus. In general, children under 12 months of age may not exhibit signs of meningitis and a low threshold should be maintained for doing a lumbar puncture. In children between the ages of 6 months and 18 months, lumbar puncture may be considered when pretreated with antibiotics and when children are deemed to be deficient in their immunizations for *Haemophilus influenzae* type B or *Streptococcus pneumoniae* or documentation for these vaccinations is incomplete.

No such guidelines exist for complex febrile seizures. The role of neuroimaging in complex febrile seizure (not status epilepticus) is limited. In a retrospective review by Teng et al. of 76 children with complex febrile seizures, none was found to have any intracranial pathology. On the other hand in a prospective study of 159 children with a first febrile seizure and a brain MRI completed within 7 days, Hesdorffer et al. found abnormalities in 20 of the 159 children. However children who had both a focal as well as a prolonged seizure were more likely to have an abnormality (n = 14) on MRI imaging such as focal cortical dysplasia or abnormality on white matter signal. This suggested that the MRI abnormality was perhaps predisposing the patient to seizures in the setting of a fever (18,19). In a more recent study evaluating the role of emergent new imaging (CT scan) in the emergency room (ER) after a complex febrile seizure (20), 268 patients with complex febrile seizures had emergent imaging completed. Of these 268 patients, only 4 patients had an abnormality: Two had intracranial hemorrhage, one had acute disseminated encephalomyelitis, and one patient had focal cerebral edema; three of these patients had obvious abnormalities like bruising suggesting nonaccidental trauma and then on neurological examination, had nystagmus or altered mental status.

The role of EEG in the workup of febrile seizures is also controversial. An EEG may remain slow for up to 7 days after a febrile seizure. In a recent case control study of 36 patients with febrile seizures who had abnormal EEG compared to 87 patients with normal EEG after febrile seizures (21), 9/36 with EEG abnormalities were more likely to have epilepsy. In a recent Cochrane review, no randomized controls trials were found to show evidence for the use of EEG after a complex febrile seizure. Guidelines do not exist to assist in the understanding of when an EEG may be valuable in these patients (22).

Lumbar puncture guidelines in complex febrile seizures are no different from those for simple febrile seizures, meaning that a lumbar puncture is indicated in any child who appears ill or has signs of meningismus or has incomplete or unclear documentation of immunization.

FEBRILE STATUS EPILEPTICUS

Febrile status epilepticus is defined as a febrile seizure lasting more than 30 minutes and may be conceived as an extreme form of a complex febrile seizure. Risk factors for developing febrile status epilepticus include younger age at onset of febrile seizure, lower temperature at onset of seizure, and longer duration of recognized temperature before onset of febrile seizure (23).

PROGNOSIS OF FEBRILE SEIZURES

After a single febrile seizure, the risk of recurrence is 30%. After two or more febrile seizures, the risk increases to 50%. Other risk factors for recurrence include young age at onset, a history of febrile seizures in a first-degree relative, low degree of fever while in the emergency department, and a brief duration between the onset of fever and the initial seizure (24,25). Risk of future epilepsy after simple febrile seizures is negligible at 1% to 2.4% and that after a complex febrile seizure is 4% to 6%. Risk factors for future epilepsy include complex febrile seizure, developmental delay, and family history of epilepsy. These risk factors are different from the risk factors for febrile seizure recurrence (younger age at onset, lower temperature at time of febrile seizure, and family history of febrile seizures) (26–28).

MANAGEMENT OF SIMPLE AND COMPLEX FEBRILE SEIZURES

Parental education is critical in further management of febrile seizures. Parents should be educated about seizure first aid and also be trained to administer rescue medication at home for seizures lasting 5 minutes. Medications used in the prehospital termination of seizures include rectal diazepam (0.3–0.5 mg/kg/dose) and buccal or intranasal midazolam (0.2–0.3 mg/kg/dose). Emergency seizure management will be the same in patients with febrile seizures as patients with afebrile seizures (29). After securing airway, breathing, and circulation in a patient still actively seizing, an intravenous benzodiazepine is administered as the first line of treatment followed by an intravenous load of a second-line drug—which may vary from hospital to hospital (at our institution we use intravenous fosphenytoin given as 20–30 phenytoin equivalents/kg/dose). Although prophylactic antipyretics may give a patient symptomatic comfort, they do not prevent the occurrence of febrile seizures (30). In addition, prophylactic anticonvulsant medications are not indicated in the treatment of febrile seizures (31).

FEBRILE SEIZURES AS THE PRESENTING FEATURE OF OTHER EPILEPSIES

Febrile seizures may be the presenting feature of Dravet syndrome, GEFS+, and PCDH19 (Table 2.2) and may also be seen in a subset of patients who develop future mesial temporal sclerosis (2,32,33). The association of febrile seizures and future hippocampal sclerosis remains a topic of much debate. Febrile seizures in school-aged children may be seen in association with a recently recognized entity called febrile infection–related epilepsy syndrome (FIRES).

FEBSTAT STUDY

Febrile status epilepticus occurs in 5% of patients with febrile seizures. The FEBSTAT study was designed to prospectively examine the association between prolonged febrile seizures and the development of hippocampal sclerosis and associated temporal lobe epilepsy, one of the

TABLE 2.2 Epilepsy Syndromes That May Start With Fever-Induced Seizures

CHARACTERISTICS	DRAVET SYNDROME	GEFS+	PCDH19	FIRES
Sex predilection	None	None	Females	None
Age of onset	Less than 1 year	Variable	Generally less than 1 year	School-aged children
Classic presenting history	Repeated hemiclonic or generalized status epilepticus	Strong family history of febrile or nonfebrile seizures in two generations	Repeated seizure clusters with fever	Repeated seizures shortly after a febrile illness that later evolve into refractory status epilepticus
Development	Initially normal, later regression possible	Usually normal throughout	Variable, initially normal, but later mostly associated with delay	Normal till onset of status epilepticus, but later significant impairment

most controversial issues in epilepsy. FEBSTAT is a prospective, multicenter study. Inclusion criteria are children, aged 1 month to 6 years of age, presenting with a febrile seizure lasting 30 minutes or longer, based on ambulance, emergency department, and hospital records, and parental interview. At baseline, procedures include an MRI study and EEG recording done within 72 hours of status, and a detailed history and neurologic examination. Baseline development and behavior are assessed at 1 month. The baseline assessment is repeated, with age-appropriate developmental testing at 1 and 5 years after enrollment as well as at the development of epilepsy and 1 year after that. Telephone calls every 3 months document additional seizures. Two other groups of children are included: a "control" group consisting of children with a first febrile seizure ascertained at Columbia University and with almost identical baseline and 1-year follow-up examinations and a pilot cohort of febrile status epilepticus from Duke University (24). Initial results of the study have been published and these results are described in the following text.

FEBSTAT identified risk factors for first febrile status epilepticus. Compared with children with simple febrile seizures, febrile status epilepticus was associated with younger age, lower temperature, and longer duration (1–24 hrs) of recognized temperature before febrile seizures, female sex, structural temporal lobe abnormalities, and first-degree family history of febrile seizure. Compared with children with other complex febrile seizures, febrile status epilepticus was associated with low temperature and longer duration (1–24 hrs) of temperature recognition before febrile seizure (23). In another paper detailing the association of hippocampal sclerosis and febrile status epilepticus (34), 226 patients were evaluated with an MRI within 7 days of febrile status epilepticus and 1 year later. In 22 children, T2 hyperintensity was noted acutely, maximum in Sommer's sector (Sommer's sector is sector CA1 in the hippocampus. It is exquisitely sensitive to hypoxic injury and is frequently involved in the pathology of temporal lobe epilepsy). On follow-up MRI, 10 of these 22 patients had hippocampal sclerosis at 12 months and reduced hippocampal volume. Compared with controls of simple febrile seizures, patients with febrile status epilepticus with normal acute MRIs had an abnormal ratio of right-to-left hippocampal volume, smaller hippocampi initially, and reduced hippocampal growth. This study could not however make immediate conclusions of these findings with relationship to future temporal lobe epilepsy.

The FEBSTAT study suggests that infection with HHV-6B is commonly associated with febrile status epilepticus (12). Of the initial cohort of patients, 136 underwent a nontraumatic lumbar puncture to confirm that febrile status epilepticus is rarely associated with pleocytosis (35).

Nordli et al. showed that out of 199 children in this study with an EEG within 72 hours of febrile status epilepticus, 45% (90) were abnormal, with the most common abnormality being focal slowing (47) or attenuation (25). Epileptiform abnormalities were present only in 6.5% (13) EEGs. In addition, focal EEG slowing or attenuation was associated with T2 signal abnormality on MRI in these patients (36).

CONTROVERSY: DO FEBRILE SEIZURES CAUSE TEMPORAL LOBE EPILEPSY?

A causal relationship between long-duration febrile seizures and temporal lobe epilepsy is difficult to demonstrate or refute in humans due to the inability to control for genetic factors or other preexisting factors (perinatal injury, other developmental anomalies). However there are several recent studies of note, which argue for a link between long-duration febrile seizures and subsequent development of temporal lobe epilepsy.

Falconer et al. (37) in a study of patients who had surgery for intractable temporal lobe epilepsy found that 30% of the patients with mesial temporal sclerosis had a preceding history of febrile seizures in childhood. Subsequently out of a cohort of 666 children with febrile seizures followed prospectively, 6% developed epilepsy (26). Berg et al. (28) evaluated 428 children prospectively and found that developmental abnormalities, complex febrile seizures, and a family history of epilepsy were associated with future unprovoked seizures in 6% of the cohort. This would suggest that a preexisting brain abnormality in addition to a genetic predisposition may predispose to complex febrile seizures and future epilepsy. The finding that hippocampal sclerosis is associated more frequently with developmental anomalies like focal cortical dysplasia and/or heterotropia suggests genetic predisposition. This is also suggested by a study of familial mesial temporal lobe epilepsy (38) in which 52 asymptomatic relatives of patients with familial mesial temporal lobe epilepsy were studied and 18 were found to have a hippocampal abnormality on MRI. A recent study looked at genome-wide association comparing 1,018 study patients with mesial temporal lobe epilepsy and hippocampal sclerosis with 7,552 controls. A sodium channel gene cluster of chromosome 2q24.3 within an intron in the *SCN1A* gene was found in a significant number of patients with mesial temporal lobe epilepsy and hippocampal sclerosis and a history of febrile seizures (39). In a review, Dube (40) pointed out that there is little evidence for short-duration febrile seizures causing an adverse impact on the human brain. In another paper, Dube et al. (41) developed an experimental animal model of prolonged febrile seizures in 10- to 11-day-old rats (an age when hippocampal development approximates that of human infants). In this model, prolonged early-life febrile seizures led to the development of spontaneously recurrent seizures in 35% of rats.

We currently do not have biomarkers to define with any degree of certainty which child with prolonged febrile seizures may be at risk for the development of future epilepsy. Future studies may help answer some of these important questions.

REFERENCES

1. Steering Committee on Quality Improvement and Management, Subcommittee on Febrile Seizures American Academy of Pediatrics. Febrile seizures: Clinical practice guideline for the long-term management of the child with simple febrile seizures. *Pediatrics.* 2008;121(6):1281–1286. doi: 10.1542/peds.2008-0939.
2. Cross JH. Fever and fever-related epilepsies. *Epilepsia.* 2012;53 Suppl 4:3–8. doi: 10.1111/j.1528-1167.2012.03608.x.
3. Graves RC, Oehler K, Tingle LE. Febrile seizures: Risks, evaluation, and prognosis. *Am Fam Physician.* 2012;85(2):149–153.
4. Berg AT, Shinnar S. Complex febrile seizures. *Epilepsia.* 1996;37(2):126–133.
5. Ng YT, Maganti R. Status epilepticus in childhood. *J Paediatr Child Health.* 2013;49(6):432–437. doi: 10.1111/j.1440-1754.2012.02559.x.
6. Berg AT, Shinnar S, Levy SR, Testa FM. Childhood-onset epilepsy with and without preceding febrile seizures. *Neurology.* 1999;53(8):1742–1748.
7. Pavlidou E, Hagel C, Panteliadis C. Febrile seizures: Recent developments and unanswered questions. *Childs Nerv Syst.* 2013;29(11):2011–2017. doi: 10.1007/s00381-013-2224-3.
8. Saghazadeh A, Mastrangelo M, Rezaei N. Genetic background of febrile seizures. *Rev Neurosci.* 2014;25(1):129–161. doi: 10.1515/revneuro-2013-0053.
9. Dube CM, Brewster AL, Baram TZ. Febrile seizures: Mechanisms and relationship to epilepsy. *Brain Dev.* 2009;31(5):366–371. doi: 10.1016/j.braindev.2008.11.010.
10. Dube C, Vezzani A, Behrens M, et al. Interleukin-1beta contributes to the generation of experimental febrile seizures. *Ann Neurol.* 2005;57(1):152–155. doi: 10.1002/ana.20358.
11. Heida JG, Moshe SL, Pittman QJ. The role of interleukin-1beta in febrile seizures. *Brain Dev.* 2009;31(5):388–393. doi: 10.1016/j.braindev.2008.11.013.
12. Epstein LG, Shinnar S, Hesdorffer DC, et al. Human herpesvirus 6 and 7 in febrile status epilepticus: The FEBSTAT study. *Epilepsia.* 2012;53(9):1481–1488. doi: 10.1111/j.1528-1167.2012.03542.x.
13. Principi N, Esposito S. Vaccines and febrile seizures. *Expert Rev Vaccines.* 2013;12(8):885–892. doi: 10.1586/14760584.2013.814781.
14. Cendes F, Sankar R. Vaccinations and febrile seizures. *Epilepsia.* 2011;52 Suppl 3:23–25. doi: 10.1111/j.1528-1167.2011.03032.x.
15. Berkovic SF, Harkin L, McMahon JM, et al. De-novo mutations of the sodium channel gene SCN1A in alleged vaccine encephalopathy: A retrospective study. *Lancet Neurol.* 2006;5(6):488–492. doi: 10.1016/S1474-4422(06)70446-X.
16. Pruna D, Balestri P, Zamponi N, et al. Epilepsy and vaccinations: Italian guidelines. *Epilepsia.* 2013;54 Suppl 7:13–22. doi: 10.1111/epi.12306.
17. Subcommittee on Febrile Seizures, American Academy of Pediatrics. Neurodiagnostic evaluation of the child with a simple febrile seizure. *Pediatrics.* 2011;127(2):389–394. doi: 10.1542/peds.2010-3318.
18. Teng D, Dayan P, Tyler S, et al. Risk of intracranial pathologic conditions requiring emergency intervention after a first complex febrile seizure episode among children. *Pediatrics.* 2006;117(2):304–308. doi: 10.1542/peds.2005-0759.
19. Hesdorffer DC, Chan S, Tian H, et al. Are MRI-detected brain abnormalities associated with febrile seizure type?. *Epilepsia.* 2008;49(5):765–771. doi: 10.1111/j.1528-1167.2007.01459.x.
20. Kimia AA, Ben-Joseph E, Prabhu S, et al. Yield of emergent neuroimaging among children presenting with a first complex febrile seizure. *Pediatr Emerg Care.* 2012;28(4):316–321. doi: 10.1097/PEC.0b013e31824d8b0b.

21. Wo SB, Lee JH, Lee YJ, et al. Risk for developing epilepsy and epileptiform discharges on EEG in patients with febrile seizures. *Brain Dev.* 2013;35(4):307–311. doi: 10.1016/j.braindev.2012.07.014.
22. Shah PB, James S, Elayaraja S. EEG for children with complex febrile seizures. *Cochrane Database Syst Rev.* 2014;1:CD009196. doi: 10.1002/14651858.CD009196.pub2.
23. Hesdorffer DC, Shinnar S, Lewis DV, et al. Risk factors for febrile status epilepticus: A case-control study. *J Pediatr.* 2013;163(4):1147–1151.e1. doi: 10.1016/j.jpeds.2013.05.038.
24. Hesdorffer DC, Shinnar S, Lewis DV, et al. Design and phenomenology of the FEBSTAT study. *Epilepsia.* 2012;53(9):1471–1480. doi: 10.1111/j.1528-1167.2012.03567.x.
25. Berg AT, Shinnar S, Darefsky AS, et al. Predictors of recurrent febrile seizures. A prospective cohort study. *Arch Pediatr Adolesc Med.* 1997;151(4):371–378.
26. Annegers JF, Hauser WA, Elveback LR, Kurland LT. The risk of epilepsy following febrile convulsions. *Neurology.* 1979;29(3):297–303.
27. Annegers JF, Hauser WA, Shirts SB, Kurland LT. Factors prognostic of unprovoked seizures after febrile convulsions. *N Engl J Med.* 1987;316(9):493–498. doi: 10.1056/NEJM198702263160901.
28. Berg AT, Shinnar S. Unprovoked seizures in children with febrile seizures: Short-term outcome. *Neurology.* 1996;47(2):562–568.
29. Appleton R, Macleod S, Martland T. Drug management for acute tonic-clonic convulsions including convulsive status epilepticus in children. *Cochrane Database Syst Rev.* 2008;(3):CD001905. doi(3):CD001905. doi: 10.1002/14651858.CD001905.pub2.
30. Offringa M, Newton R. Prophylactic drug management for febrile seizures in children (review). *Evid Based Child Health.* 2013;8(4):1376–1485. doi: 10.1002/ebch.1921.
31. Offringa M, Newton R. Prophylactic drug management for febrile seizures in children. *Cochrane Database Syst Rev.* 2012;4:CD003031. doi: 10.1002/14651858.CD003031.pub2.
32. Scheffer IE, Zhang YH, Jansen FE, Dibbens L. Dravet syndrome or genetic (generalized) epilepsy with febrile seizures plus?. *Brain Dev.* 2009;31(5):394–400. doi: 10.1016/j.braindev.2009.01.001.
33. van Harssel JJ, Weckhuysen S, van Kempen MJ, et al. Clinical and genetic aspects of PCDH19-related epilepsy syndromes and the possible role of PCDH19 mutations in males with autism spectrum disorders. *Neurogenetics.* 2013;14(1):23–34. doi: 10.1007/s10048-013-0353-1.
34. Lewis DV, Shinnar S, Hesdorffer DC, et al. Hippocampal sclerosis after febrile status epilepticus: The FEBSTAT study. *Ann Neurol.* 2014;75(2):178–185. doi: 10.1002/ana.24081.
35. Frank LM, Shinnar S, Hesdorffer DC, et al. Cerebrospinal fluid findings in children with fever-associated status epilepticus: Results of the consequences of prolonged febrile seizures (FEBSTAT) study. *J Pediatr.* 2012;161(6):1169–1171. doi: 10.1016/j.jpeds.2012.08.008.
36. Nordli DR,Jr, Moshe SL, Shinnar S, et al. Acute EEG findings in children with febrile status epilepticus: Results of the FEBSTAT study. *Neurology.* 2012;79(22):2180–2186. doi: 10.1212/WNL.0b013e3182759766.
37. Falconer MA, Serafetinides EA, Corsellis JA. Etiology and pathogenesis of temporal lobe epilepsy. *Arch Neurol.* 1964;10:233–248.
38. Kobayashi E, Li LM, Lopes-Cendes I, Cendes F. Magnetic resonance imaging evidence of hippocampal sclerosis in asymptomatic, first-degree relatives of patients with familial mesial temporal lobe epilepsy. *Arch Neurol.* 2002;59(12):1891–1894.
39. Kasperaviciute D, Catarino CB, Matarin M, et al. Epilepsy, hippocampal sclerosis and febrile seizures linked by common genetic variation around SCN1A. *Brain.* 2013;136(Pt 10):3140–3150. doi: 10.1093/brain/awt233.
40. Dube CM, McClelland S, Choy MK, et al. Fever, febrile seizures and epileptogenesis. In: Noebels JL, Avoli M, Rogawski MA, Olsen RW, Delgado-Escueta AV, eds. *Jasper's Basic Mechanisms of the Epilepsies.* 4th ed. Bethesda, MD:National Center for Biotechnology Information (US); 2012.
41. Dube C, Richichi C, Bender RA, et al. Temporal lobe epilepsy after experimental prolonged febrile seizures: Prospective analysis. *Brain.* 2006;129(Pt 4):911–922. doi: 10.1093/brain/awl018.

Epileptic and Nonepileptic Paroxysmal Events in Childhood

Jorge Vidaurre, MD

Paroxysmal events (epileptic and nonepileptic) are commonly encountered in general pediatric and neurology practices. Epileptic events or seizures refer to a transient occurrence of signs and/or symptoms due to abnormal excessive or synchronous neuronal activity in the brain (1). Paroxysmal nonepileptic events (PNEs) also manifest as a transient occurrence of stereotyped or somewhat stereotyped clinical episodes, but they are not associated with paroxysmal, excessive cortical activity.

In children admitted to epilepsy units for long-term video-electroencephalogram (EEG) monitoring, about 22% to 43% may receive the diagnosis of PNEs (2–4). This diagnosis is even more common in children who are neurologically impaired (4,5), as hyperkinetic movement disorders, spasticity, attention deficit, and staring are more prevalent complaints. Children with autism and developmental delay with or without cerebral palsy may represent a diagnostic challenge (3).

A detailed history and physical examination is helpful in clarifying the etiology of these episodes, but often this clinical differentiation is not an easy task and specific tests such as long term video-EEG or polysomnograms are needed, in order to arrive at a specific diagnosis (6,7). Furthermore, epileptic and nonepileptic events may coexist in the same patient, making diagnosis even more challenging.

The use of video-EEG can distinguish the nature of these paroxysmal events in most cases (4,8,9).

Epileptic and nonepileptic events share many common characteristics that can make differentiation difficult (Table 3.1), even for the more experienced neurologist. Clinicians have to rely often on the history provided by parents, as the events are not directly witnessed during the short clinic visit.

TABLE 3.1 Common Features of Epileptic and Nonepileptic Events

Intermittent, periodic occurrence
Sudden change in what is considered normal behavior for the child
Daytime and nighttime occurrence
Stereotyped or somewhat stereotyped symptomatology
Usually short in duration
Cause of concern for parents

Identification and accurate classification of the event is extremely important, as treatment is based on the presumptive etiology. Many children referred to tertiary epilepsy centers are misdiagnosed as epileptic and placed unnecessarily on antiepileptic medication (2,4,10). The incorrect diagnosis of epilepsy can add significant stress to the family and impose unnecessary limitations on the child.

The clinical manifestations of PNEs are highly variable. These may include hypermotor features (paroxysmal movement disorders, shuddering attacks, benign sleep myoclonus), behavioral or motor arrest (staring, apnea), alteration in consciousness (syncope, breath-holding events), sensory phenomena (hallucinations, migraine), mixed manifestations (syncope with convulsive features), or other symptoms (cyclic vomiting).

Some PNEs may occur exclusively during wakefulness (psychogenic nonepileptic seizures [PNESs], shuddering attacks) and others take place during sleep (parasomnias).

Age of presentation is an important factor in the differential diagnosis, as certain PNEs are prevalent in specific age groups, for example, "benign sleep myoclonus" is observed in neonates and young infants and PNES occurs mainly in older children and adolescents.

As a result of this highly variable clinical presentation and symptomatology, it is easy to perceive the difficulties in making an accurate diagnosis during the first clinic visit. Short periods of inattention in children with attention deficit disorder (ADD) or autism can be confused with absence seizures, and parasomnias may be difficult to distinguish from seizures of frontal lobe origin. On the other hand, epileptic syndromes such as "benign occipital epilepsy" presenting with episodes of vomiting or headaches can be misdiagnosed as gastroesophageal reflux disorder or migraine.

This chapter presents a review of some of the most frequent nonepileptic events encountered in clinical practice. The clinical characteristics and features that may help in correct identification of the episodes are described.

EVENTS WITH MOTOR MANIFESTATIONS AS THE MAIN CLINICAL FEATURE

Benign Neonatal Sleep Myoclonus

Benign neonatal sleep myoclonus (BNSM) is a benign condition characterized by repetitive, usually synchronous myoclonus involving the extremities. The jerks occur exclusively during sleep and remit when the child is aroused. This condition usually starts in the first 2 weeks of life and resolves spontaneously by 3 months of age with no neurological sequelae (11).

The true prevalence is unknown as cases may be underrecognized (12,13). The jerks involve the distal portion of the upper extremities (flexion of fingers, wrist, and elbow) and usually spare the face (11,14,15). The myoclonic jerks are more frequent during quiet sleep (15) and may occur in short clusters, recurring every few seconds (16). The jerks do not stop with restraint, but can be activated by rocking the baby in a head-to-toe direction (17,18).

It is important to differentiate this benign condition, as BNSM can be confused with neonatal seizures and the patients placed on anticonvulsants (18). The diagnosis should be made by history and careful clinical observation. The occurrence of myoclonus during sleep and its disappearance by arousal in a neonate should raise the suspicion for this benign condition.

Jitteriness

Jitteriness is one of the most common involuntary movements encountered in full-term babies. Jitteriness consists of rhythmic tremors of equal amplitude around a fixed axis. The etiology of the condition is not clearly defined in the majority of cases, but it has been associated with electrolyte abnormalities or maternal drug use. Jitteriness is observed very early in the neonatal period and diminishes markedly by the second week of life.

The prevalence can be about 44% in large urban centers (19). There is a positive association of maternal marijuana and possibly cocaine use with neonatal jitteriness (19,20). These infants also demonstrate visual inattention and irritability compared with nonjittery infants. The jittery movements can be differentiated from seizures because they are commonly stimulus sensitive and may terminate with passive flexion of the baby. Rarely, jitteriness can occur immediately after the neonatal period (21).

Benign Myoclonus of Early Infancy

Benign myoclonus of early infancy (BMEI) was described for the first time in 1976 by Fejerman (22,23). The first descriptions included children with events resembling infantile spasms without abnormalities in the EEG. The clinical entity consisted of jerks of the neck and upper limbs leading to flexion or rotation of the head and abduction of limbs and no changes in consciousness. Patients with brief tonic flexion of the limbs, shuddering, and loss of tone or negative myoclonus have also been included as part of the syndrome. Age of presentation is usually between 3 and 8 months.

Newer attempts to redefine the clinical spectrum of the syndrome include different types of motor phenomena such as myoclonic jerks, spasms and brief tonic contractions, shuddering, and atonia.

BMEI can be confused with "epileptic" infantile spasms. For most cases, this differentiation is not difficult. There is lack of hypsarrhythmia or EEG abnormalities in BMEI in contrast to epileptic infantile spasms, which often have a characteristic EEG pattern. Also in contrast to infantile spasms, development in BMEI is normal, and the events subside by 6 to 30 months of age (24).

Shuddering Attacks

Shuddering attacks are benign nonepileptic events of infancy consisting of rapid "shivering" of the shoulders, head, and occasionally the trunk.

The attacks may involve mild stiffening of the upper extremities with very fine low-amplitude tremors of 8 to 10 cycles per second (cps), usually lasting less than 5 seconds (25). The child may adopt a characteristic posture of flexion of the head, elbows, trunk, and knees with abduction of the elbows and knees (26). Parents describe the event "as if water was poured down the child's back." Shivering attacks usually occur during playtime and may be precipitated by excitement.

It is believed that prevalence of events is low, but in a large series of children with nonepileptic events, shuddering attacks represented 7% of all cases (3). The pathophysiology is not understood, but a relationship with essential tremor has been postulated (26), and propranolol has been used as treatment (27). Further studies did not find an association between essential tremor and shuddering attacks (28).

The distinction between seizures, especially brief generalized and myoclonic seizures should not represent a diagnostic challenge. Shuddering attacks have precipitating factors and there is no alteration in consciousness or postictal state.

Stereotypies

Similar to tics, stereotypies are repetitive, purposeless, ritualistic movements that can be exacerbated by stress, excitement, or even boredom. Stereotypies usually affect the body and arms (arm flapping, body rocking). They can occur in normal children as well as in children with autism spectrum disorder (29) and syndromes associated with mental retardation.

The presence of precipitating factors and the fact that they can stop if the child is distracted can help in differentiating these movements from epileptic events.

Tics

Tic disorder is another common condition affecting about 1% of the population. Tics are sudden, rapid, brief movements (motor tics) or sounds (vocal tics). Tics may be simple or complex, involving different muscle groups or presenting with a complex sequence of movements. On occasions, tics can cause self-injury.

Tics are classified as transient tic disorder (duration of symptoms lasting less than 1 year) or chronic motor or vocal tics (lasting more than 1 year). Tourette syndrome is the most common cause of tics and includes motor and one or more vocal tics, although not necessarily concurrent. Tics must occur intermittently for more than 1 year (30). Children diagnosed with Tourette may face different comorbidities, including attention deficit hyperactivity disorder, obsessive-compulsive disorder, and behavioral difficulties (31).

The motor manifestations of tics are florid. The movements usually start on the face (blinking or gestures) and later they may involve the trunk and extremities. The nature of movements can be tonic, clonic, or even myoclonic, creating diagnostic confusion.

Some features are helpful in making the distinction between tics and epileptic events. Tics are often preceded by a sensation of discomfort, which is alleviated after execution of the tic (32). Patients can also suppress their tics. Tics can occur multiple times a day and become more frequent during periods of stress, boredom, or excitement.

Independently, the prognosis of children with Tourette is favorable. The worst period is around 10.6 years of age (33), with improvement or disappearance of tics in the majority of affected patients.

Treatment with behavioral therapy or habit reversal is promising (34). Medications are used in selected cases, especially if tics are causing problems with self-esteem or injury.

Paroxysmal Dyskinesias

The paroxysmal dyskinesias as a group can, at times, be confused with epileptic events, as they share common features including the following:

1. Paroxysmal, intermittent episodes of involuntary movements

2. Events may be preceded by premonitory symptoms or "auras"

3. Symptoms may respond to antiepileptic medications

In contrast to epilepsy, affected children do not have alteration in consciousness during the attacks and the EEG is normal.

The paroxysmal dyskinesias can be classified by the circumstances in which they occur as follows:

Paroxysmal kinesigenic dyskinesia (PKD), typically affects children from middle childhood to early adolescence. The etiology may be idiopathic or secondary to other neurological conditions, such as stroke or multiple sclerosis. PKD is characterized by involuntary movements (usually dystonia chorea or ballismus). The attacks are short in duration and they are precipitated by movement. There is no loss of consciousness during the episodes, and generally patients respond well to antiepileptic drug treatment (35,36). Premonitory symptoms, usually abnormal gastric sensations, are reported by patients. In some pedigrees, PKD has been associated with infantile convulsions (37).

Paroxysmal nonkinesigenic dyskinesia (PNKD) is a disorder of early childhood, but can manifest in the early 20s. The attacks may be longer than the episodes observed in PKD, lasting hours or days (38), and do not have to be associated with movement. Problems with speech have also been reported at the time of the attack, but there are no changes in the level of consciousness. Patients may respond better to clonazepam than to sodium channel blockers (38). Paroxysmal exertion-induced dyskinesia is a movement disorder triggered by prolonged exercise (39) and affects mainly the legs, with attacks lasting about 5 to 30 minutes.

Paroxysmal hypnogenic dyskinesia consists of attacks of chorea or dystonia occurring in non–rapid eye movement (NREM) sleep. The frequency is variable and duration is usually less than 1 minute. Frontal lobe seizures, especially "autosomal dominant frontal lobe epilepsy" may present with similar clinical features (40,41), and many cases of paroxysmal hypnogenic dyskinesias may actually represent epileptic events. Distinction between a true movement disorder and epilepsy may be difficult in those cases, as frontal lobe seizures may lack an ictal EEG correlate and the interpretation is difficult, due to excessive movement artifact. A high index of suspicion for seizures is recommended for nocturnal dystonic events, especially if episodes are stereotyped in nature.

Psychogenic Nonepileptic Seizures

PNESs are paroxysmal events, involving clear changes in behavior or consciousness, similar to epileptic seizures, but without associated abnormal cortical discharges. The prevalence of PNES is estimated between 2 and 33 per 100,000 (42) and comprises about 20% to 30% of the patients referred for diagnostic video-EEG monitoring (43).

PNES can be encountered in young children, but it is more prevalent in adolescents (43). There also appears to be a female predominance in the latter group, whereas in younger patients, boys can be more commonly affected.

There are signs that can help in differentiating nonepileptic from epileptic seizures (44):

1. High frequency of seizures

2. Resistance to antiepileptic drugs

3. Specific triggers

4. Occurrence in the presence of an audience or in a physician's office

5. Multiple complaints, including fibromyalgia and chronic pain

There are also specific features of the episode that can help in distinguishing PNESs from epileptic seizures. These features are irregular and asynchronous motor phenomena, waxing and waning symptoms, pelvic thrusting, weeping, preservation of awareness with generalized motor activity, or eye closure during the events.

Clinical manifestations of PNES may be different in the pediatric population. Quiet unresponsiveness or "catatonic" state is a common manifestation in children (10,43). Tremor is also a common feature (10,45), in addition to negative emotions (45), eye closure or opening, and events with minor motor activity. Pelvic thrusting and major motor activity are more prevalent in adults (46).

Many children have associated psychiatric comorbidities including other conversion/mood disorders, anxiety and school refusal, along with psychosocial stressors, including physical and sexual abuse (47).

Video-EEG is an important tool in making an early diagnosis and therefore designing a treatment plan (Figure 3.1), which includes psychological support. The prognosis of PNES in children is more favorable (48).

Sandiffer Syndrome

Gastroesophageal reflux in infants can cause symptoms that are different from those in adults. The symptoms are variable and consist of crying, irritability, sleep difficulties, and back arching (49). Sandiffer syndrome is a more extreme posturing of the head and neck, manifesting as intermittent spells of opisthotonic posturing associated with reflux and hiatal hernia (50). The occurrence of the events during or after feedings is a clue to the diagnosis.

Hyperekplexia

Hyperekplexia is a disorder associated with an exaggerated startle response with delayed habituation, elicited at times by minor auditory or tactile stimuli (nose tapping or air blowing on the

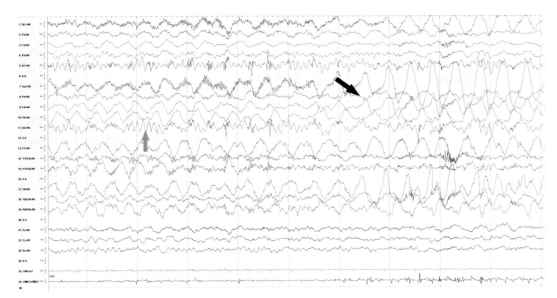

FIGURE 3.1 Ten-year-old boy with typical PNES captured on video-EEG monitoring. EEG shows a clear posterior dominant rhythm (green arrow), despite movement artifact (black arrow). Clinical episode consisted of asymmetric shaking of extremities, associated with pelvic thrusting. Patient remained with eyes closed during the event. Average montage, amplitude 7 uV/mm, 10-seconds screen.

Abbreviations: EEG, electroencephalogram; PNES, psychogenic nonepileptic seizures.

face), in association with other symptoms such as hyperalert gaze, marked stiffness, violent rhythmic jerks, and breath-holding episodes (51). This is a relatively benign disorder, but in severe cases, the symptoms can cause apnea or interfere with feedings. The condition can be easily mistaken for epilepsy, as nocturnal myoclonus can be part of the clinical picture (52). In hyperekplexia, the EEG is normal and patients usually improve with clonazepam at doses of 0.1–0.2 mg/kg/day (53). This neurological condition can be inherited in an autosomal dominant fashion. Most mutations have been identified in the *GLRA1* gene encoding the alpha 1 subunit of the glycine receptor (54,55).

Self-Gratification Disorder

Self-gratification disorder or infantile masturbation is considered a variant of normal behavior and an important consideration in the differential diagnosis of seizures. Symptoms may include dystonic posturing, sweating, grunting, and rocking (56). This is a benign and self-limited behavior that often disappears by 2 years of age (57).

EVENTS WITH SENSORY MANIFESTATIONS AS THE MAIN CLINICAL FEATURE

Migraine

Migraines, especially when preceded by an aura, can be mistaken for seizures. This is not surprising, as auras represent a focal cortical and/or brainstem dysfunction. Occasionally, migraine auras may not be followed by a headache, creating even more confusion.

The most common aura is visual. Auras consist of scintillating scotomata or flickering, zigzag patterns in the center of the visual field with gradual progression to the periphery (58). Less frequently, auras may also manifest as paresthesias affecting one side of the body, motor deficits, confusion, or cerebellar symptoms, such as syncope, vertigo, and ataxia. Impairment of body image and visual analysis of the environment (Alice in Wonderland syndrome) have been reported (59).

There are certain characteristics that are helpful in distinguishing migraines from epileptic events. In migraines, the aura develops gradually for over more than 4 minutes, and two or more symptoms occur in succession. Headaches follow the aura with a symptom-free period of about 60 minutes (60). A positive family history of migraine is usually encountered.

Seizures of occipital origin may manifest with visual symptomatology, but circular shapes appear to predominate and the duration of symptoms is short, from 5 to 30 seconds (61). The postictal headache may be diffuse rather than unilateral (62).

Panic Attacks

Panic attacks are primarily a psychiatric disorder, consisting of recurrent episodes of a sudden, unpredictable overwhelming sensation of fear with a myriad of symptoms including dizziness, shortness of breath, nausea, depersonalization, and paresthesias. During the attack, fear of dying and autonomic symptoms, such as palpitations, are usually present. Patients may interpret typical symptoms of anxiety as dangerous, creating an exaggerated response.

Seizures can also manifest with anxiety or fear, especially seizures of temporal or even parietal lobe origin (63), at times making the differentiation between panic attacks and seizures more difficult. Both can occur spontaneously without warning, but ictal fear usually is brief, lasting a few seconds, in contrast to the prolonged duration of panic attacks, usually lasting minutes to hours (64).

Hallucinations

Hallucinations can occur in children and may be visual, auditory, or involve abnormal sensations. Hallucinations are not necessarily an indication of psychosis. They can be related to physical abuse or the use of psychotropic medications, and a detailed history becomes necessary. As mentioned earlier, hallucinations associated with seizures usually consist of simple forms, smells, or sounds, and they are of short duration. The events are also stereotyped and brief (seconds), only rarely persist longer (65).

EVENTS ASSOCIATED WITH CHANGES IN THE LEVEL OF CONSCIOUSNESS OR ALERTNESS AS THE MAIN CLINICAL FEATURE

Staring Events

Staring spells are among the most common nonepileptic events observed in the pediatric population, making up to 15% of the patients referred for video-EEG monitoring (3). These events consist of vague facial expression, behavioral arrest, and fixed vision at one point. Children may not react to hand waving but the spell can be interrupted by stronger stimulation (3).

A typical scenario involves a child usually sitting or lying in bed quietly at the time of the event. These episodes occur more frequently in children with developmental delay or neurological handicap and epilepsy. Parents of children with ADD or autism may frequently report staring events, and the diagnosis of absence or complex partial seizures may be entertained. A detailed medical history is helpful in differentiating epileptic from nonepileptic events. The presence of automatisms, aura, upward eye movements, limb twitches, and urinary incontinence favors epileptic seizures (66,67). The lack of interruption of playing, responsiveness to touch, and initial identification by a teacher or health care professional rather than by a parent favors nonepileptic staring (67).

Breath-Holding Spells

Breath-holding spells (BHSs) are common pediatric conditions, which may occur in up to 27% of children (68,69). BHSs have a distinctive sequence of clinical features. There is a precipitating event, which is usually a mild trauma (commonly to the head) or provocation, resulting in crying. Subsequently, the child becomes silent during the expiratory phase, followed by color changes and loss of consciousness. The child may adopt an opisthotonic posture with upward eye deviation. After the event is over, the child may go to sleep. Two clinical types are recognized, based on skin color changes: cyanotic and pallid type. Cyanotic spells are more common with a ratio of 5:3 (70). Mixed types can also occur.

BHS presents in children between 6 months to 4 years of age, but younger and older patients have been reported. Median age of onset is between 6 and 12 months and the frequency of attacks is variable, with a median frequency of daily to weekly attacks (70). The attacks usually resolve by 3 to 4 years of age.

The pathophysiology is not completely understood, but involves a vagal mediated cardiac inhibition with significant bradycardia and asystole in the pallid type. This can be elicited by ocular compression, a procedure not recommended in current practice. The EEG during an attack shows generalized rhythmic slowing, followed by electrical attenuation and slowing again, with subsequent recovery of normal background activity (Figure 3.2) (71).

The cyanotic type may involve increased intrathoracic pressure due to a Valsalva maneuver with associated hypocapnia (72), but bradycardia can also be present, and the two types of spells can occur in a single patient, suggesting some common mechanisms. An autosomal dominant mode of inheritance with reduced penetrance is postulated (73).

The attacks usually are short, but frightening to parents. Longer events can produce "reflex anoxic seizures" and, in rare cases, status epilepticus. This may create confusion and BHS may be deemed to be epileptic in nature. The presence of precipitating factors, crying, and family history of similar events favors the diagnosis of BHS.

The treatment is directed mainly at reassurance about the benign nature of the events. The relationship between BHS, anemia, and effectiveness of iron therapy has been documented (74–76). Piracetam is another drug that showed to be safe and effective in controlling the spells (77,78). For patients with severe and frequent spells associated with seizures and prolonged asystole, cardiac pacemakers have been used (79).

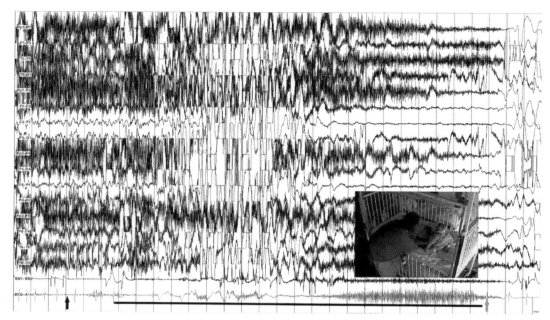

FIGURE 3.2 Twenty-month-old boy with pallid breath-holding events. EEG demonstrates bradycardia (black arrow) after episode of crying, followed by prolonged, 20-seconds asystole (black line). EEG during that period shows generalized background slowing, followed by diffuse electrical suppression, associated with opisthotonic posturing of the child (inserted picture). After the event, heart rate returns to baseline (gray arrow). Longitudinal montage, amplitude 150 peak-to-peak, 30-seconds screen.

Syncope

Syncope is a transient, abrupt loss of consciousness due to reduction in global cerebral perfusion. The most common cause of syncope is "vasovagal." The true incidence of syncope is difficult to estimate due to variation in definition and underreporting in the general population (80). The median peak of the first syncope is around 15 years of age. Convulsive movements may be described in all types of syncope related to cerebral hypoxia and this may lead to a misdiagnosis of seizures (81). The EEG may show a pattern of slowing—attenuation–slowing or a "slow pattern" (Figure 3.3A–B). Stiffening and loss of consciousness develop during the slow phase and persist during the flat portion of the EEG. Myoclonic jerks occur when the EEG is slow (82). Clues in the differential diagnosis include precipitating factors, premonitory symptoms, and postictal events, such as tongue biting (83).

Situations commonly encountered in syncope are upright posture, emotionally induced events, and being in crowded places. The myoclonic jerks observed in syncopal episodes usually occur after loss of consciousness, whereas in epilepsy they appear at the same time (81). In syncope, motor manifestations are usually short-lived and postictal symptoms are not common.

If syncopal attacks occur during exercise or there is family history of heart disease or the presence of palpitations, an EKG should be ordered. A tilt table test is not necessary to make the diagnosis in most instances (81).

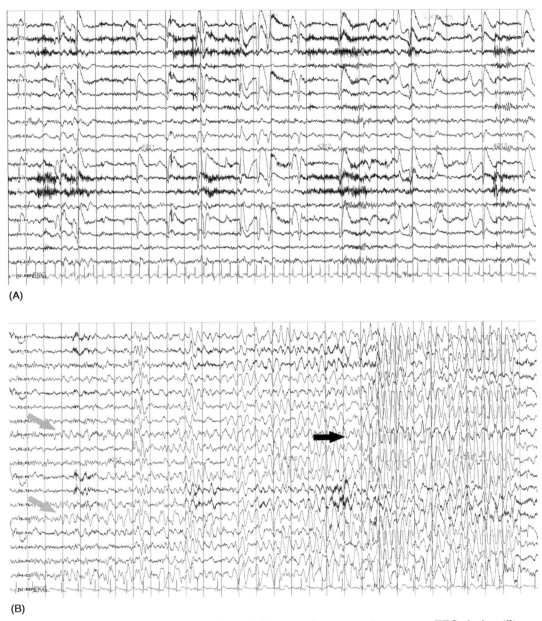

(A)

(B)

FIGURE 3.3B (A) Sixteen-year-old girl with history of vasovagal syncope. EEG during tilt table tests shows a normal background at the time patient was in the upright position. HR: 112. Bipolar montage, amplitude 7 uV/mm, 30-seconds screen. (B) This tracing is a continuation from the previous EEG on Figure 3.3A. EKG lead shows bradycardia (HR 60) immediately after patient was tilted. EEG demonstrates posterior slowing (gray arrows) followed by generalized higher-amplitude delta activity (black arrow). Patient had transient alteration of consciousness with associated upward eye deviation and pallor. Bipolar montage, amplitude 7 uV/mm, 30-seconds screen.

Abbreviations: EEG, electroencephalogram; HR, heart rate.

Narcolepsy/Cataplexy

Cataplexy is a symptom associated with the diagnosis of narcolepsy. The disorder is characterized by muscle weakness triggered by emotions. There is a strong association with centrally mediated hypocretin (orexin) deficiency and with HLA-DQB1*0602 (84).

Children who present with a lack of responsiveness due to excessive sleepiness can be incorrectly diagnosed as having absence seizures, and cataplexy may be misdiagnosed as atonic or other types of epileptic attacks. Videotape recordings of the events can be helpful in clarifying the etiology of the episodes (85).

SLEEP-RELATED EVENTS

The parasomnias as a group are among the most frequent sleep disorders encountered in the pediatric population.

The most common parasomnias in children are the following:

Disorders of arousal (from NREM sleep): These events usually occur in the first half of the night, 1 to 2 hours after falling asleep. NREM sleep disorders are highly prevalent in children between the ages of 3 and 13 years and usually disappear by adolescence (86,87). Disorders of arousal may be mistaken for epileptic seizures and they include:

A. Sleepwalking. During sleepwalking, children may walk or wander around the room. They can go to the parent's room or other places in the house. During the episode, children may be partially responsive.

B. Night terrors. During these events, the child may wake up and scream with a frightened look. Autonomic symptoms including tachycardia, pupillary dilatation, and sweating accompany the event.

C. Confusional arousals consist of partial awakenings in which the child remains confused and unresponsive, despite appearing to be awake.

Parasomnias associated with REM sleep: One of the common parasomnias that occur in REM sleep in children is nightmares. These are frightening dreams in which the child usually has a recollection of the event.

▓ Other parasomnias such as sleep enuresis can also create confusion, as parents may interpret these events as nighttime seizures, especially in children with epilepsy.

▓ There are other paroxysmal events, such as cyclic vomiting, tremors, and rage attacks, which occur less frequently and can also be mistaken for epileptic events.

▓ As mentioned earlier, a clinical history with attention to detail is extremely important to formulate an appropriate diagnosis and differentiate between epileptic and nonepileptic events.

▓ With the advent of new technology and widespread use of iPhones, these episodes can now be captured on digital videos, thus facilitating the diagnosis.

▓ There will always be cases in which this differentiation is not easy to accomplish, and other tests including video-EEG may be required in order to make a specific diagnosis.

REFERENCES

1. Fisher RS, van Emde Boas W, Blume W, et al. Epileptic seizures and epilepsy: definitions proposed by the International League Against Epilepsy (ILAE) and the International Bureau for Epilepsy (IBE). *Epilepsia*. 2005;46(4):470–472.
2. Kotagal P, Costa M, Wyllie E, Wolgamuth B. Paroxysmal nonepileptic events in children and adolescents. *Pediatrics*. 2002;110(4):e46.
3. Bye AM, Kok DJ, Ferenschild FT, Vles JS. Paroxysmal non-epileptic events in children: a retrospective study over a period of 10 years. *J Paediatr Child Health*. 2000;36:244–248.
4. Desai P, Talwar D. Nonepileptic events in normal and neurologically handicapped children: a video-EEG study. *Pediatr Neurol*. 1992;8(2):127–129.
5. Canavese C, Canafoglia L, Costa C, et al. Paroxysmal non-epileptic motor events in childhood: a clinical and video-EEG-polymyographic study. *Dev Med Child Neurol*. 2012;54:334–338.
6. Derry CP, Duncan JS, Berkovic SL. Paroxysmal motor disorders of sleep: the clinical spectrum and differentiation from epilepsy. *Epilepsia*. 2006;47:1775–1791.
7. Tinuper P, Provini F, Bisulli F, et al. Movement disorders in sleep: guidelines for differentiating epileptic from non-epileptic motor phenomena arising from sleep. *Sleep Med Rev*. 2007; 11:255–267.
8. Holmes GL, Sackellares JC, McKiernan J, et al. Evaluation of childhood pseudoseizures using EEG telemetry and video tape monitoring. *J Pediatr*. 1980;97:554–558.
9. Reilly C, Menlove L, Fenton V, Das KB. Psychogenic nonepileptic seizures in children: a review. *Epilepsia*. 2013;54:1715–1724.
10. Dhiman V, Sinha S, Rawat VS, et al. Children with psychogenic non-epileptic seizures (PNES): a detailed semiologic analysis and modified new classification. *Brain Dev*. 2014;36:287–293.
11. Paro-Panjan D, Neubauer D. Benign neonatal sleep myoclonus: experience from the study of 38 infants. *Eur J Paediatr Neurol*. 2008;12:14–18.
12. Ramelli GP, Sozzo AB, Vella S, Bianchetti MG. Benign neonatal sleep myoclonus: an under-recognized, non-epileptic condition. *Acta Paediatr*. 2005;94:962–963.
13. Mauer VO, Rizzi M, Bianchetti MG, Ramelli GP. Benign neonatal sleep myoclonus: a review of the literature. *Pediatrics*. 2010;125:e919–e924.
14. Coulter DL, Allen RJ. Benign neonatal sleep myoclonus. *Arch Neurol*. 1982; 39:191–192.
15. Caraballo R, Yépez I, Cersósimo R, Fejerman N. [Benign neonatal sleep myoclonus]. *Rev Neurol*. 1998;26:540–544.
16. Resnick TJ, Moshé SL, Perotta L, Chambers HJ. Benign neonatal sleep myoclonus. Relationship to sleep states. *Arch Neurol*. 1986;43:266–268.
17. Alfonso I, Papazian O, Aicardi J, Jeffries HE. A simple maneuver to provoke benign neonatal sleep myoclonus. *Pediatrics*. 1995;96:1161–1163.
18. Daoust-Roy J, Seshia SS. Benign neonatal sleep myoclonus. A differential diagnosis of neonatal seizures. *Am J Dis Child*. 1992;146:1236–1241.
19. Parker S, Zuckerman B, Bauchner H, et al. Jitteriness in full-term neonates: prevalence and correlates. *Pediatrics*. 1990;85:17–23.
20. Fried PA, Makin JE. Neonatal behavioural correlates of prenatal exposure to marihuana, cigarettes and alcohol in a low risk population. *Neurotoxicol Teratol*. 1987;9:1–7.
21. Shuper A, Zalzberg J, Weitz R, Mimouni M. Jitteriness beyond the neonatal period: a benign pattern of movement in infancy. *J Child Neurol*. 1991;6:243–245.
22. Fejerman N. Mioclonias benignas de la infancia temprana. Communicacion preliminar. *Actas I, V Jornadas Rioplatenses de Neurologia Infantil. Neuropediatria Lantinoamericana*. 1976:131–134.
23. Fejerman N. Mioclonias benignas de la infancia temprana. *Rev Hosp Niño (Lima)*. 1977;19:130–135.
24. Caraballo RH, Capovilla G, Vigevano F, et al. The spectrum of benign myoclonus of early infancy: Clinical and neurophysiologic features in 102 patients. *Epilepsia*. 2009;50(5):1176–1183.
25. Holmes GL, Russman BS. Shuddering attacks. Evaluation using electroencephalographic frequency modulation radiotelemetry and videotape monitoring. *Am J Dis Child*. 1986;140(1):72–73.
26. Vanasse M, Bedard P, Andermann F. Shuddering attacks in children: an early clinical manifestation of essential tremor. *Neurology*. 1976;26(11):1027–1030.

27. Barron TF, Younkin DP. Propranolol therapy for shuddering attacks. *Neurology.* 1992;42(1):258–259.
28. Jan MM. Shuddering attacks are not related to essential tremor. *J Child Neurol.* 2010;25(7):881–883.
29. Goldman S, Wang C, Salgado MW, et al. Motor stereotypies in children with autism and other developmental disorders. *Dev Med Child Neurol.* 2009;51(1):30–38.
30. Jankovic J, Kurlan R. Tourette syndrome: evolving concepts. *Mov Disord.* 2011;26(6):1149–1156.
31. Freeman RD, Fast DK, Burd L, et al. An international perspective on Tourette syndrome: selected findings from 3,500 individuals in 22 countries. *Dev Med Child Neurol.* 2000;42(7):436–447.
32. Kwak C, Dat Vuong K, Jankovic J. Premonitory sensory phenomenon in Tourette's syndrome. *Mov Disord.* 2003;18(12):1530–1533.
33. Bloch MH, Peterson BS, Scahill L, et al. Adulthood outcome of tic and obsessive-compulsive symptom severity in children with Tourette syndrome. *Arch Pediatr Adolesc Med.* 2006;160(1):65–69.
34. McGuire JF, Piacentini J, Brennan EA, et al. A meta-analysis of behavior therapy for Tourette Syndrome. *J Psychiatr Res,* 2014;50:106–112.
35. Bruno MK, Hallett M, Gwinn-Hardy K, et al. Clinical evaluation of idiopathic paroxysmal kinesigenic dyskinesia: new diagnostic criteria. *Neurology.* 2004;63(12):2280–2287.
36. Sun W, Li J, Zhu Y, et al. Clinical features of paroxysmal kinesigenic dyskinesia: report of 24 cases. *Epilepsy Behav.* 2012;25(4):695–699.
37. Cuenca-Leon E, Cormand B, Thomson T, Macaya A. Paroxysmal kinesigenic dyskinesia and generalized seizures: clinical and genetic analysis in a Spanish pedigree. *Neuropediatrics.* 2002;33(6):288–293.
38. Demirkiran M, Jankovic J. Paroxysmal dyskinesias: clinical features and classification. *Ann Neurol.* 1995;38(4):571–579.
39. Plant GT, Williams AC, Earl CJ, Marsden CD. Familial paroxysmal dystonia induced by exercise. *J Neurol Neurosurg Psychiatry.* 1984;47(3):275–279.
40. Scheffer IE, Bhatia KP, Lopes-Cendes I, et al. Autosomal dominant nocturnal frontal lobe epilepsy. A distinctive clinical disorder. *Brain.* 1995;118(Pt 1):61–73.
41. Ferini-Strambi L, Sansoni V, Combi R. Nocturnal frontal lobe epilepsy and the acetylcholine receptor. *Neurologist.* 2012;18(6):343–349.
42. Benbadis SR, Allen Hauser W. An estimate of the prevalence of psychogenic non-epileptic seizures. *Seizure.* 2000;9(4):280–281.
43. Wyllie E, Benbadis S, Kotagal P. Psychogenic seizures and other nonepileptic paroxysmal events in children. *Epilsepy Behav.* 2002;3:46–50.
44. Benbadis S. The differential diagnosis of epilepsy: a critical review. *Epilepsy Behav.* 2009; 15(1):15–21.
45. Szabó L, Siegler Z, Zubek L, et al. A detailed semiologic analysis of childhood psychogenic nonepileptic seizures. *Epilepsia.* 2012;53(3):565–570.
46. Alessi R, Vincentiis S, Rzezak P, Valente KD. Semiology of psychogenic nonepileptic seizures: age-related differences. *Epilepsy Behav.* 2013;27(2):292–295.
47. Wyllie E, Glazer JP, Benbadis S, et al. Psychiatric features of children and adolescents with pseudo-seizures. *Arch Pediatr Adolesc Med.* 1999;153(3):244–248.
48. Wyllie E, Friedman D, Lüders H, et al. Outcome of psychogenic seizures in children and adolescents compared with adults. *Neurology.* 1991;41(5):742–744.
49. Vandenplas Y, Salvatore S, Hauser B. The diagnosis and management of gastro-oesophageal reflux in infants. *Early Hum Dev.* 2005;81(12):1011–1024.
50. Kinsbourne M. Hiatus hernia with contortions of the neck. *Lancet.* 1964;1(7342):1058–1061.
51. Shahar E, Raviv R. Sporadic major hyperekplexia in neonates and infants: clinical manifestations and outcome. *Pediatr Neurol.* 2004;31(1):30–34.
52. Hayashi T, Tachibana H, Kajii T. Hyperekplexia: pedigree studies in two families. *Am J Med Genet.* 1991;40(2):138–143.
53. Nigro MA, Lim HC. Hyperekplexia and sudden neonatal death. *Pediatr Neurol.* 1992;8(3):221–225.
54. Bode A, Wood SE, Mullins JG, et al. New hyperekplexia mutations provide insight into glycine receptor assembly, trafficking, and activation mechanisms. *J Biol Chem.* 2013;288(47):33745–33759.
55. Elmslie FV, Hutchings SM, Spencer V, et al. Analysis of GLRA1 in hereditary and sporadic hyperekplexia: a novel mutation in a family cosegregating for hyperekplexia and spastic paraparesis. *J Med Genet.* 1996;33(5):435–436.

56. Nechay A, Ross LM, Stephenson JB, O'Regan M. Gratification disorder ("infantile masturbation"): a review. *Arch Dis Child*. 2004;89(3):225–226.
57. Jan MM, Al Banji MH, Fallatah BA. Long-term outcome of infantile gratification phenomena. *Can J Neurol Sci*. 2013;40(3):416–419.
58. Russell MB, Olesen J. A nosographic analysis of the migraine aura in a general population. *Brain*. 1996; 119(Pt 2):355–361.
59. Golden GS. The Alice in Wonderland syndrome in juvenile migraine. *Pediatrics*. 1979;63(4):517–519.
60. Winner P, Martinez W, Mate L, Bello L. Classification of pediatric migraine: proposed revisions to the IHS criteria. *Headache*. 1995;35(7):407–410.
61. Panayiotopoulos CP. Elementary visual hallucinations, blindness, and headache in idiopathic occipital epilepsy: differentiation from migraine. *J Neurol Neurosurg Psychiatry*. 1999;66(4):536–540.
62. Andermann F, Zifkin B. The benign occipital epilepsies of childhood: an overview of the idiopathic syndromes and of the relationship to migraine. *Epilepsia*. 1998;39 Suppl 4:S9–S23.
63. Alemayehu S, Bergey GK, Barry E, et al. Panic attacks as ictal manifestations of parietal lobe seizures. *Epilepsia*. 1995;36(8):824–830.
64. Spitz MC. Panic disorder in seizure patients: a diagnostic pitfall. *Epilepsia*. 1991;32(1):33–38.
65. Lüders H, Acharya J, Baumgartner C, et al. Semiological seizure classification. *Epilepsia*. 1998;39(9):1006–1013.
66. Carmant L, Kramer U, Holmes GL, et al. Differential diagnosis of staring spells in children: a video-EEG study. *Pediatr Neurol*. 1996;14(3):199–202.
67. Rosenow F, Wyllie E, Kotagal P, et al. Staring spells in children: descriptive features distinguishing epileptic and nonepileptic events. *J Pediatr*. 1998;133(5):660–663.
68. Bridge EM, Livingston S, Tietze C. Breath-holding spells: Their relationship to syncope, convulsions, and other phenomena. *J Pediatr*. 1943;23:539–561.
69. DiMario FJ Jr. Breath-holding spells in childhood. *Am J Dis Child*. 1992;146(1):125–131.
70. DiMario FJ Jr. Prospective study of children with cyanotic and pallid breath-holding spells. *Pediatrics*. 2001;107(2):265–269.
71. Breningstall GN. Breath-holding spells. *Pediatr Neurol*. 1996;14(2):91–97.
72. Lombroso CT, Lerman P. Breathholding spells (cyanotic and pallid infantile syncope). *Pediatrics*. 1967;39(4):563–581.
73. DiMario FJ Jr, Sarfarazi M. Family pedigree analysis of children with severe breath-holding spells. *J Pediatr*. 1997;130(4):647–651.
74. Daoud AS, Batieha A, al-Sheyyab M, et al. Effectiveness of iron therapy on breath-holding spells. *J Pediatr*. 1997;130(4):547–550.
75. Colina KF, Abelson HT. Resolution of breath-holding spells with treatment of concomitant anemia. *J Pediatr*. 1995;126(3):395–397.
76. Holowach J, Thurston DL. Breath-holding spells and anemia. *N Engl J Med*. 1963;268:21–23.
77. Donma MM. Clinical efficacy of piracetam in treatment of breath-holding spells. *Pediatr Neurol*. 1998;18(1):41–45.
78. Sawires H, Botrous O. Double-blind, placebo-controlled trial on the effect of piracetam on breath-holding spells. *Eur J Pediatr*. 2012;171(7):1063–1067.
79. Kelly AM, Porter CJ, McGoon MD, et al. Breath-holding spells associated with significant bradycardia: successful treatment with permanent pacemaker implantation. *Pediatrics*. 2001;108(3):698–702.
80. Kenny RA, Bhangu J, King-Kallimanis BL. Epidemiology of syncope/collapse in younger and older Western patient populations. *Prog Cardiovasc Dis*. 2013;55(4):357–363.
81. Ikiz MA, Cetin II, Ekici F, et al. Pediatric syncope: is detailed medical history the key point for differential diagnosis? *Pediatr Emerg Care*. 2014;30(5):331–334.
82. van Dijk JG, Thijs RD, van Zwet E, et al. The semiology of tilt-induced reflex syncope in relation to electroencephalographic changes. *Brain*. 2014;137(Pt 2):576–585.
83. Lempert T. [Syncope. Phenomenology and differentiation from epileptic seizures]. *Nervenarzt*. 1997;68(8):620–624.
84. Mignot E, Lin L, Rogers W, et al. Complex HLA-DR and -DQ interactions confer risk of narcolepsy-cataplexy in three ethnic groups. *Am J Hum Genet*. 2001;68(3):686–699.
85. Macleod S, Ferrie C, Zuberi SM. Symptoms of narcolepsy in children misinterpreted as epilepsy. *Epileptic Disord*. 2005;7(1):13–17.

86. Laberge L, Tremblay RE, Vitaro F, Montplaisir J. Development of parasomnias from childhood to early adolescence. *Pediatrics*. 2000;106(1 Pt 1):67–74.
87. Petit D, Touchette E, Tremblay RE, et al. Dyssomnias and parasomnias in early childhood. *Pediatrics*. 2007;119(5):e1016–e1025.

EEG Interpretation in Childhood Epilepsies

Charuta N. Joshi, MBBS, FRCPC
Thoru Yamada, MD, FACNS

In this chapter we address the electroencephalography (EEG) of pediatric epilepsies. The epilepsies of premature babies or neonates are beyond the scope of this chapter.

PAROXYSMAL DISCHARGES AND SEIZURE DIAGNOSIS

In evaluating the EEG of a patient with possible seizures, we may see *interictal epileptiform discharges (IEDs)* and/or nonspecific paroxysmal discharges, with or without focal or diffuse slowing. IEDs, represented by spike or spike-wave discharges, are the most sensitive and specific markers for the diagnosis of seizures. In a routine EEG (a recording of approximately 30 min) the chance of recording a clinical seizure (ictal) event is rather rare, unless the patient is having frequent seizures or is in status epilepticus. Thus, we often rely primarily on IEDs for the diagnosis of epilepsy.

The likelihood of detecting IEDs varies, depending on seizure type, age, and seizure frequency. An EEG that includes sleep or is recorded after sleep deprivation increases the yield of IEDs. Generally, greater seizure frequency is associated with higher yield of IEDs (1). IEDs are also recorded more often in children than in adults. Detection of IEDs differs, depending on the origin of the epileptiform activity: If a relatively small area of cortex is involved as the epileptogenic zone, IEDs may not be detected by scalp electrodes. Also, epileptiform activity arising from deep brain structures such as the medial temporal lobe, subfrontal lobe, or interhemispheric medial cortex may not be readily recorded by scalp electrodes.

The specificity of IEDs is determined by the incidence of IEDs in the normal population (false-positive), compared with that in patients with epilepsy. IEDs are found in 1.9% to 3.5%

of healthy children (2,3) and 0.5% of healthy adults (4). Specificity also varies depending on the type of IEDs: Only about 40% of the patients with benign rolandic spikes of childhood or *benign epilepsy of childhood with centrotemporal spikes (BECTS)* and 50% of patients with *childhood epilepsy with occipital paroxysms (benign occipital spikes of childhood)* have a history of seizures (5). Also IEDs elicited by photic stimulation and generalized spike-wave discharges are less correlated with seizure history compared to focal spikes. Multifocal IEDs and focal IEDs, especially at the midline, frontal, and anterior temporal regions are highly (75%–95%) correlated with clinical seizures (5,6). Overall, the incidence of detecting IEDs during the first EEG in adult epilepsy patients is about 30% to 50% (7,8). In children less than 10 years old, the incidence is about 80%. Overall, repeating the EEG once increases the yield an additional 20% to 30% (7,8).

THE EPILEPSIES

Certain forms of epileptic seizure disorders have special clinical and EEG characteristics irrespective of their etiologies. The International Classification of Epilepsies and Epileptic Syndromes were proposed by the Committee on Classification and Terminology of the International League Against Epilepsy (9). This classification is based on two principles, distinguishing first between localized (focal) and generalized epilepsies and second between idiopathic and symptomatic etiologies.

Normal or near-normal background activity is characteristic of idiopathic epilepsy, and slowing of background activity or multifocal epileptiform activity are suggestive of symptomatic epilepsy. Focal background abnormality and/or focal polymorphic delta activity are likely correlated with symptomatic epilepsy.

Localized (Focal) Epilepsies and Syndromes

In the localized epilepsies and syndromes, examples of the idiopathic type include benign childhood epilepsy with centrotemporal spikes (rolandic spikes or BECTS and childhood epilepsy with occipital paroxysms (benign childhood occipital lobe epilepsy). Symptomatic localized epilepsies and syndromes include frontal, parietal, and temporal or occipital lobe seizures that are secondary to focal pathology.

The localization of an epileptogenic focus often determines the character of the seizures. To some extent, it is possible to speculate on the clinical manifestation of seizures based on the localization and waveform of epileptiform activity. Conversely, it may be possible to postulate the localization and waveforms of epileptiform activity based on clinical seizure types.

Benign Epilepsy of Childhood With Centrotemporal Spikes

Spikes maximally recorded from central or midtemporal electrodes have been described as BECTS or *benign rolandic epilepsy*. The waveform is more commonly "sharp" rather than a true spike, having a triphasic configuration with a prominent negative peak, preceded and followed by small positive peaks. The negative field centered at the central or midtemporal electrode is commonly associated with positive fields in the frontal region (Figure 4.1A–B). These discharges are often unilateral but one-third of the patients have bilateral independent foci. Sleep (non–rapid eye movement [non-REM]) greatly increases the spikes and about one-third

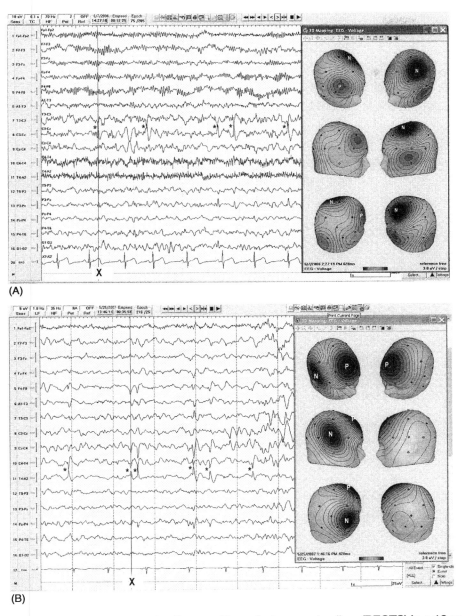

FIGURE 4.1 (A) Benign childhood epilepsy with centrotemporal spikes (BECTS) in a 12-year-old girl with a history of nocturnal generalized tonic-clonic convulsions with postictal aphasia and right arm weakness (Todd's paralysis). Electroencephalogram (EEG) showed spikes maximum at C3 (marked by *). Note the maximum negative (N) field at C3 and positive (P) field at contralateral frontal regions shown by three-dimensional (3D) topographic mapping (maps were made at the negative peak marked by X). (B) Benign childhood epilepsy with centrotemporal spikes (BECTS) in a 10-year-old boy with a history of nocturnal generalized tonic-clonic convulsions. Electroencephalogram (EEG) showed spikes maximum at T4 (marked by *). Note the maximum negative (N) field at T4 and positive field (P) at contralateral frontal region shown by three-dimensional (3D) topographic mapping (maps were made at the negative peak marked by X).

Source: From Ref. (74). Yamada T, Meng E. *Practical Guide for Clinical Neurophysiologic Testing: EEG.* Philadelphia, PA: Wolters Kluwer/Lippincott Williams & Wilkins, 2010; with permission.

of the patients have spike discharges only in sleep (10). Also, unilateral spikes in the awake state may progress to bilaterally independent spikes in sleep. Rolandic spikes tend to decrease progressively with age and eventually disappear by the midteen years (11). The onset of seizures usually occurs between 4 years and adolescence. Consistent with the dramatic increase of spike discharges in sleep, about 80% of seizures occur exclusively in sleep (12).

Clinically, seizures initially consist of unilateral paresthesias of tongue, lips, cheek, and gum and/or unilateral tonic-clonic activity of facial and pharyngeal/laryngeal muscles contralateral to the side of the spike focus. The ictal discharges often start with an initial electrodecremental pattern followed by rhythmic spike bursts with subsequent spike-wave discharges. The seizure ends without postictal slowing, unless the seizure evolves to a generalized tonic-clonic convulsion, which is not uncommon.

Not all spike discharges from central regions are benign. Some features help to distinguish benign rolandic epilepsy from symptomatic (nonbenign) epilepsy. As shown in Figures 4.1A–B, benign rolandic spikes are tangentially oriented with a negative field just behind the rolandic fissure, either at or close to the central or midtemporal electrode, and a positive field over the frontal region. In symptomatic epilepsy, spikes have often radially oriented distribution; thus the negative field spreads diffusely over a wide scalp region (12). Focal slowing (corresponding to the side of spikes) is absent in benign rolandic epilepsy but it is often present in symptomatic epilepsy (Figure 4.2). When a rolandic spike is maximum at the midtemporal electrodes, differentiation of temporal lobe epilepsy with spikes at T3/T4 electrode from benign rolandic epilepsy can be more difficult. In this case, additional electrodes between C3/C4 and T3/T4 (C5/C6 according to the expanded 10-20 system) help to distinguish the two: Rolandic spikes are maximum at C5/C6, whereas symptomatic temporal lobe seizures likely have a maximum at T3 or T4 (13).

Childhood Epilepsy With Occipital Spikes

There are two types of seizures categorized in this entity: late onset, originally described by Gastaut (14) (*Gastaut type*) and early onset, more recently described by Panayiotopoulos (15), and now referred to as *Panayiotopoulos syndrome*. Affected children are neurologically normal in both types. Family history of epilepsy is positive in more than one-third of the patients for the late-onset type but negative for the early-onset type. In the late-onset variant, age of seizure onset ranges from 15 months to 17 years with a peak age of 7 to 9 years (16). In the early-onset variant, onset is between 1 and 14 years with a peak age of 3 to 6 years (17).

In the late-onset type, seizures almost always begin with visual symptoms (blindness, scintillating scotoma, visual hallucinations, or illusions). The seizure is usually brief, lasting only a few to several seconds. Half of the patients complain of severe migraine-like headache associated with nausea and vomiting (14). Thus, differentiation from migraine headache may be sometimes difficult. The prognosis is good overall but less favorable than that of BECTS.

In the early-onset type, seizures lack characteristic visual symptoms but consist of a variety of autonomic symptoms including "feeling sick," paleness, nausea, vomiting, cyanosis, myosis, or mydriasis, and cardiopulmonary irregularities. The seizure lasts much longer (5–10 min) than the late-onset type and often ends with a hemiconvulsion, Jacksonian march, or generalized motor activity. About one-third of the seizures occur in sleep. Nearly all patients become seizure-free by age 12 years (17).

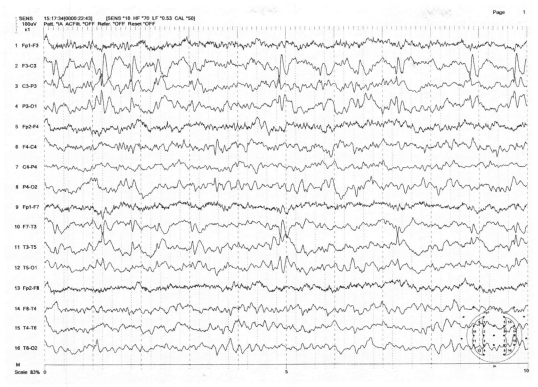

FIGURE 4.2 Spike discharges at left central and midtemporal region in a 6-year-old boy with a history of focal seizure involving the right arm. Note the spike discharges maximum at left central and midtemporal region and also the increased delta and decreased background activity over the left hemisphere. This is unlikely to be benign childhood epilepsy with centrotemporal spikes (BECTS).

Source: From Ref. (74). Yamada T, Meng E. *Practical Guide for Clinical Neurophysiologic Testing: EEG.* Philadelphia, PA: Wolters Kluwer/Lippincott Williams & Wilkins, 2010; with permission.

EEG abnormalities are indistinguishable between the Gastaut or the Panayiotopoulos type of seizures. Spikes consist of high-amplitude surface negativity (200–300 µV), often followed by a small positive and negative slow wave (Figure 4.3). These occur singly or more commonly in serial, semirhythmic bursts with a unilateral or bilaterally independent appearance. Eye opening tends to abolish the spike wave and eye closing may precipitate the burst. However, neither repetitive photic stimulation nor hyperventilation precipitates epileptiform discharges (16). As with BECTS, sleep (non-REM) increases the discharges, but less prominently as compared to BECTS.

About one-fourth to one-third of the patients have other epileptogenic abnormalities including generalized spike-waves or BECTS (16,18) (Figure 4.4). The ictal EEG consists of rhythmic spike discharges starting from one occipital region evolving into rhythmic theta-delta that spreads to the contralateral occipital region (Figure 4.5).

Benign childhood occipital lobe epilepsy must be differentiated from other occipital spikes. Many patients with congenital or acquired amblyopia are found to have occipital spikes, but the morphology of the spike is much faster ("needlelike spike") than that of benign childhood occipital epilepsy (19). Occipital spikes may also occur in idiopathic generalized seizure patients

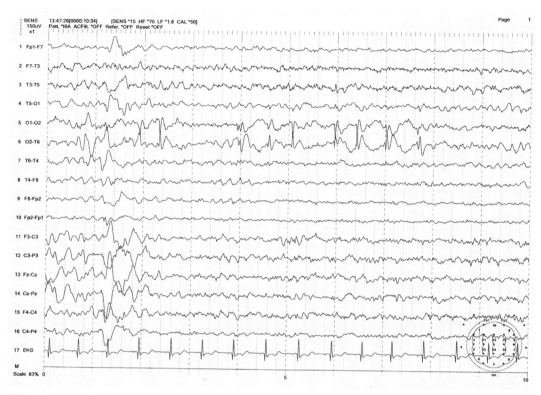

FIGURE 4.3 Childhood epilepsy with occipital paroxysms (benign occipital lobe epilepsy) in a 4-year-old boy whose seizures manifest as seeing "flashing light." Note the high-amplitude occipital spikes at O2 electrode.

Source: From Ref. (74). Yamada T, Meng E. *Practical Guide for Clinical Neurophysiologic Testing: EEG.* Philadelphia, PA: Wolters Kluwer/Lippincott Williams & Wilkins, 2010; with permission.

with photoparoxysmal response (20) (Figure 4.6A–B). Patients may have localization-related seizures with vivid visual hallucinations (21). Although many "pure" simple partial seizures fail to show ictal discharges, partial seizures of occipital origin tend to show well-localized ictal EEG activity and the patient often is able to describe his/her visual hallucinatory event in detail.

Generalized Epilepsies

Idiopathic generalized epilepsies and syndromes include absence seizures (childhood and juvenile) and juvenile myoclonic epilepsy (JME). West syndrome and Lennox-Gastaut syndrome (LGS) are examples of generalized epilepsy of a symptomatic type.

Primary Generalized Epilepsies

Generalized epileptiform discharges appear in both hemispheres simultaneously with similar configuration, symmetric amplitude, and synchronous timing between homologous electrodes. Timing between anterior and posterior discharges may differ slightly within the same hemisphere. When discharges consistently have a higher amplitude in one hemisphere or generalized discharges are consistently preceded by focal discharges, this suggests a focal onset to a secondarily generalized seizure type, but clear-cut differentiation between a primary and secondary

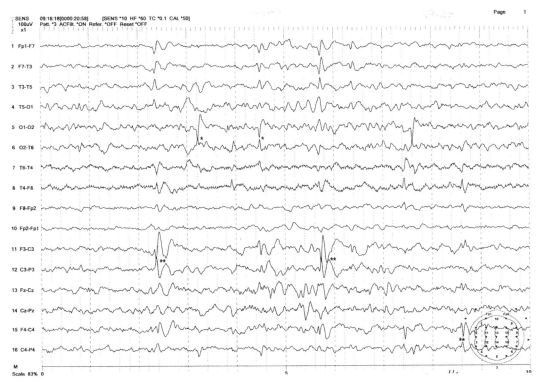

FIGURE 4.4 Two coexisting types of benign paroxysm—benign rolandic spike of childhood (BECTS) and childhood epilepsy with occipital paroxysm (benign occipital childhood epilepsy) in a 10-year-old girl with a history of generalized tonic-clonic seizures. Note the two independent BECTS at C3/T3 and C4/T4.

Source: From Ref. (74). Yamada T, Meng E. *Practical Guide for Clinical Neurophysiologic Testing: EEG.* Philadelphia, PA: Wolters Kluwer/Lippincott Williams & Wilkins, 2010; with permission.

generalized seizure pattern is not always clear-cut. Distinction between ictal and interictal patterns in absence seizures is also not as clear as that of a focal seizure. Often, the EEG associated with a clinical seizure may be simply a longer and more rhythmic repetition than interictal IEDs.

ABSENCE EPILEPSY The discovery of 3 Hz spike-wave bursts in association with petit mal or absence seizures by Gibbs, Davis, and Lennox (22) in 1935 was the first major epoch in the history of EEG and the electrographic diagnosis of epilepsy. This is characterized by rhythmic cycles of spike-wave complexes at a frequency of about 3 Hz, usually lasting a few to several seconds. The spike-wave complexes are generally maximum in the frontal region and may start with a frequency 3 to 3.5 Hz and end with a frequency 2 to 3 Hz (Figure 4.7). The initial complex may have a polyspike-wave pattern. Although the bursts seem to be synchronous between the two hemispheres, detailed analysis with a faster sweep recording shows that the spikes in one hemisphere may randomly precede those in the other hemisphere by a few milliseconds (23). The discharges tend to be inhibited by eye opening or increased vigilance. Hyperventilation often precipitates the bursts associated with clinical absence seizures in 50% to 80% of the patients (24). Intermittent photic stimulation induces spike-wave bursts in about one-fifth of the

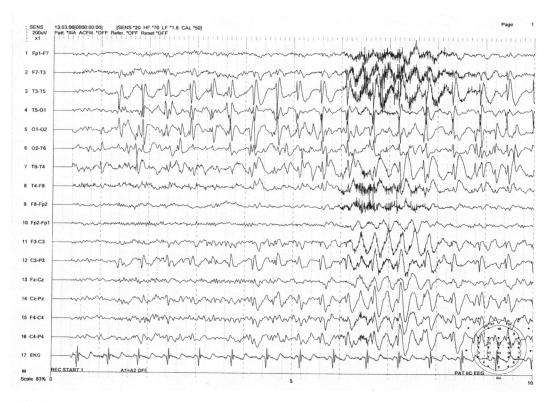

FIGURE 4.5 Ictal discharges in childhood epilepsy with occipital paroxysm (benign occipital childhood epilepsy) in an 11-year-old girl with ictal manifestation of blindness, nausea, and migraine-like headache. Note the rhythmic spike-wave discharges initially originating from O1 electrode with subsequent spread to other electrodes. Also there were independent spikes at T6 electrode, which became synchronized with the occipital spikes as the seizure progressed.

Source: From Ref. (74). Yamada T, Meng E. *Practical Guide for Clinical Neurophysiologic Testing: EEG.* Philadelphia, PA: Wolters Kluwer/Lippincott Williams & Wilkins, 2010; with permission.

patients with absence epilepsy (25). Non-REM sleep also increases the number of spike-wave complexes, which tend to become more irregular with polyspike-wave patterns (26). REM sleep decreases the number of bursts to a frequency slightly less than the waking state (26). Valproic acid and ethosuximide, commonly used medications for absence seizures, tend to decrease the number of spike-wave bursts (27) and also attenuate activation by photic stimulation (28).

In patients with absence epilepsy, background activity is usually normal, but slowing can occur in a minority of patients. Generally, about 20% to 40% of patients with absence seizures show 3 Hz rhythmic delta bursts in the occipital regions (occipital intermittent rhythmic delta activity [OIRDA]) (Figure 4.8), and the incidence of OIRDA is much higher in children between 6 and 10 years (29). Visible clinical seizures can usually be observed when spike-wave bursts last more than 4 to 5 seconds. Symptoms are characterized by staring, impaired responsiveness, and behavior arrest. Impaired responsiveness can occur with spike-wave bursts as short as 3 seconds. Responsiveness returns abruptly to normal at the end of the spike wave. Detailed psychophysiological testing of such patients found decreased reaction time even during a brief spike-wave burst without an associated overt clinical seizure (30). Automatisms with

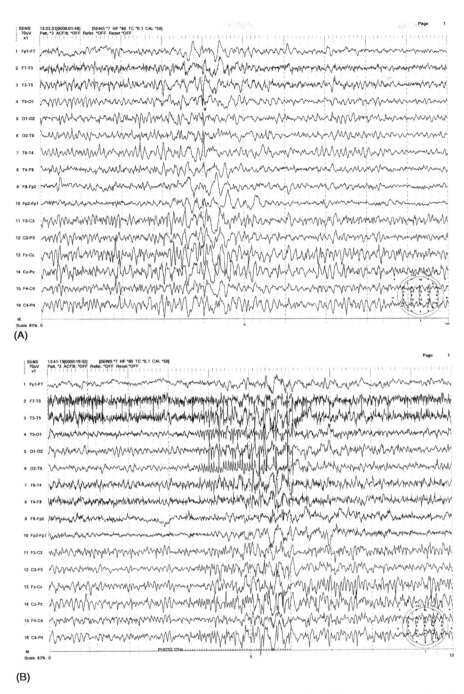

FIGURE 4.6 (A) Occipital spikes in a 34-year-old man with a history of generalized tonic-clonic convulsions since childhood. Note the spike discharges are maximum at O1 electrode (indicated by *). (B) This patient also had a photoparoxysmal response at 17 Hz with the initial occipital polyspikes time-locked to the flashes, followed by generalized irregular spike-wave bursts.

Source: From Ref. (74). Yamada T, Meng E. *Practical Guide for Clinical Neurophysiologic Testing: EEG.* Philadelphia, PA: Wolters Kluwer/Lippincott Williams & Wilkins, 2010; with permission.

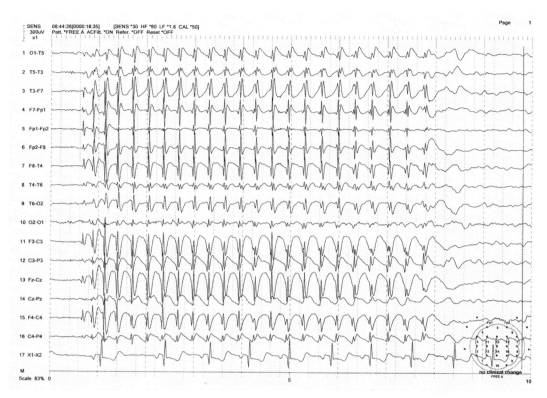

FIGURE 4.7 Spike-wave bursts of 3 Hz associated with absence seizure in a 7-year-old boy (childhood absence). Note that spike-wave bursts started with a frequency slightly faster than 3 Hz and ended with a frequency slightly slower than 3 Hz.

Source: From Ref. (74). Yamada T, Meng E. *Practical Guide for Clinical Neurophysiologic Testing: EEG.* Philadelphia, PA: Wolters Kluwer/Lippincott Williams & Wilkins, 2010; with permission.

lip smacking, chewing, fumbling, or mild myoclonus (eyelid twitches) resembling a temporal lobe seizure may be seen (31). The frequency of eyelid twitches is usually 3 Hz coinciding with 3 Hz spike waves. Some patients may have prominent eyelid myoclonus with faster frequency of 4 to 10 Hz. This is referred to as Jeavons syndrome (eyelid myoclonia with absences) (32). Some patients may have decreased postural tone. It is the technologist's role to examine the presence or absence of impaired responsiveness and to note the patient's behavior changes during spike-wave bursts. Absence seizures are classified into two types based on the age of onset.

Childhood Absence Epilepsy Onset of epilepsies is from 3 to 12 years. EEG and clinical presentation can assist in predicting the prognosis. Patients with an EEG showing 3 Hz OIRDA have a smaller risk of developing tonic-clonic seizures in the future (33). Absence seizures without myoclonus have a higher chance of remission than those with myoclonus (34).

Juvenile Absence Epilepsy The onset of juvenile absence epilepsy (JAE) is around 10 to 12 years or even later. The spike-wave bursts tend to be of a slightly faster frequency than 3 Hz and may have polyspike components (Figure 4.9). This group of patients is more likely to develop generalized tonic-clonic seizures or myoclonic seizures (35).

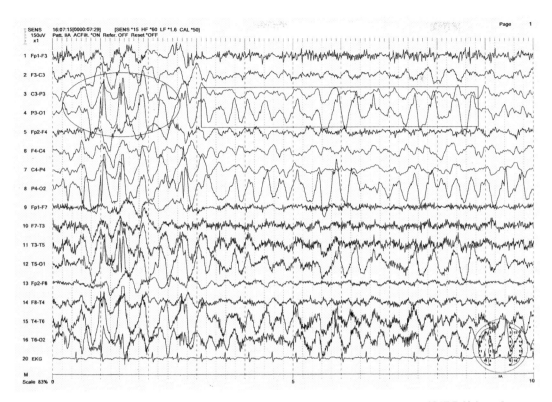

FIGURE 4.8 An example of occipital intermittent rhythmic delta activity (OIRDA) in a 9-year-old boy with a history of absence seizures. Note the occipital dominant 3 Hz spike-wave burst (shown by oval circle) mixed with 3 Hz OIRDA (shown by rectangular box).

Source: From Ref. (74). Yamada T, Meng E. *Practical Guide for Clinical Neurophysiologic Testing: EEG.* Philadelphia, PA: Wolters Kluwer/Lippincott Williams & Wilkins, 2010; with permission.

GENERALIZED TONIC-CLONIC EPILEPSIES Multiple spike-wave (polyspike-wave) bursts lasting less than 1 to several seconds are usually an interictal expression of a generalized seizure (Figure 4.10A–B). The interictal EEG of idiopathic (primary) generalized tonic-clonic epilepsies consists of a variety of waveforms, which are more irregular and of a faster frequency than the 3 Hz rhythmic spike-wave discharges seen in absence seizures. In addition, spike-wave bursts often include multiple spikes (polyspike). Spike-wave bursts are usually, but not always, symmetric and synchronous. Asymmetric bursts, however, do not necessarily exclude the possibility of primary generalized epilepsy. In fact, it is often difficult to differentiate primary from secondary generalized epilepsy, especially in the case of frontal lobe epilepsy. In some patients, focal spike discharges, such as "rolandic spikes," may coexist with generalized spike-wave bursts. In such cases, it is not possible to determine if the patient has a seizure of focal onset with secondary generalization or has both partial and primary generalized epilepsy. There are two features, which may help point toward a diagnosis of primary generalized epilepsy. One is a photoparoxysmal response (Figure 4.11A–B), and the other is generalized spike-wave bursts resembling K-complexes (Figure 4.12A–B). Like K-complexes, spike-wave bursts act as an arousal pattern. In some, generalized spike-wave bursts may be precipitated

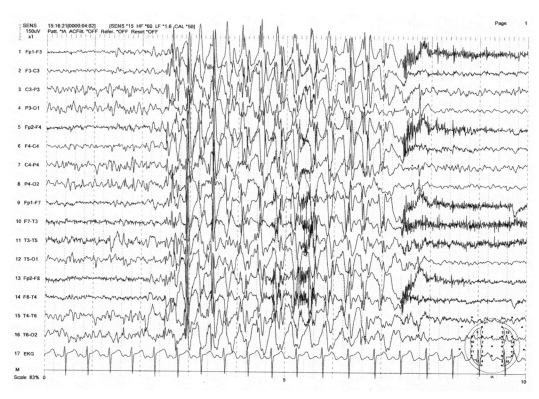

FIGURE 4.9 Spike-wave bursts of 3 Hz with initial polyspike component in an 18-year-old girl (juvenile absence). The patient had absence seizures in the past and recently started having generalized tonic-clonic convulsions.

Source: From Ref. (74). Yamada T, Meng E. *Practical Guide for Clinical Neurophysiologic Testing: EEG.* Philadelphia, PA: Wolters Kluwer/Lippincott Williams & Wilkins, 2010; with permission.

by arousal stimuli, similar to the K-complex. In some patients, especially in children who tend to have "spiky" K-complexes, the differentiation between the two could be difficult. These features were studied in detail by Niedermeyer, who introduced the concept of "dyshormia" in which primary generalized spike-wave bursts and K-complexes share the same generating mechanism producing generalized burst activity (36).

Onset of the ictal event in a generalized seizure consists of low-voltage, rhythmic beta-range fast activity, with progressively increasing amplitude and decreasing frequency (Figure 4.13A–B). This is followed by generalized spike-wave bursts, which become progressively slower in frequency and less rhythmic toward the end of the seizure. The EEG becomes suppressed during the immediate postictal period and is then followed by the appearance of postictal delta activity. Clinically, the initial fast activity corresponds with the tonic phase and the subsequent spike-wave bursts coincide with the clonic phase of the seizure. During the ictal events, EEG activities are largely obscured by muscle and movement artifacts, making it difficult to differentiate a genuine seizure from a pseudoseizure. The presence of postictal flattening or slowing provides evidence of a genuine seizure. Conversely, immediate normalization of the EEG favors a pseudoseizure, especially when the patient is unconscious or confused.

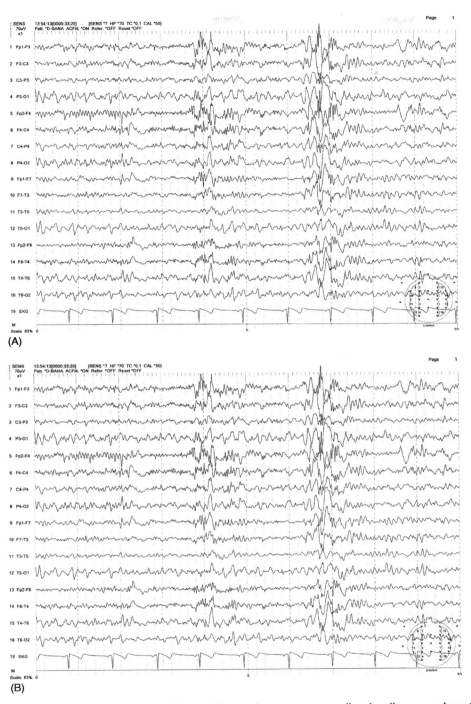

FIGURE 4.10 Somewhat irregular, bilaterally synchronous generalized spike-wave bursts of 4 to 6 Hz, maximum at midline (A) in a 30-year-old woman with a history of generalized tonic-clonic convulsions as well as myoclonic seizures since childhood. The patient also had more irregular polyspike-wave bursts during stage two sleep (B).

Source: From Ref. (74). Yamada T, Meng E. *Practical Guide for Clinical Neurophysiologic Testing: EEG.* Philadelphia, PA: Wolters Kluwer/Lippincott Williams & Wilkins, 2010; with permission.

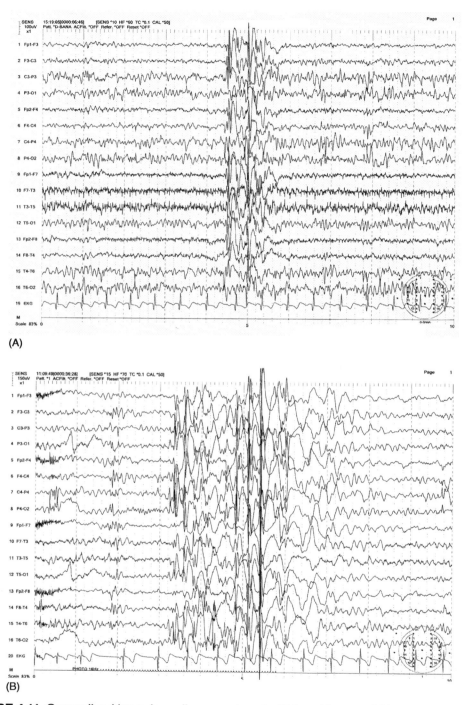

FIGURE 4.11 Generalized irregular spike-wave bursts (A) in a 10-year-old boy with a history of absence seizures and a recent grand mal seizure. Photic stimulation produced photoparoxysmal response at 16 Hz frequency flashes with generalized irregular spike-wave bursts (B).

Source: From Ref. (74). Yamada T, Meng E. *Practical Guide for Clinical Neurophysiologic Testing: EEG.* Philadelphia, PA: Wolters Kluwer/Lippincott Williams & Wilkins, 2010; with permission.

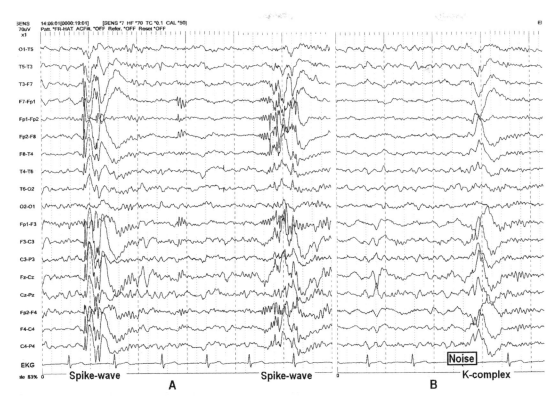

FIGURE 4.12 (A) Bilaterally diffuse synchronous and symmetric spike-wave bursts with bifrontal dominance in a 31-year-old man with a history of grand mal seizures since childhood. Note that the spike-wave bursts were followed by spindles. (B) With the exception of the spikes, the epileptiform bursts had similar waveform and distribution with K-complex induced by noise.

Source: From Ref. (74). Yamada T, Meng E. *Practical Guide for Clinical Neurophysiologic Testing: EEG.* Philadelphia, PA: Wolters Kluwer/Lippincott Williams & Wilkins, 2010; with permission.

JUVENILE MYOCLONIC EPILEPSY This was originally described by Janz as *impulsive petit mal* (37) and may be referred to as *juvenile myoclonic epilepsy of Janz*. JME is the most common type of seizure among idiopathic generalized epilepsies. Close to half of the patients have a family history of epilepsy (37). As the name implies, seizures usually begin in adolescence. The majority of patients (>90%) also have generalized tonic-clonic convulsions. Both myoclonic and generalized tonic-clonic convulsions tend to occur within 1 to 2 hours after awakening. A history of absence seizures coexists with or precedes myoclonic seizures in about one-third of the patients (38).

Interictal EEG patterns consist of generalized polyspike and polyspike-wave discharges with frontocentral predominance (Figure 4.14A). These patterns are not distinguishable from other idiopathic generalized epilepsies but may include more polyspike components. Like other idiopathic seizures, background activity is usually normal. Spike-wave or polyspike-wave bursts are usually faster than the typical 3 Hz spike-waves seen in absence seizures, but in some patients, 2.5 to 3 Hz spike-wave bursts may occur that are indistinguishable from typical absence seizures.

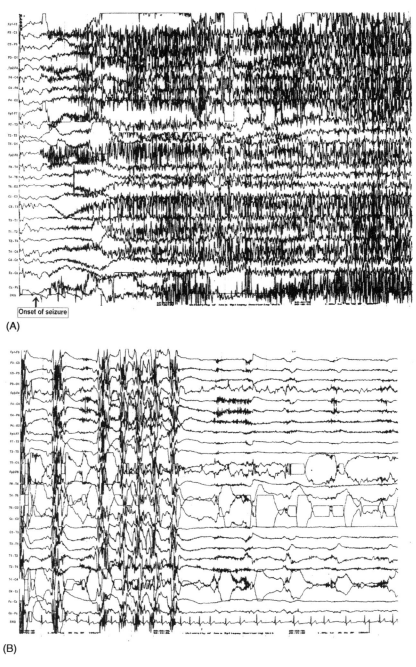

(A)

(B)

FIGURE 4.13 (A) A generalized ictal event in a 25-year-old man with a history of grand mal seizures since childhood. Note the sudden flattening of electroencephalography (EEG) activity at the onset, followed by beta activity peeking through the massive electromyogram (EMG) artifact during the tonic phase of seizure. (B) Toward the end of the seizure, ictal discharges changed to periodic spike-wave discharges, which were contaminated by muscle artifact (clonic phase). Afterward, there was postictal suppression of EEG activity.

Source: From Ref. (74). Yamada T, Meng E. *Practical Guide for Clinical Neurophysiologic Testing: EEG.* Philadelphia, PA: Wolters Kluwer/Lippincott Williams & Wilkins, 2010; with permission.

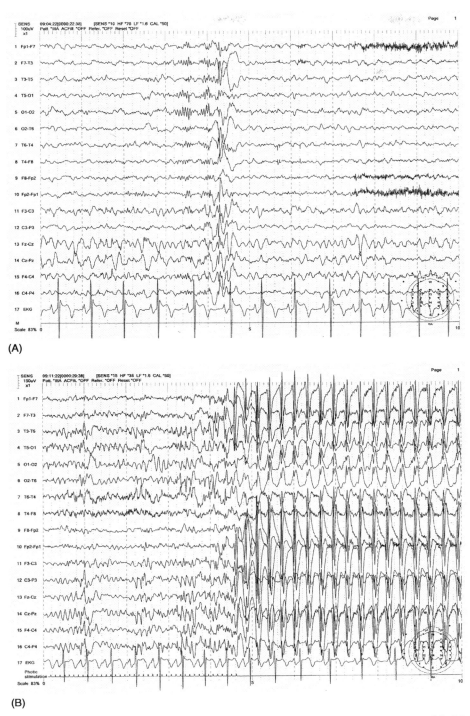

(A)

(B)

FIGURE 4.14 (A) An example of juvenile myoclonic epilepsy (JME) in a 14-year-old girl. Brief irregular (non-3 Hz) spike-wave discharges in sleep. (B) Photic stimulation–induced 3 Hz spike-wave bursts.

Source: From Ref. (74). Yamada T, Meng E. *Practical Guide for Clinical Neurophysiologic Testing: EEG.* Philadelphia, PA: Wolters Kluwer/Lippincott Williams & Wilkins, 2010; with permission.

Hyperventilation may activate epileptiform activity in JME but less often as compared to absence seizures. About 30% to 40% of the patients also have photoparoxysmal seizures (Figure 4.14B) (39). Photosensitive epilepsy is three to four times more common in girls than in boys (39). In contrast to other types of epilepsy, epileptiform activity tends to decrease in sleep but markedly increases shortly after awakening. The ictal pattern is indistinguishable from interictal epileptiform activity in most cases but may have a greater number of polyspikes with higher amplitude.

Symptomatic Generalized, Multifocal Seizures or Syndromes

Lennox-Gastaut Syndrome

W.G. Lennox (40) and later H. Gastaut (41) described the clinical and electroencephalographic features of this disorder. *LGS* represents characteristic triads comprising (a) severe generalized seizures, (b) mental retardation, and (c) an EEG showing slow spike-and-wave (SSW) complexes. The SSW complexes consist of biphasic or triphasic sharp or spike waves followed by high-voltage (300–400 µV or greater) slow waves (Figure 4.15). Frequency of SSW complexes is between 1.5 and 2.5 Hz and is slower and often more irregular than the 3 Hz spike-wave complexes associated with idiopathic absence epilepsy. The bursts are usually bilaterally

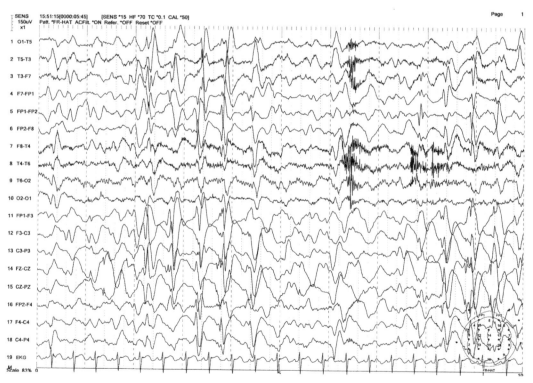

FIGURE 4.15 Generalized 2 Hz spike-wave bursts in an 18-year-old mentally disabled male with a history of intractable generalized tonic-clonic, tonic, and atypical absence seizures (Lennox-Gastaut syndrome). Note the high-voltage slow (2 Hz) spike-and-wave complexes associated with abundant irregular delta-theta activity in this awake EEG.

Source: From Ref. (74). Yamada T, Meng E. *Practical Guide for Clinical Neurophysiologic Testing: EEG.* Philadelphia, PA: Wolters Kluwer/Lippincott Williams & Wilkins, 2010; with permission.

synchronous but may show shifting or persistent asymmetries. Asymmetric bursts may be associated with a unilateral lesion (42). In contrast to idiopathic absence epilepsy, which is usually associated with normal background activity, background activity in LGS is slow in more than 70% of the patients (43). Unlike the 3 Hz spike-wave discharges of absence seizures, both hyperventilation and photic stimulation are less effective in eliciting spike-wave discharges (44). In sleep, SSW complexes may become polyspike-wave discharges (44). Also paroxysmal fast activity is common during sleep (45). In addition to SSW, focal or multifocal epileptiform discharges may be seen in some patients (46).

Median age of seizure onset in LGS is about 1 year and SSW complexes appear by 3 years. Greater than 75% have more than one type of seizure. The most common seizures are tonic seizure and atypical absence. Tonic seizures tend to appear at an earlier age and consist of sudden flexion of the hips, upper trunk, and neck, as well as arm abduction, elevation, or semiflexion. Because the seizure resembles infantile spasms, it can be considered a mature form of infantile spasms (47). Tonic seizures are associated with paroxysmal fast activity, often preceded by EEG flattening. The clinical distinction between typical and atypical absence seizures is not always clear but some features distinguish them. In atypical absence, impairment of consciousness is incomplete, rendering the transitions between normal activity and seizure activity unclear. Other symptoms such as eyelid or mouth myoclonus, changes in muscle tone, excessive salivation, and automatisms are common in atypical absence.

Ictal EEG change in atypical absence may be difficult to distinguish from the interictal pattern because both are represented by SSW complexes. The ictal pattern, however, tends to be more rhythmic, more widely distributed, and lasts longer than the interictal event (44). Other seizure types in LGS include clonic or tonic-clonic, atonic, myoclonic, and infantile spasms. The least common seizure is partial complex seizure.

INFANTILE SPASMS, SALAAM SPASMS, AND WEST SYNDROME Gibbs and Gibbs (48) first coined *hypsarrhythmia* (*hyps* means mountainous) to characterize the EEG pattern of "very high-voltage" (usually greater than 500 μV) irregular, asynchronous delta slow waves associated with multifocal spikes (Figure 4.16A). Spikes may be obscured by high-amplitude delta activity. The chaotic high-amplitude slow wave activity may be intermittently replaced by a relatively low-amplitude pattern (partial flattening) lasting 1 to 2 seconds. Because of exceedingly high-amplitude slow waves, waveforms are typically truncated in a recording using routine sensitivity (S = 7). Also, spikes are often hidden among large slow waves, and multifocal spikes are better visualized by using a shorter time constant (higher low-frequency filter) (Figure 4.16B). Typical hypsarrhythmia is common in younger infants, and over time the degree of abnormality tends to lessen to produce more organized activity with greater synchrony and symmetry and lower amplitude (49). The pattern may become modified, in which generalized sharp and slow-wave bursts become more synchronous within one hemisphere or between the two hemispheres (50). In cases of large focal lesions such as cysts or porencephaly, the hypsarrhythmic pattern may be unilateral (asymmetric hypsarrhythmia) or associated with persistent focal spikes or sharp waves (Figure 4.17). These variations may be classified as *modified hypsarrhythmia*. The hypsarrhythmic pattern is much more common in non-REM sleep than in the awake state or REM sleep (51). In non-REM sleep, bursts may become associated with longer attenuation periods. Hypsarrhythmia is commonly, but not always, associated with the clinical syndrome of *infantile spasms* or *West syndrome* (52). Infantile spasms

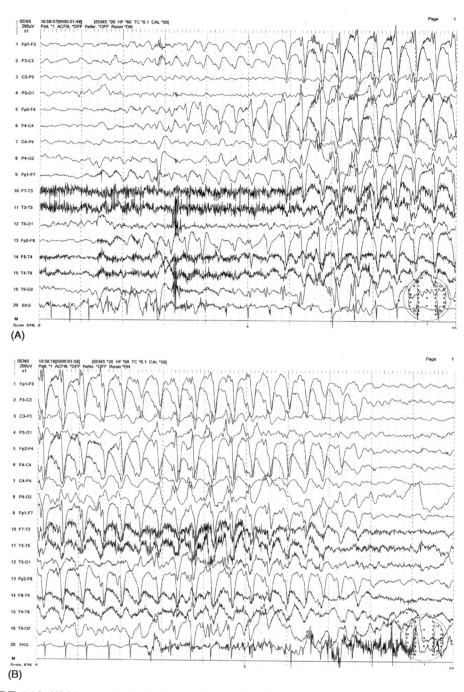

FIGURE 4.16 (A) Hypsarrhythmia in an 18-month-old microcephalic boy with infantile spasms. Note the high-amplitude irregular delta activity mixed with multifocal spikes and characteristic brief episodes of quiescence between bursts. (B) The evidence of multifocal and scattered spikes are better visualized by eliminating slow waves using a shorter time constant (0.03 seconds) or lower filter setting of 5 Hz (A and B are the same EEG samples).

Source: From Ref. (74). Yamada T, Meng E. *Practical Guide for Clinical Neurophysiologic Testing: EEG.* Philadelphia, PA: Wolters Kluwer/Lippincott Williams & Wilkins, 2010; with permission.

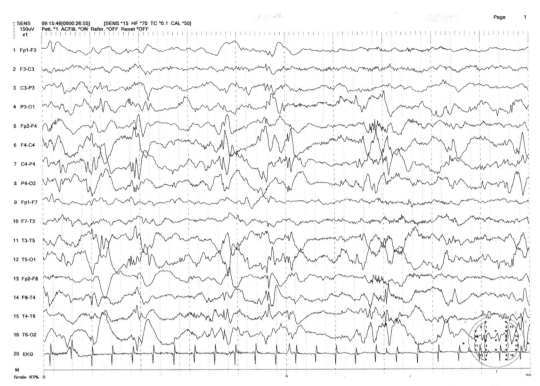

FIGURE 4.17 Modified hypsarrhythmia in an 8-month-old girl with a history of group B streptococcal meningitis at 2 weeks of age. The patient had frequent body jerks representing infantile spasms. Note the high-amplitude irregular spike-wave discharges from the right hemisphere, with brief flattening periods between bursts.

Source: From Ref. (74). Yamada T, Meng E. *Practical Guide for Clinical Neurophysiologic Testing: EEG.* Philadelphia, PA: Wolters Kluwer/Lippincott Williams & Wilkins, 2010; with permission.

may also be seen in patients with *Aicardi syndrome* with a distinct EEG pattern characterized by completely asynchronous burst suppression and multifocal spikes (Figure 4.18) (53). Seizures consist of brief flexion of the neck, trunk, and extremities. This sudden flexed motion is called a *jackknife seizure or salaam attack.* Seizures tend to occur in clusters shortly after awakening. The most common ictal EEG pattern associated with flexion spasms is sudden cessation of paroxysmal activity replaced by low-voltage fast activity or flattening of EEG activity, termed an *electrodecremental seizure* (Figure 4.19A–B). Other ictal patterns include frontal-dominant, high-amplitude rhythmic delta bursts or, less commonly, generalized spike- or sharp-wave complexes.

The majority (>95%) of infantile spasms begin before the age of 1 year. Etiologies are diverse and include hereditary metabolic disorders, intrauterine infection, cerebral dysgenesis, tuberous sclerosis, hypoxic encephalopathy, etc. After adrenocorticotropic hormone (ACTH) or prednisone therapy, more than 60% of the patients improve dramatically with normalization of the EEG (54). Hypsarrhythmia disappears by 5 years; the EEG becomes normal in about half of the patients, while others continue to show various epileptiform discharges, focal, multifocal, or generalized including an SSW pattern (LGS). Normalization of the EEG does not necessarily indicate a normal neurologic state; nearly 90% of the patients remain disabled by epilepsy and other neurological deficits including severe mental impairment.

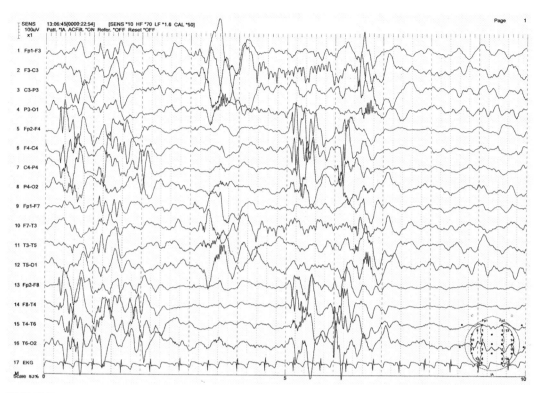

FIGURE 4.18 Electroencephalogram (EEG) of Aicardi syndrome in a 15-month-old girl with infantile spasms and hypsarrhythmic EEG. Note the gross asynchrony of EEG patterns between the two hemispheres.

Source: From Ref. (74). Yamada T, Meng E. *Practical Guide for Clinical Neurophysiologic Testing: EEG.* Philadelphia, PA: Wolters Kluwer/Lippincott Williams & Wilkins, 2010; with permission.

Landau-Kleffner Syndrome

This syndrome, first described by Landau and Kleffner (55), is diagnosed based on characteristic clinical presentation and EEG abnormalities. Landau-Kleffner syndrome (LKS) affects 3- to 9-year-old children who were previously in good health. The first clinical sign is aphasia, which progressively worsens. Speech becomes progressively less intelligible and is eventually limited to only a few words (56). Hyperactivity and personality changes may appear as the aphasia worsens. About two-thirds of the patients have seizures of various types, including myoclonus, partial motor, akinetic/atonic, atypical absence, and generalized tonic-clonic convulsions (56).

The EEG in LKS is characterized by abundant epileptiform activity that is extremely variable in both location and volume; because of the characteristic deterioration of speech function, one may assume that the dominant hemisphere (left) is primarily affected. In some cases, the epileptiform activity indeed affects preferentially the left temporal region. But surprisingly, the majority of cases show variable patterns ranging from unifocal to multifocal and generalized spike waves. In the early stages of the illness, epileptiform activity may appear only in sleep. As the disease progresses, EEG abnormalities change considerably in terms of location, abundance, and pattern. Eventually, spikes and spike-wave discharges become more or less continuous, resulting in an

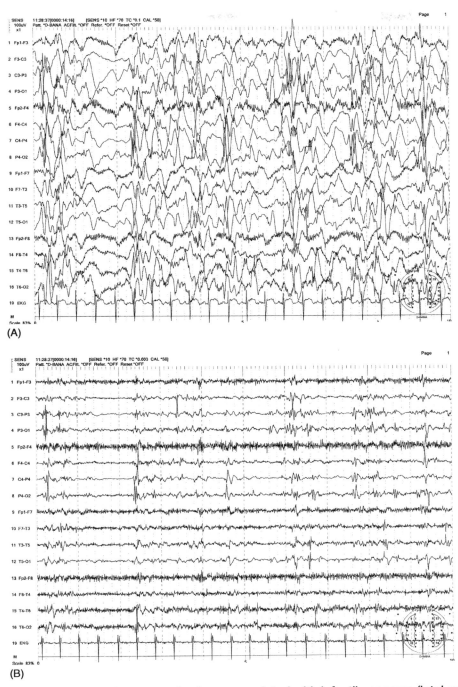

FIGURE 4.19 (A) Electrodecremental seizure associated with infantile spasms (ictal event) in a 2.5-year-old child with a history of hypoxic encephalopathy and severe developmental delay. Note the sudden flattening of electroencephalographic (EEG) activity accompanied by beta activity with concomitant increase of muscle tone artifact associated with body and arm jerks. (B) Interictal hypsarrhythmic pattern of this patient.

Source: From Ref. (74). Yamada T, Meng E. *Practical Guide for Clinical Neurophysiologic Testing: EEG.* Philadelphia, PA: Wolters Kluwer/Lippincott Williams & Wilkins, 2010; with permission.

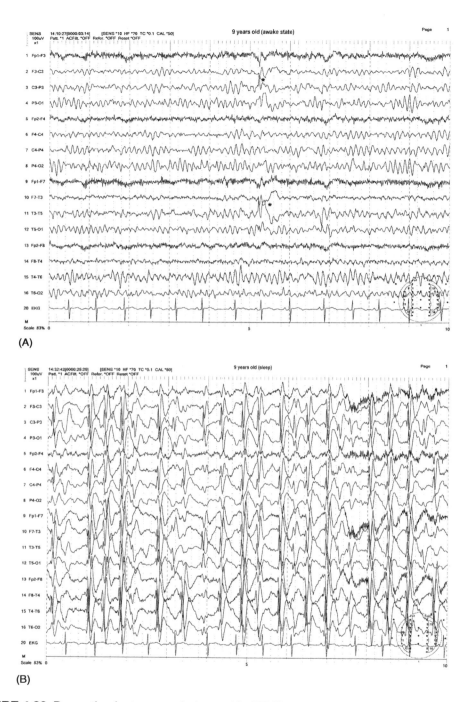

FIGURE 4.20 Dramatic electroencephalographic (EEG) change from awake (A) to asleep (B) state in a 9-year-old boy with the diagnosis of Landau-Kleffner syndrome. Note the sporadic sharp wave discharges from the left hemisphere (indicated by the * in A) in the awake state and the more or less continuous generalized spike-wave bursts becoming electrographic status epilepticus in sleep (B).

Source: From Ref. (74). Yamada T, Meng E. *Practical Guide for Clinical Neurophysiologic Testing: EEG.* Philadelphia, PA: Wolters Kluwer/Lippincott Williams & Wilkins, 2010; with permission.

appearance of "electrographic status epilepticus" in sleep (Figure 4.20A–B). This EEG feature is similar to that seen in the syndrome of continuous spikes and waves during slow-wave sleep (CSWS) (57). In fact, LKS and CSWS overlap in both clinical and electrographic features.

Despite the severe degree of clinical as well as EEG abnormalities, many patients recover, with normal EEG and seizure remission, but some degree of language dysfunction may persist (56,58).

Continuous Spike and Wave During Slow-Wave Sleep

CSWS was first described by Patry (59). The syndrome is characterized by continuous spike and wave activity during non-REM sleep (56,60) and is sometimes referred to as *epilepsy with electrical status epilepticus during slow sleep* (*ESES*) (Figure 4.21A–B) (60). The age of onset ranges from 1 to 12 years, but most occur around 8 years. Two-thirds of the patients are neurologically normal before onset. In time, most patients have frequent seizures (generalized tonic-clonic, atypical absence, and atonic) and have a significant decline in IQ with deterioration in language, impaired memory, reduced attention span, and behavioral changes with aggression or psychosis (56,60).

Epileptiform activity consists of generalized SSWs (1.5–2.5 Hz) as well as focal or multifocal spikes, which are sporadic in the waking state. In sleep, spike-wave bursts become nearly continuous (CSWS pattern), occupying more than 85% of the total non-REM sleep time (60). The CSWS pattern persists for 1 to several years. Similar to LKS, the EEG then tends to normalize and seizures remit spontaneously in most patients. However, recovery of neurological deficit and behavior is often incomplete and about one-half of the patients remain profoundly impaired (56,60).

Subacute Sclerosing Panencephalitis

Subacute sclerosing panencephalitis (SSPE) is a sequel of the measles infection and has become extremely rare because of mandatory immunization. The periodic burst activity in SSPE consists of high-amplitude slow waves mixed with sharp waves, occasionally including spike discharges, maximum in the frontocentral region (Figure 4.22A). The bursts repeat at 4- to 15-second intervals (61) and tend to be more prominent during the awake state. Because of the relatively slow periodicity, a slower sweep speed (20–30 sec/page) makes it easier to rate the repetition (Figure 4.22B). Patients with SSPE often have myoclonus coinciding with the EEG bursts. Background activity becomes slow as the disease progresses. The origin of the periodic discharges has been debated as either thalamic (62) or cortical (63).

Progressive Myoclonic Epilepsy

There are several clinical entities that account for progressive myoclonic epilepsies. They are myoclonic epilepsies with ragged red fibers (MERRF syndrome) (64), Lafora disease (65), Unverricht-Lundborg disease (Baltic myoclonic epilepsy) (66), neuronal ceroid lipofuscinosis (Batten disease) (67), and sialidosis (cherry-red spot myoclonus syndrome) (68). These syndromes are characterized by myoclonic seizures, progressive ataxia, and dementia secondary to degenerative central nervous system (CNS) disease with metabolic derangement. In all forms of progressive myoclonic epilepsies, epileptiform activity consists of generalized spike-waves, polyspike-waves, and multifocal spikes. Background activity becomes progressively slower as

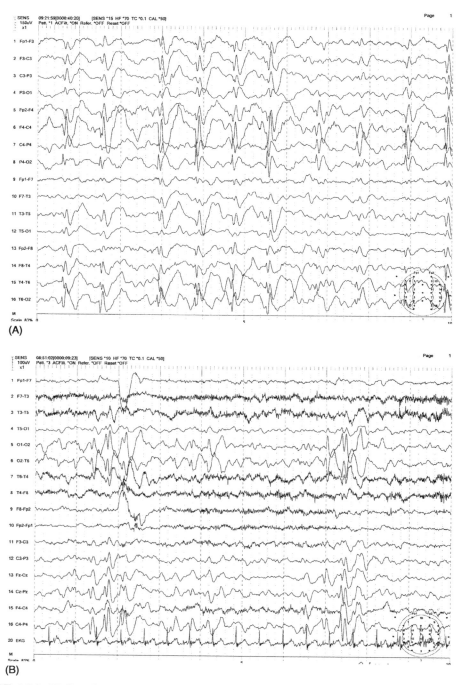

FIGURE 4.21 (A) Continuous spike-wave discharges during slow-wave sleep (CSWS) in a 7-year-old with a history of generalized tonic-clonic seizures mostly during sleep and atypical absence associated with drop attacks. Note the continuous right-greater-than-left parasagittal-dominant spike-wave bursts in sleep. (B) These discharges are much less prominent in the awake state.

Source: From Ref. (74). Yamada T, Meng E. *Practical Guide for Clinical Neurophysiologic Testing: EEG.* Philadelphia, PA: Wolters Kluwer/Lippincott Williams & Wilkins, 2010; with permission.

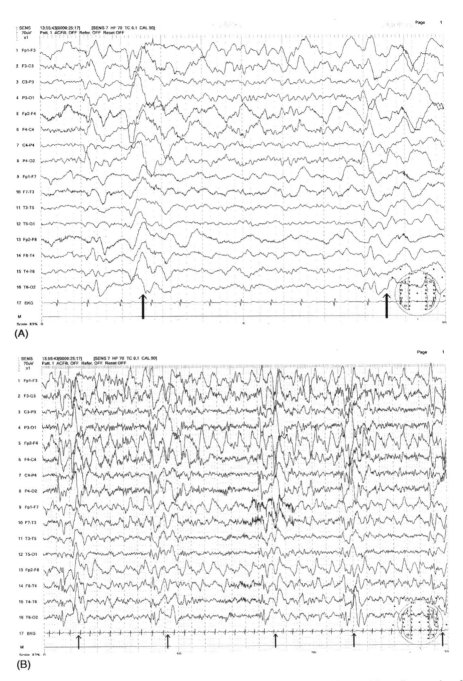

FIGURE 4.22 (A) Generalized periodic discharges in a 15-year-old boy with a diagnosis of subacute sclerosing panencephalitis (SSPE). Note the two bursts of irregular delta waves occurring in about 5-second intervals (indicated by arrows). (B) Because of slow recurrence, the periodicity was not clear with the routine sweep speed of 10 seconds/page, but this became more evident (indicated by arrows) with a slower sweep speed of 30 seconds/page. (The first 10 seconds in Figure B are actually represented by Figure A at a faster sweep of 10 seconds/page.)

Source: From Ref. (74). Yamada T, Meng E. *Practical Guide for Clinical Neurophysiologic Testing: EEG.* Philadelphia, PA: Wolters Kluwer/Lippincott Williams & Wilkins, 2010; with permission.

the disease process progresses. Photoparoxysmal responses are common in patients with Lafora disease, Unverricht-Lundborg disease, and Batten disease. In Batten disease, single or low-frequency intermittent photic stimulation characteristically produces prominent spike discharges at occipital electrodes with a one-to-one relationship with the light flash (67) (Figure 4.23).

Rasmussen Encephalitis

These seizures consist of refractory focal motor seizures or prolonged episodes of epilepsia partialis continua, associated with progressive hemiatrophy with contralateral hemiparesis (69,70). EEG shows more or less continuous ictal spike discharges associated with focal motor seizures or epilepsia partialis continua. In some cases, no ictal discharges may be detected despite obvious clinical seizures if the seizure discharges arise from a deep source or limited cortical zone. The diagnostic criteria were outlined by a recent European conference based on clinical, EEG, and MRI findings. This consists of (a) clinical focal seizures with or without epilepsia partialis continua and unilateral cortical deficit, (b) EEG showing unilateral slowing with or without epileptiform activity and unilateral seizure onset, and (c) MRI demonstrating unihemispheric cortical atrophy and at least one either gray or white matter hyperintensity or atrophy of the caudate (70). The treatments include autoimmune treatment, limited cortical excisions, lobectomies, or hemispherectomies, but hemispherectomy seems to be the most effective treatment (70).

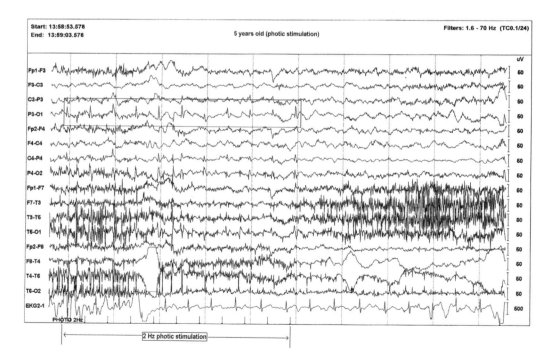

FIGURE 4.23 Photic stimulation–induced spikes in a 5-year-old boy with a diagnosis of Batten disease. The time-locked spikes with slow photic stimulation is characteristic of this diagnosis.

Source: From Ref. (74). Yamada T, Meng E. *Practical Guide for Clinical Neurophysiologic Testing: EEG.* Philadelphia, PA: Wolters Kluwer/Lippincott Williams & Wilkins, 2010; with permission.

Autosomal Dominant Nocturnal Frontal Lobe Epilepsy

Clinical manifestations of this epilepsy include sudden awakening with violent movement, dystonic or tonic posturing, and hyperactive behavior. The event resembles night terror or nocturnal paroxysmal dystonia. EEG may be normal or may show frontal slowing or spikes. The ictal EEG may show rhythmic frontal-dominant discharges, but more importantly there may be no overt EEG changes associated with the event (71).

Multifocal Independent Spikes Syndrome

This is defined by three or more independent spike foci arising from various locations (72) (Figure 4.24) and commonly appears between age 4 and 7 years. This could occur after hypsarrhythmia or LGS. EEG is usually associated with slow background activity and multifocal spikes in the awake state which may become more frequent and more synchronized in sleep. The clinical seizures often appear as tonic spasms, but generalized tonic-clonic seizures or focal seizures are possible (73). The EEG, especially with normal background activity, may show dramatic improvement in time with normal neurologic finding.

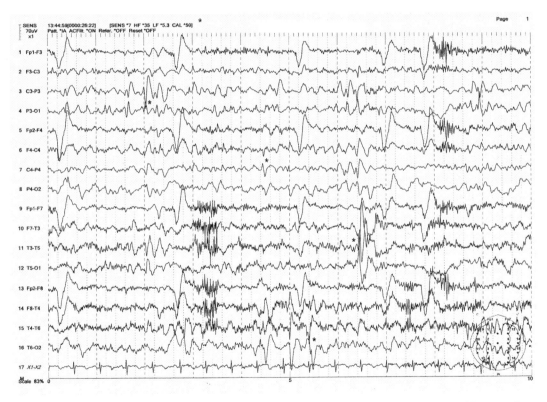

FIGURE 4.24 Multifocal sharp and spike discharges in a 4-year-old boy with a history of partial complex seizures and generalized tonic-clonic convulsions. There are at least four spike foci appearing as single or repetitive transients from P3, C4, T3, and T6 electrodes (shown by * marks) independently.

Source: From Ref. (74). Yamada T, Meng E. *Practical Guide for Clinical Neurophysiologic Testing: EEG.* Philadelphia, PA: Wolters Kluwer/Lippincott Williams & Wilkins, 2010; with permission.

REFERENCES

1. Gotman J, Marciani MG. Electroencephalographic spiking activity, drug levels, and seizure occurrence in epileptic patients. *Ann Neurol.* 1985;17:597–603.
2. Eeg-Olofsson O, Petersen I, Sellden U. The development of electroencephalogram in normal children from the age of 1 though 15 years. Paroxysmal activity. *Neuropaediatric.* 1971;2:375–404.
3. Cavazzuti GB, Cappella L, Nalin A. Longitudinal study of epileptiform EEG patterns in normal children. *Epilepsia.* 1980;21:43–55.
4. Bennet DR. Spike wave complexes in "normal" flying personnel. *Aerosp Med.*1967;38:1276–1282.
5. Kellaway P. The incidence, significance, and natural history of spike foci in children. In Henary CE, ed. *Current Clinical Neurophysiology: Update on EEG and Evoked Potentials.* Amsterdam: Elsevier;1981:151–175.
6. Ehle A, Co S, Jones MG, Clinical correlates of midline spike. An analysis of 21 patients. *Arch Neurol.* 1981;38:355–357.
7. Marsan CA, Zivin LS. Factors related to the occurrence of typical paroxysmal abnormalities in the EEG records of epileptic patients. *Epilepsia.* 1970;11:361–381.
8. Salinsky M, Kanter R, Dasheiff RM. Effectiveness of multiple EEGs in supporting the diagnosis of epilepsy: an operation curve. *Epilepsia.* 1989;28:331–334.
9. Berg AT, Berkovic SF, Brodie MJ, et al. Revised termimology and concept for seizures and epilepsies: report of the ILAE Commission on Classification and Terminology, *Epilepsia.* 2010;51:676–685.
10. Blom S, Heijbel J. Benign epilepsy of children with centro-temporal EEG foci: Discharge rate during sleep. *Epilepsia.* 1975;16:133–140.
11. Loiseau P, Ducke B, Cordova S, et al. Prognosis of benign childhood epilepsy with centro temporal spikes: a follow up study of 168 patients. *Epilepsia.* 1988;29:229–235.
12. Gregory DL, Wong PK. Topographic analysis of the centrotemporal discharges in benign rolandic epilepsy of childhood. *Epilepsia.* 1984;25:705–711.
13. Legarda S, Jayakar P, Duchowny M, et al. Benign rolandic epilepsy: high central and low central subgroups. *Epilepsia.* 1994;35:1125–1129.
14. Gastaut H. A new type of epilepsy: benign partial epilepsy of childhood with occipital spike-waves. *Clin Electroencephalogr.* 1982;13:13–22.
15. Panayiotopoulos CP. Benign childhood epileptic syndromes with occipital spikes: new classification proposed by the International League Against Epilepsy. *J Child Neurol.* 2000;15:548–552.
16. Gastaut H. Zifken BG. Benign epilepsy of childhood with occipital spike and wave complexes. In: Andermann F, Lugaresi E, eds. *Migraine and Epilepsy.* Boston, MA: Butterworth;1987:47–81.
17. Panayiotopoulos CP. Early-onset benign childhood occipital seizure susceptibility syndrome; syndrome to recognize *Epilepsia.* 1999;40:621–630.
18. Ferrie CD, Beaumanoir A, Guerrini R, et al. Early-onset benign occipital seizure susceptibility syndrome. Epilepsia. 1997;38:285–293.
19. Kellaway P. The incidence, significance and natural history of spike foci in children: In: Henry CE, ed. *Current clinical neurophysiology: update on EEG and evoked potentials.* Amsterdam: Elsevier;1981:151–175.
20. Guerrini R, Dravet C, Genton P, et al. Idiopathic photosensitive occipital lobe epilepsy. *Epilepsia.* 1995;36:883–891.
21. Cooper GW, Lee SI. Reactive occipital epileptiform activity: is it benign? *Epilepsia.* 1991;32: 63–68.
22. Gibbs FA, Davis H, Lennox WG. The electroencephalogram in epilepsy and in conditions of impaired consciousness. *Arch Neurol Psychiatry.* 1935;34:1133–1148.
23. Rodin E, Ancheta O. Cerebral electrical fields during petit mal absences. *Electroencepharogr Clin Neurophysiol.* 1987;66:457–466.
24. Sato S, Dreifuss FE, Perry JK, et al. Long-term follow-up of absence seizures. *Neurology.* 1983;33:1590–1595.
25. Wolf P. Juvenile absence epilepsy In: Roger J, Bureau M, Dravet C, et al, eds. *Epileptic syndrome in infancy, childhood and adolescence.* London: John Libbey; 1992:307–312.
26. Sato S, Dreifuss FE, Penry JK. The effect of sleep on spike-wave discharge in absence seizures. *Neurology.* 1973;23:1335–1345.
27. Sato, White BG, Penry JK, et al. Valproic acid versus ethosuximide in the treatment of absence seizures. *Neurology.* 1982;32:157–163.

28. Harding GF, Herrick CE, Jeavons PM. A controlled study of the effect of sodium valproate on photosensitive epilepsy and its prognosis. *Epilepsia*. 1978;19:555–565.
29. Holmes GL, McKeever M, Adamson M. Absence seizures in children: clinical and electroencephalographic features. *Ann Neurol*. 1987;21:268–273.
30. Browne TR, Penry JK, Porter RJ, et al. Responsiveness before, during and after spike-wave paroxysms. *Neurology*. 1974;24:659–665.
31. Penry JK, Dreifuss FE. A study of automatisms associated with the absence of petit mal. *Epilepsia*. 1969;10:417–418.
32. Camfield CS, Camfields PR, Sadler M, et al. Paroxysmal eyelid movements: a confusing feature of generalized photosensitive epilepsy. *Neurology*. 2004;63:40–42.
33. Loiseau P. Childhood absence epilepsies. In: Roger J, Dravert C, Bureau M, et al, eds. *Epileptic Syndrome in Infancy and Adolescence*. London: John Libbey;1985:106–120.
34. Sato S, Dreifuss FE, Perry JK, et al. Long-term follow-up of absence seizures. *Neurology*. 1983;33:1590–1595.
35. Wolf P, Juvenile absence epilepsy. In: Roger J, Dravert C, Bureau M, et al, eds. *Epileptic Syndrome in Infancy and Adolescence*. London: John Libbey;1992:307–312.
36. Niedermeyer E. Generalized seizure discharges and possible precipitating mechanisms. *Epilepsia*. 1966;7:23–29.
37. Janz D, Christian W. Impulsive-petit mal. *Dtsch Z Nervenheik*. 1957;176:346–386.
38. Delgado – Escueta AV, Enrile-Bascal F. Juvenile myoclonic epilepsy of Janz. *Neurology*. 1984;34:285–294.
39. Wolf P, Groosses R. Relation of photosensitivity to epileptic syndrome. *J Neurol Neurosurg Psychiatry*. 1986;49:1386–1391.
40. Lennox WG. *Epilepsy and related disorders*. Boston, MA: Little Brown; 1960
41. Gastaut H, Broughton R. *Epileptic Seizures*. Springfield, IL: Charles C Thomas; 1972.
42. Gastaut H, Roger J, Soulayrol R, et al. Epileptic encephalopathy of children with diffuse slow spikes and waves (alias "petit mal variant") or Lennox syndrome. *Ann Pediatr*. 1966;13:489–499.
43. Blume WT. Lennox-Gastaut syndrome. In: Luders H, Lesser RP, eds. *Epilepsy: electroclinical syndromes*. London: Springer – Verlag;1987:73–92.
44. Markand ON. Slow spike-wave activity in EEG and associated clinical feature: often called "Lennox" or "Lennox-Gastaut" syndrome. *Neurology*. 1977;27:746–757.
45. Beaumanoir A. The Lennox – Gastaut syndrome: a personal study. *Electroencepharogr Clin Neurophysiol Suppl*. 1982;35:85–99.
46. Blume WT, David RB, Gomez MR. Generalized sharp and slow wave complexes. Associated clinical features and long-term follow up. *Brain*. 1973;96:289–306.
47. Egli M, Mothersill I, O'Kane N, et al. The axial spasm—the predominant type of drop seizure in patients with secondary generalized epilepsy. *Epilepsia*. 1985;26:401–415.
48. Gibbs FA, Gibbs JD. *Atlas of Encephalography*. Cambridge, MA: Addison-Wesley; 1952
49. Kellaway P, Frost JD Jr, Hrachovy RA. Infantile spasms. In: Morselli PD, Pippinger KF, Penry JK,eds. *Antiepileptic drug therapy in pediatrics*. New York, NY: Raven Press; 1983:115–136.
50. Hrachovy RA, Frost JD Jr, Kellaway P. Hypsarrythmia: variations on theme. *Epilepsia*. 1984;25:317–325.
51. Watanabe K, Negoro T, Aso K et al. Reappraisal of interictal electroencephalogram in infantile spasms. *Epilepsia*. 1993;34: 679–685.
52. West WJ. On a particular form of infantile convulsions. *Lancet*. 1841;1:724–725.
53. Fariello RG, Chen RW, Doro JM et al. EEG recognition of Aicardi's syndrome. *Arch Neurol*. 1977;34:563–566.
54. Hrachovy RA, Frost JD Jr, Kellaway P, Zion TE. Double–blind study of ACTH vs prednisone therapy in infantile spasms. *J Pediatr*. 1983;103:641–645.
55. Landau WM, Kleffner FR. Syndrome of acquired aphasia with convulsive disorder in children. *Neurology*. 1957;7:523–530.
56. Beaumanoir A. EEG data: In Beaumanoir A, Bureau M, Deonnat T, et al, eds. *Continuous spike and waves during slow sleep electrical status epileptics during slow sleep*. London: John Libbey; 1995:217–223.

57. Hirsch E, Marescaux C, Maquet P, et al. Landau-Kleffner syndrome: a clinical and EEG study of five cases. *Epilepsia*. 1990;31:756–767.
58. Deonna T, Peter C, Ziegler AL. Adult follow-up of the acquired aphasia – epilepsy syndrome in childhood. Report of 7 cases. *Neuropediatrics*. 1989;20:132–138.
59. Patry G, Lyagoubi S, Tassinari CA. Subclinical "electrical status epilepticus" induced by sleep in children. A clinical and electroencephalographic study of six cases. *Arch Neurol*. 1971;24:242–252.
60. Tassinari CA, Bureau M, Dravet C, et al. Epilepsy with continuous spikes and waves during slow wave sleep—otherwise described as ESES (epilepsy with electrical status epilepticus during slow sleep). In Roger J, Bureau M, Dravet C, et al, eds. *Epileptic syndrome in infancy, childhood and adolescence*. London: John Libbey; 1992:245–256.
61. Rabending G, Radermecker FJ. Subacute sclerosing panencephalitis (SSPE). In Remmon A (ed-in-chief). *Handbook of Electroencephalopathy and Clinical Neurophysiology*. Vol 15A. Amsterdam: Elsevier;1977:28–35.
62. Radermecker J, Poser CM. The significance of repetitive paroxysmal electroencephalographic pattern. Their specificity in subacute sclerosing leukoencephalitis. *World Neurol*. 1960;1:422–433.
63. Storm van Leeuwen W. Electroencephalographical and neurophysiological aspects of subacute sclerosing leuco-encephalitis. *Psychiatr Neurol Neurochir*. 1964;67:312–322.
64. Ohtsuka Y, Amano R, Oka E, et al. Myoclonus epilepsy with ragged-red fibers: a clinical and electrophysiological study on two siblings cases. *J Child Neurol*. 1993;8:366–372.
65. Reese K, Toro C, Malow B, et al. Progression of the EEG in Lafora-body disease. *Am J EEG Technol*. 1993;33:229–235.
66. Roger J, Genton P, Bureau M, et al. Progressive myoclonus epilepsies in childhood and adolescence. In Roger J, Bureau M, Dreifuss FF, et al, eds. *Epileptic syndromes in infancy, childhood and adolescence*. 2nd ed. London: Libbey; 1992:381–400.
67. Pampiglione G, Harden A. So-called neuronal ceroid lipofuscinosis. Neurophysiological studies in 60 children. *J Neurol Neurosurg Psychiatry*. 1977;40:323–330.
68. Engel J Jr, Rapin I, Giblin DR. Electroencephalographical studies in two patients with cherry red spot-myoclonus syndrome. *Epilepsia*. 1977;18:73–87.
69. Rasmussen T, Olszewski J, Lloyd-Smith D. Focal seizures due to chronic localized encephalitis. *Neurology*. 1958;8:435–445.
70. Bien CG, Granata T, Antozzi C, et al. Pathogenesis, Diagnosis, and treatment of Rasmussen encephalitis. A European consensus statement. *Brain*. 2005;128:454–471.
71. Raju P, Sarco DP, Poduri A, et al. Oxcarbazepine in children with nocturnal frontal lobe epilepsy. *Pediat Neurol*. 2007;37:345–349.
72. Blume WT. Clinical and electroencephalographic correlates of the multiple independent spike foci in children. *Ann Neurol*. 1978;4:541–547.
73. Yamatogi Y, Ohtahara S. Multiple independent spike foci with epilepsy, with special reference to a new epileptic syndrome of "severe epilepsy with multiple independent spike foci in children". *Epilepsy Res*. 2006;70(S1):541–547.
74. Yamada T, Meng E. *Practical Guide for Clinical Neurophysiologic Testing: EEG*. Philadelphia, PA: Wolters Kluwer/Lippincott Williams & Wilkins, 2010.

The Evaluation of Pediatric Sleep Disorders

Deborah C. Lin-Dyken, MD
Mark Eric Dyken, MD

Sleep is a major component of a child's life. About half of early childhood is spent sleeping. Rapid changes occur in the development and maturation of the neurologic structures responsible for sleep in the early years of life, resulting in a fairly predictable progression of sleep patterns. However, disruption of these processes can lead to developmental, behavioral, and cognitive consequences, which can be either helped or hindered by a caregiver's responses and actions. In addition, a child's sleep difficulties can have effects on other family members, including parents and siblings and can impair the child's daytime functioning in school and social and emotional development. It is important, therefore, to understand what is normal and abnormal in childhood sleep, and when sleep disorders occur how to appropriately assess and treat them in an attempt to significantly improve not only the child's life but also those of their families (1).

Common sleep concerns for children include not enough sleep, disrupted sleep, and, less commonly, too much sleep. These problems can present as difficulties with sleep initiation and maintenance, sleep at inappropriate times, and abnormal activity or behaviors during sleep. All of these can lead to daytime behavioral problems, including inattention, irritability, and learning difficulties.

Evaluation of pediatric sleep disorders consists of obtaining a detailed pediatric sleep history, performing a sleep-focused physical examination, and in select cases, obtaining and interpreting a pediatric polysomnogram (PSG). Each of these components, as well as case studies of common pediatric sleep disorders, are discussed in the following text.

HISTORY

In addition to a standard pediatric medical history, a sleep history should also be reviewed. Obtaining a history of the presenting sleep problem in children requires interviewing the caretakers, who are typically the parents. This often adds a layer of complexity that is typically not seen in adult patients, who usually give their own history. Often the pediatric patient is not concerned about sleep, but rather it is the parents who are voicing the complaint.

A helpful mnemonic device for gathering a history of sleep symptoms is BEARS (Bedtime, Excessive daytime sleepiness, Awakenings, Regularity, Snoring) (2). Starting with dinnertime is a useful way to start asking a sleep history, including inquiring if any caffeinated beverages are consumed, the time that dinner is usually eaten, and how is it structured—ie, does the family sit down together at the table? Following dinner, what activities does the child do? When does the child start the bedtime ritual, and what does the child do? Many children have a bath as a part of the bedtime activities, but for some, this may be very stimulating and cause them to have difficulties settling down. Also, sometimes children can get a "second wind" or *schlafbereitschaft*. This is a brief burst of energy that usually lasts around 20 minutes and occurs just before sleep readiness. Often parents allow their children to watch TV before going to sleep, and many children even have TVs in their bedrooms. Evening TV shows are frequently stimulating and can increase sleep latency. A much better strategy is to encourage parents to spend time reading bedtime stories together with their children. When does the child typically fall asleep and how long does that take from the time lights are turned off? If they do not fall asleep immediately, what do they do during that time? What conditions are needed for the child to fall asleep, and are they able to initiate sleep on their own or do they need the presence of the parent or someone (or something) else?

Questions should also be asked of the sleep environment. Is the child in a crib, toddler bed, a bunk bed, or a regular bed? Does the child share a bed or bedroom, and if so with whom? Does he or she sleep with pets? How dark and how quiet is the bedroom? Most children sleep better in a darkened environment, but some anxious children may do better with a dim night light. What is the temperature of the room? An ideal bedroom should be a bit on the cool side but not uncomfortably cold. How close, or far, is the child's bedroom from the parents' room? This can indicate how easy or difficult it may be for the parents to hear what happens in the child's room at night.

Do the children sleep through the night? If not, when and how often do they wake up? What do they do during the waking? Do they go back to sleep on their own, or do the parents have to put them back to sleep? Do they snore and if so, how loud is it? Do they gasp, choke, or stop breathing? Do they wet the bed? Are they quiet or restless? Do they sleep in unusual positions? When do they wake up? Do they wake up on their own, or do parents have to wake them up? How easy or difficult is it to wake the child up? How long does it take for the child to become wide awake? Is the child refreshed upon awakening or still tired? How many hours do the children sleep at night? Do they nap during the day and if so, at what times and for how long? While young children typically nap during the day, pediatric sleepiness scales have been published and can help provide an objective measure of daytime sleepiness (3).

Finally, a detailed sleep diary should be kept. While this may need to be completed by the parents and some of it may have to be their best estimates, it can still provide significant information, especially over an extended period of time, typically about 2 weeks. The sleep diary should be in a graph form, with times noted for in bed, asleep, awake, and out of bed. Any unusual events, such as sleepwalking, should be noted.

PHYSICAL EXAMINATION

While many, if not most, children with sleep problems have normal physical and neurological examinations, there are several important findings that should be assessed. Vital signs and measurements (height, weight, head and neck circumference, heart rate, blood pressure, and respiratory rate) should be obtained and plotted on standardized growth charts. The body mass index (BMI; weight in kilograms [kg]/square of height in meters) should be calculated and also plotted, as both obesity and relative emaciation can associate with obstructive sleep apnea (OSA) in certain childhood syndromes. A detailed oropharyngeal evaluation should be performed, with attention to the tonsil size, palate elevation, posterior airway size, tongue size and thickness, and dentition. The Mallampati scales are often used to describe the posterior airway size (4). The nasopharynx should also be examined, with attention to nasal obstruction and septal deviation. Any significant craniofacial features should be noted, such as jaw size, midface hypoplasia, or "adenoidal facies" (5). In addition to the neck circumference, any neck masses or thyroid enlargement should also be assessed. Cardiopulmonary evaluation should note any respiratory abnormalities such as wheezing, rales, or rhonchi, and a persistently split S2 can indicate pulmonary hypertension (6). Breathing patterns, including mouth breathing and nasal speech should be noted if present. The neurological examination should also include a brief developmental assessment as well as any behavior concerns, such as tiredness, hyperkinesis, or attention problems.

POLYSOMNOGRAPHY

PSG describes a procedure of objective, simultaneous recording of many different physiologic parameters (electroencephalogram [EEG], electrooculogram [EOG], and electromyogram [EMG]) during sleep (7). In 1875, Caton performed the first EEG animal studies, and in 1929 Berger published recordings from humans (8–11). The first continuously recorded all-night EEG sleep studies by Loomis et al. in 1937 were followed by the discovery of rapid eye movement (REM) sleep by Aserinsky and Kleitman in 1953, which showed the utility of the EOG (12,13). In 1967, Jovet's associating REM sleep with hypotonia justified the present use of EMG for PSG (14). In 1968 the combination of EEG, EOG, and EMG allowed for formal PSG and the first published standardized technique for scoring sleep stages by Rechtschaffen and Kales (15). Presently, PSG analysis allows the differentiation of three specific non–rapid eye movement (NREM) sleep stages; stage N1 (NREM 1), stage N2 (NREM 2), stage N3 (NREM 3), and stage R, REM sleep (16).

For children younger than 2 months of age, the PSG is scored using the accepted criteria of Anders, Parmalee, and Emdee (17). Four EEG patterns are described during full-term neonatal sleep: (a) low voltage irregular (LVI); low voltage (14–35 μV), fast theta (5–8 Hz) with significant slow (1–5 Hz) activity, (b) high voltage slow (HVS); continuous, rhythmic 50–150 μV, slow activity, (c) trace alternant (TA); 3- to 8-second bursts of HVS, separated by similar periods of attenuated mixed frequency activity, with occasional rapid low-voltage and 2 to 4 Hz sharp wave activity, and (d) mixed (M); LVI and HVS mixed, with little periodicity.

Clinical observations and EEG patterns define (a) quiet (NREM) sleep; eyes closed (behavioral/physiological quiescence) and EEG pattern of HVS, TA, or M, (b) active (REM) sleep; eyes closed (rapid eye movements, with facial, limb, and body movements) and EEG pattern of LVI and M (rarely HVI), and (c) indeterminate sleep (not meeting the criteria for quiet or active sleep) often during the transition from active to quiet sleep (17). Infant sleep onset is associated with active (REM) sleep (50% of a newborn's total sleep time); LVI is an EEG pattern unique to this stage of sleep. Although quiet (NREM) sleep is characterized by an HVS pattern on EEG, the TA pattern is unique to this sleep stage in younger infants.

In children, 2 to 3 months post-term, standard child/adult nomenclature for stages W (wake), N1, N2, N3, and R can often be used, as V-waves (defining stage N1 sleep) often appear within 2 to 3 months, sleep spindles and K-complexes (defining stage N2 sleep) appear within 2 to 3 and 4 to 6 months, respectively, and slow wave activity (SWA; defining stage N3 sleep) appears within 2 to 5 months. The occipital EEG, dominant posterior rhythm (DPR) during restful wakefulness upon eye closure, attenuates with eyes open and when falling asleep. The DPR at 3 to 4 months is 3.5 to 4.5 Hz; at 5 to 6 months, 4 to 6 Hz; and by 3 years, 7.5 to 9.5 Hz (normal adult values, 8–13 Hz, are defined as alpha rhythm).

In addition to V-waves and loss of DPR, stage N1 sleep is also defined by a general low-voltage, mixed frequency pattern on EEG, with slow roving eye movements on EOG and occasionally hypnagogic hypersynchrony. In stage R sleep there is a general low-voltage mixed frequency pattern that appears around 3 Hz at 7 weeks post-term, 4 to 5 Hz at 5 months, 4 to 6 Hz at 9 months, 5 to 7 Hz at 1 to 5 years, and from 5 to 10 years, 8 to 13 Hz, with a variable heart and respiratory rate, relatively frequent phasic muscle twitches, grimaces, and vocalizations. In a sleeping child, 2 to 6 months old, if there are no sleep spindles, K-complexes, SWA, or characteristics of stage R sleep, the sleep stage can be given the general designation N (NREM).

A PSG study should last a minimum of 6 hours, but optimally 8 or more hours for children, who typically sleep longer than adults. They should be conducted during the child's normal sleep times, ie, beginning in the early evening and lasting through to the next morning. Proper patient and parent preparation is crucial and will alleviate anxiety about the procedure and improve compliance. A tour of the laboratory can significantly ease tension for both the child and the parent. The sleep laboratory environment should be child-friendly, but also simulate a home environment as much as possible and should be light and sound attenuated. Patient setup should be done in a separate room from the sleep room to avoid unpleasant conditioning effects. The technician working with pediatric patients should be comfortable with children and parents, and realize that it may take more time, effort, and patience to gain a child's trust and cooperation. Rushing or forcing children to do something they do not want to do is rarely successful and usually counterproductive. Often, using distraction (watching a video or TV show) during electrode application can be helpful, along with providing a small incentive, such as a small toy, for completion of the setup.

SPECIFIC SLEEP DISORDERS

The third edition of the International Classification of Sleep Disorders (ICSD), published in 2014, describes 7 major categories of sleep disorders with 2 appendices, describing approximately

TABLE 5.1 Topic Outline From the International Classification of Sleep Disorders, Third Edition

1. Sleep-related breathing disorders
    i. Obstructive sleep apnea disorders
        a. Obstructive sleep apnea, pediatric

2. Central disorders of hypersomnolence   i. Narcolepsy

3. Parasomnias
    i. NREM-related parasomnias
        a. Confusional arousals
        b. Sleepwalking
        c. Sleep terrors
    ii. REM-related parasomnias
        a. REM sleep behavior disorder
        b. Recurrent isolated sleep paralysis

4. Sleep-related movement disorders
    i. Sleep-related bruxism
    ii. Sleep-related rhythmic movement disorder

5. Sleep-related medical and neurological disorders   i. Sleep-related epilepsy

Source: Adapted from American Academy of Sleep Medicine. *International Classification of Sleep Disorders*, 3rd ed. Darien IL: American Academy of Sleep Medicine, 2014.

75 different diagnoses (18). This chapter addresses major diagnoses for which clinical neurophysiological monitoring techniques are useful (see Table 5.1).

SLEEP-RELATED BREATHING DISORDERS

Obstructive Sleep Apnea

In 1978, utilizing the PSG, Guilleminault et al. coined the term *apnea index* (the average number of apneas and hypopneas per hour of sleep) to precisely define the presence and severity of OSA (19). In 2007 the American Academy of Sleep Medicine (AASM) published the first pediatric standard definition for hypopnea, allowing for the routine reporting of the apnea-hypopnea index (AHI; the average number of apneas plus hypopneas per hour of sleep) in children (20). Today, the AHI is "the key measure used for case identification, for quantifying disease severity, and for defining disease prevalence in normal and clinical populations" (21).

PSG monitoring for OSA mandates the use of transcutaneous or end-tidal PCO_2 (partial pressure of carbon dioxide) monitoring for children less than 13 years (16). There are specific recommended standards for scoring obstructive respiratory events in children less than 18 years of age although depending on the child's relative physical level of maturity, the sleep scoring expert can choose to use adult standards for patients greater than 13 years (16). An obstructive apnea in a child is scored when there is a 90% reduction of amplitude on the thermal airflow channel for a duration of two missed breaths when compared to baseline but continued respiratory effort. An obstructive hypopnea is defined as greater than 30% reduction in the nasal pressure transducer channel from baseline, for a duration of greater than two missed breaths, with greater than 3% oxygen desaturation or the event is associated with an arousal.

CENTRAL DISORDERS OF HYPERSOMNOLENCE

Narcolepsy

Narcolepsy is defined in the ICSD as either type 1 or type 2 (with and without cataplexy, respectively), and is associated with periods of irrepressible sleep or sleepiness for at least 3 months (18). In type 1 there is one or both of the following:

1. Cataplexy and a mean sleep latency (MSL) of less than or equal to 8 minutes and two or more sleep-onset REM periods (SOREMPs) on a mean sleep latency test (MSLT; 4–5 day-time 20-min nap attempts separated by approximately 2-hour intervals, performed the day following overnight PSG). A SOREMP within 15 minutes of sleep onset on the preceding PSG may replace one SOREMP on the MSLT.

2. Cerebrospinal fluid (CSF) hypocretin-1 concentration less than or equal to 110 pg/mL (or < 1/3 of normal mean values).

Type 2 follows these criteria except there is no cataplexy and the CSF hypocretin-1 has either not been measured or is greater than 110 pg/mL or greater than one-third of the mean normal.

The onset of type 1 narcolepsy is usually after 5 years, peaking at 15 years. Typically, sleepiness is followed within a year by cataplexy, with hypnagogic hallucinations, sleep paralysis, and insomnia potentially gradually developing over years. In young children, sleepiness can present as excessively long night sleep or as a resumption of previously discontinued daytime naps.

Almost all patients with cataplexy are positive for the human leukocyte antigen (HLA) subtype DQB1*0602, compared with 12% to 38% of the general population. Although anticipation of reward is a common precipitant, cataplexy may present atypically in young children where it can be severe at disease onset and may occur with weakness of face, eyelids, mouth, and tongue protrusion ("cataplectic facies") not clearly associated with emotion (22).

Hyperactive behavior, poor school performance, inattentiveness, lack of energy, and hallucinations can lead to psychiatric misdiagnosis of depression and schizophrenia. In addition, depending upon the child's verbal capabilities, sleep paralysis and hypnagogic hallucinations can be difficult to confirm. Finally, precocious puberty, obesity, REM sleep behavior disorder (RBD; and REM without atonia) can also manifest at symptom onset.

There are no normative MSLT values for children less than 6 years. As such, CSF hypocretin-1 measurements may prove invaluable as 90% to 95% of type 1 patients have undetectable or low CSF hypocretin-1 levels. In children, the minimum 7 hours of sleep recommended for adults on the preceding PSG should be longer.

There is evidence that in type 1 narcolepsy during prolonged "global" cataplectic attacks (with quadriparesis and areflexia), the PSG can show a "REM sleep pattern" with EOG bursts of rapid eye movements, atonic EMG electrical silencing, and EEG patterns with low-voltage mixed frequency activity and sporadic sawtooth waves (Figure 5.1) (23–27). In patients with frequent attacks, provoking and documenting the clinical exam and PSG findings during a cataplectic attack can prove useful.

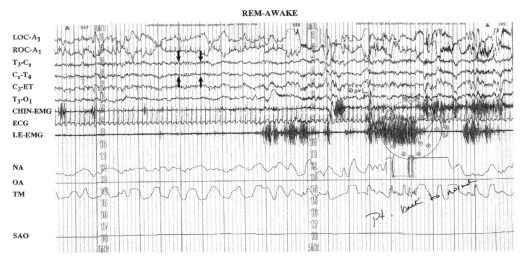

REM-AWAKE

FIGURE 5.1 PSG rapid eye movement (REM) patterns generated by a 17-year-old boy with narcolepsy type 1 clearly contrast with his normal waking study (top left) and show general atonia on EMG, with REM on EOG (top right and bottom left and right). While preparing for a routine diagnostic overnight PSG the patient complained of paralysis and stated in a very hypophonic, rather dysarthric manner "I think I'm having a hypnagogic hallucination," while demonstrating a classic REM-PSG pattern with a marked paucity of muscle tone on chin EMG, with EEG sawtooth waveforms, and rapid eye movements on the EOG (bottom left). This patient's REM patterns were indistinguishable when visual comparisons were made between studies recorded during events that represented cataplexy (top right), sleep paralysis with a hypnagogic hallucination (bottom left), and normal sleep (bottom right).

Abbreviations: EOG, electrooculogram; EMG, electroencephalogram; LOC, left outer canthus; PSG, polysomnography; ROC, right outer canthus.

Source: Adapted from Ref. (24). Dyken ME, Yamada T, Lin-Dyken DC, et al. Diagnosing narcolepsy through the simultaneous clinical and electrophysiologic analysis of cataplexy. *Arch Neurol.* 1996;53:456–460; with permission.

PARASOMNIAS

The ICSD describes parasomnias as undesired physical phenomena, associated with sleep, often with central nervous system (CNS) activation, evidenced as an elevation of autonomic and skeletal muscle activity, and occasionally an experiential element (18).

In the ICSD, parasomnias have been divided into four major categories: the NREM-related parasomnias, the REM-related parasomnias, other parasomnias, and isolated symptoms and normal variants (Table 5.1).

As suggested by the ICSD classification scheme, many parasomnias associate specifically with stages N3 and R sleep (28,29). Normally, there is a preponderance of stage N3 sleep in the first third of the night, and stage R sleep in the last third of the sleeping period (Figure 5.2) (28). This makes the sleep history helpful, because when a parasomnia consistently occurs soon after sleep onset, or just before waking, the differential diagnosis narrows.

Although a single PSG may not capture a suspected parasomnia, PSG correlates often suggest the diagnosis. When a parasomnia is captured, attention should focus on the PSG data and the clinical presentation immediately prior to, during, and following the event. The differential

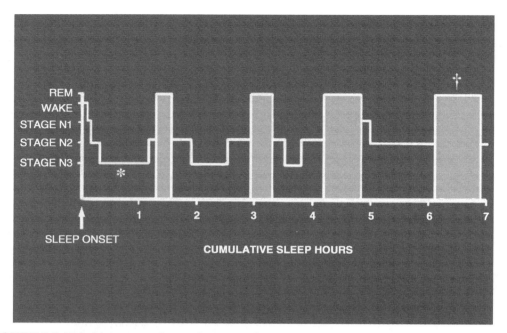

FIGURE 5.2 This histogram shows the general progression of sleep stages throughout a relatively normal night of sleep in a young adult, with the majority of consolidated stage N3 sleep occurring early in the night (as depicted by the asterisk) and the majority of consolidated/relatively prolonged stage R sleep occurring in the early morning hours (as depicted by the dagger) relatively close to the expected waking time.

Source: Modified from the educational slide set "Sleep Disorders;" Scope Publications, The Upjohn Company, 1983.

diagnosis frequently includes seizures and a variety of sleep-related movement disorders not otherwise classified as parasomnias. The documentation of a specific sleep stage, an ictal (seizure) EEG pattern, and behaviors characteristic of a parasomnia or seizure with split-screen, video-PSG is mandated for accurate diagnosis.

NREM-Related Parasomnias

Confusional Arousals

Confusional arousals in children classically occur early in the night during the first or second period of N3 sleep (27,28). They can last minutes to hours and can occur during daytime naps (30). Although confusional arousals are common and benign in children, they may predispose to adolescent sleepwalking (31). Violent behavior can occur if there is an attempt to awaken them. Two variants of the adolescent/adult type disorder include morning sleep inertia (sleep drunkenness) occurring primarily from light NREM sleep and abnormal sexual, at times assaultive, behavior (sexsomnia) (32,33).

The prevalence of confusional arousals from age 3 to 13 years has been reported at 17.3% (30). Predisposing factors include stress, anxiety, sleep deprivation, untreated OSA, and bipolar and depressive disorders (30). A genetic predisposition may be exacerbated by stressors that include sleep deprivation and drug use (34).

Sleepwalking

The PSG tracing in Figure 5.3 shows sleepwalking from stage N3 sleep (see technician's note, "get up walking"). Sleepwalking classically occurs at the end of the first or second period of stage N3 sleep (29,31). The differential diagnosis includes seizures and other sleep-related movement disorders not considered parasomnias. Adolescent sleepwalking may be preceded by early childhood confusional arousals (31). As a single PSG may not capture sleepwalking, the history and PSG capture of confusional arousals support a sleepwalking diagnosis.

Sleepwalking can be precipitated by stress and major depressive disorders (MDDs). Reynolds et al. reported that almost 90% of the patients with MDD show some sleep-related EEG disturbance, most commonly, alterations in N3 sleep (35). Espa et al., in a controlled study of 11 subjects with sleepwalking or sleep terrors, showed increased slow-wave sleep "intensity" with increased total time and percentage of total sleep time and fragmentation of stage N3 sleep (36). Increased stage N3 sleep intensity was hypothesized to inhibit full arousal from N3 sleep, predisposing to sleepwalking and sleep terrors.

Sleep Terrors

The PSG tracing in Figure 5.4 captures a classical stage N3 sleep terror from a 16-year-old girl with recurrent sleep spells with combative behavior (during one she fell down the stairs and

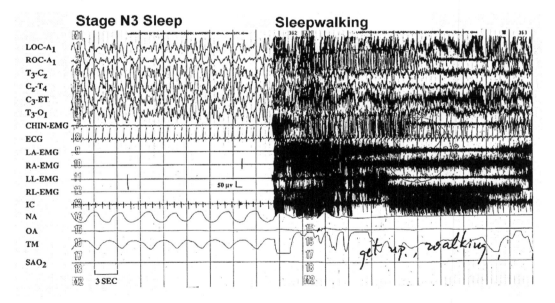

FIGURE 5.3 This PSG tracing captures a classical sleepwalking event from stage N3 sleep (see the technician's note, "get up walking").

Abbreviations: A1, left ear; C, central; ECG, electrocardiogram; EMG, electromyogram; ET, ears tied; IC, intercostal EMG; LA, left arm; LL, left leg; LOC, left outer canthus; NA, nasal airflow; O, occipital; OA, oral airflow; RA, right arm; RL, right leg; ROC, right outer canthus; SAO$_2$, oxygen saturation; T; temporal, TM, thoracic movement.

Source: Modified from Ref. (28). Dyken ME, Yamada T, Lin-Dyken DC. Polysomnographic assessment of spells in sleep: nocturnal seizures versus parasomnias. *Semin Neurol.* 2001;21:377–390; with permission.

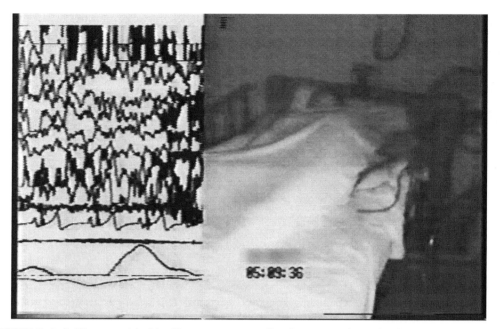

FIGURE 5.4 A 16-year-old girl with recurrent spells of nocturnal combative behaviors for which she was amnestic. This figure shows the split screen video analysis of the PSG, which captured a classical sleep terror that began in stage N3 sleep.

Source: From Ref. (37). Dyken ME, Lin-Dyken DC, Boyle J. Vignette 8; Sleep terrors, In: Chokroverty S, Thomas RJ, eds. *Atlas of Sleep Medicine: Second Edition.* Philadelphia: Elsevier Saunders; 2014:386–387; with permission.

chipped a few teeth) (37). During the PSG spell she tore off electrodes, and the technician's restraining efforts exacerbated combative physical activity and screaming, for which the patient was later amnestic.

Sleep terrors differ from confusional arousals in that they are often associated with significant autonomic hyperactivity and signs of fear, frequently with bloodcurdling screams. Sleep terrors (*pavor nocturnus* in children) are abrupt episodes from sleep, associated with motor agitation, vocalization, and extreme fear, often with screaming and crying (29,31). Autonomic hyperactivity is often evidenced by diaphoresis, mydriasis, tachypnea, and tachycardia (31). Although patients appear alert, attempts at interaction are usually unsuccessful and may prolong the spell (29,31).

The onset of sleep terrors ranges between 4 and 12 years of age, with a prevalence in up to 6.5% (31). Although they usually resolve in adolescence, the prevalence may reach 2.6% in the adult population up to 65 years (31). Precipitants include medications, stress, illness, insufficient sleep, and altered sleep schedule or environment. Sleep terrors are usually not associated with psychopathology in children (31,38). Although patients are generally amnestic for spells of sleep terror, some can recall feeling fear or threat as an episode resolves. This can lead to clinophobia (fear of going to bed) and sleep-onset insomnia (psychophysiological; conditioned insomnia), a stress that could exacerbate further sleep terrors (39).

Diagnostic aids include a sleep diary, actigraphy, and PSG. PSG can provide a definitive diagnosis if a typical event is captured arising out of N3 sleep (29,31,39). However, a PSG may not capture the sleep terror. Some experts believe PSG documentation of confusional arousals supports the diagnosis of sleep terrors when clinically suspected (29).

Treatment centers on patient, family, and caregiver education. Detailed description should be given regarding gently directing the patient back to bed, and avoiding attempts to awaken them as this generally exacerbates fear, confusion, and the potential for injury (39,40). The family should avoid discussing the events with the patient in the mornings after the events occur as it could engender psychosocial stress (40). Scheduled awakenings should be considered if episodes occur at a consistent time during the night (39,41). This involves gently awakening the patient 15 to 30 minutes prior to the usual onset of the episode (39,41). Medications are rarely used. If the events become dangerous or highly disruptive, imipramine or low-dose clonazepam (starting dose, 0.5 mg) at bedtime has been reported to be potentially beneficial (39).

REM-Related Parasomnias

REM Sleep Behavior Disorder

RBD occurs in REM sleep in association with violent, directed behavior, frequently leading to injury, followed by spontaneous report of detailed dreams corresponding with observed movements (isomorphism) (28,42,43). Although, primarily affecting elderly males, it has been reported in children and adolescents (44).

In adults, RBD may be the initial manifestation of a synucleinopathy, a group of neuro-degenerative disorders that includes Parkinson's disease (PD), and in children RBD has been linked to juvenile PD (43,45). In children, RBD has also been associated with various neurological disorders with putative brainstem lesions, including infiltrating tumors of the pons and cerebellar astrocytomas (46,47).

In normal REM sleep, large-amplitude movements do not occur because uninhibited REM-on cells in the brainstem with caudally directed neuronal tracts lead to atonia (48,49). In RBD, a lesion may affect the brainstem structure in humans, analogous to the subcoeruleus area (SCA) in the cat (Figure 5.5) (49,50). From animal studies, it has been hypothesized that degeneration of the SCA disrupts descending tracts that normally cause atonia/paresis, thus allowing violent behaviors during REM ("dreaming/paralyzed") sleep.

PSG criteria for RBD demands the presence of REM without atonia, as characteristic behaviors are captured in only 8% of adults (Figure 5.5) (42,43,51). RBD is also associated with periodic limb movements in sleep (75% of adult patients) (43). Clonazepam can control RBD in up to 90% of adults, and in an account of five cases of childhood RBD, 0.25 mg led to complete resolution of nighttime disturbances (52–54). It has been speculated that clonazepam may act preferentially through serotonergic-like inhibition of excitatory motor systems (54).

Recurrent Isolated Sleep Paralysis

Although classically associated with narcolepsy, at least one episode of sleep paralysis occurs in 40% of the general population (18,55). Isolated events may last minutes, while spells that tend to recur can last hours (56). Sleep paralysis can be precipitated by stress, sleep deprivation, and apnea (57). Sleep paralysis can associate with hallucinations that include the presence of an

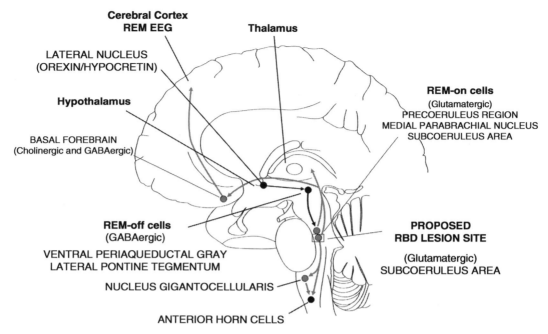

FIGURE 5.5 This parasagittal section of the brain and brainstem shows the suspected pathology explaining RBD, based upon the recently proposed "flip-flop" model of sleep state transitions by Saper et al. (48). In normal REM sleep, glutamatergic REM-on cells in what would be considered the SCA in cats and the sublaterodorsal nucleus in rats (an area presently not well defined in humans), directly and indirectly (through the nucleus gigantocellularis, one of the ventromedial groups of the reticular nuclei in the medulla oblongata) cause hyperpolarization of anterior horn cells in the spinal cord, resulting in atonia. From animal studies, it has been hypothesized that in RBD, degeneration of the SCA disrupts descending tracts that would normally lead to atonia/paresis, thus allowing violent behaviors during REM (dreaming/paralyzed) sleep. Black circles and lines indicate nuclei and neuronal tracts normally inhibited during REM sleep; gray circles and lines indicated nuclei and neuronal tracts normally activated during REM sleep; rectangle indicates proposed lesion site in RBD.

Abbreviations: GABA, gamma-aminobutyric acid; RBD, rapid eye movement sleep behavior disorder; SCA, subcoeruleus area.

Source: From Ref. (49). Dyken ME, Afifi AK, Lin-Dyken DC. Sleep-related problems in neurologic diseases. *Chest.* 2012;141:528–544; with permission.

intruder (an incubus), or an out-of-body experience (58). In severe cases, therapy has included tricyclic antidepressants and selective serotonin reuptake inhibitors (56).

SLEEP-RELATED MOVEMENT DISORDERS

Restless Legs Syndrome and Periodic Limb Movements in Sleep

Restless legs syndrome (RLS) is classically described as a sleep-related movement disorder although it is a sensorimotor problem defined by the waking symptoms (defined by the acronym *URGE*) that includes the **u**rge to move the legs, that is worsened by **r**est, relieved by **g**oing (movement of the limb), and is worst in the **e**vening (18,31). It is only associated with sleep-related movements that are known as periodic limb movement in sleep (PLMs) in 80% to 90% of the cases (18,31). Disruption of sleep onset and maintenance can lead to insomnia, sleepiness, memory and motivational problems, and potentially to anxiety and depression.

Pediatric prevalence rates for RLS are 2% to 4% (moderate to severe in approximately 0.5% to 1%) (18). Boys and girls are affected equally until the late teens where the prevalence is approximately two times greater in women (18). Pediatric RLS is highly familial, with up to 92% of the cases reporting affected family members.

The typical age of onset for the periodic limb movement disorder (PLMD; where PLMs significantly affects sleep) is unknown, but it has been reported to occur as early as infancy. There is potential concern that PLMs-associated overactivity of the sympathetic nervous system may lead to a higher risk of vascular disease (59). About 70% of the children with RLS demonstrate greater than 5 PLMs per hour on PSG study (18,31).

Therapy has been based largely on a dopamine deficiency for the hypothesis regarding the etiology of RLS and PLMs (60). There is also a high prevalence of iron deficiency with these problems, which may be explained by the fact that iron is a cofactor for tyrosine hydroxylase in dopamine production (61). In such cases iron replacement is recommended, otherwise dopaminergic therapy is generally considered the treatment of choice (61,62).

Sleep-Related Bruxism

Sleep bruxism is stereotypic teeth-grinding movements during sleep, often seen in normal children, with a prevalence up to 17% (31). It is divided into a primary form (most often seen in healthy children) and a secondary form (often seen in children with disabilities) (63). Up to 50% of the patients have a family history of bruxism. Bruxism is associated with two types of jaw contractions: tonic/isolated sustained contractions and rhythmic masticatory muscle activity, which appears as a series of repetitive jaw clenchings (31). Bruxism can lead to dental damage, temporal-mandibular injuries, facial pain, headaches, and insomnia, although the natural course is usually benign (64,65).

Sleep-Related Rhythmic Movement Disorder

Rhythmic movements of the body during drowsy wakefulness and sleep are common in normal infants and children, occurring in 59% of the infants at 9 months, in 33% of the children at 18 months, and in 5% by 5 years (31). The formal diagnosis of sleep-related rhythmic movement disorder (RMD) can only be considered if the movements interfere with sleep, impair daytime function, or result in injury. Most patients with sleep-related rhythmic movements are normal, but in older children there may be a higher association with intellectual disabilities, and there have been reports of soft-tissue injuries, with significant injury being rare (66).

In RMD, the subtypes of movements include body rocking, headbanging, and head rolling (less commonly body rolling, leg banging, or leg rolling), often in association with rhythmic humming or inarticulate oral sounds (31). The movement frequency is between 0.5 and 2.0 movements per second and the duration of repetitive movements is generally less than 15 minutes (18).

One study of six children with RMD found that 3 weeks of controlled sleep restriction with the concomitant use of hypnotics during the first week of therapy led to an almost complete

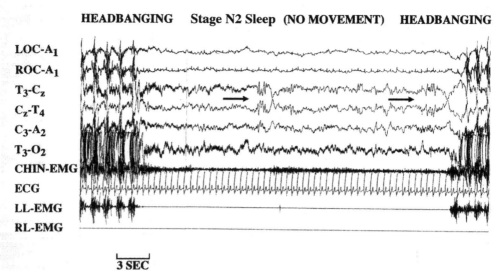

FIGURE 5.6 Immediately after and before respective episodes of headbanging, a young girl with rhythmic movement disorder stopped moving for a period of time, which allowed the recognition of stage N2 (NREM) sleep with characteristic K-complexes (as depicted by the 2 black arrows) with negative sharp waves followed by positive components (total duration lasting ≥ 0.5 seconds).

Abbreviations: A_1, left ear; A_2 right ear; C, central; ECG, electrocardiogram; EMG, electromyogram; LL, left leg; LOC, left outer canthus; O, occipital; RL, right leg; ROC, right outer canthus; T, temporal.

Source: From Ref. (66). Dyken ME, Lin-Dyken DC, Yamada T. Diagnosing rhythmic movement disorder with video-polysomnography. *Pediatr Neurol.* 1997;16:37–41; with permission.

resolution of pathological movements (67). The authors of that paper believed their results suggested that the RMD is a voluntary, self-soothing behavior.

In 1997, a video-PSG study of children 1 to 12 years of age, referred for the evaluation of violent nocturnal behavior, characterized the movement, responsiveness, and sleep stage during each spell (66). Thirty-seven periods of headbanging, body rocking, and leg banging occurred during sleep; 26 were associated with stage N2 sleep, one appeared in stage N3 sleep, one occurred in stage REM sleep, whereas only nine events were recognized in N1 sleep (see Figure 5.6).

SLEEP-RELATED MEDICAL AND NEUROLOGICAL DISORDERS

Sleep-Related Epilepsy

Nocturnal frontal lobe epilepsy (NFLE) is a sleep-related epilepsy with a mean age of onset of 14 +/− 10 years, characterized by seizures that occur predominately during sleep, with 34% of the patients reporting occasional seizures (similar to their sleep seizures) during wakefulness (68). The neurological examination is normal in up to 92% of all cases and although there are no major clinical differences between the sporadic and the autosomal dominantly inherited form of NFLE, diurnal behavioral problems including impulsivity, aggression, and hyperactivity have been reported in some forms of NFLE in relation to mutations of the subunits of the nicotinic acetylcholine receptor (69).

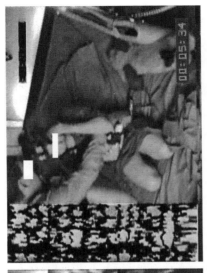
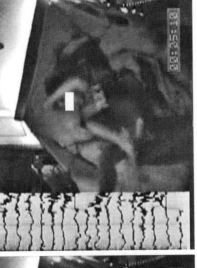
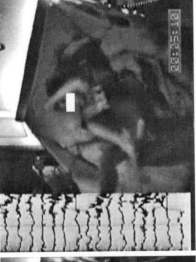

FIGURE 5.7 Sleep-related epilepsy. Of the 40 stereotypical spells captured during a 10-year-old girl's sleep video-EEG, only one showed rhythmic theta activity from the right frontal region (as shown by the arrows in the EEG channels enclosed by the rectangular boxes in the first picture frame) prior to a clinical spell, which was characterized by a sudden frightened awakening and yelling for "Daddy" (see the second picture frame), followed by crouching on bended hands and knees and subsequently (see the third picture frame) clutching her father.

Source: From Ref. (70). Dyken ME, Lin-Dyken DC. Seizure, parasomnia or behavioral disorder? In: Culebras A, ed. *Case Studies in Sleep Neurology; Common and Uncommon Presentations.* New York, NY: Cambridge University Press; 2010;193–199; with permission.

NFLE is associated with brief hypermotor seizures, with marked autonomic activation and stereotypical arousals with emotive vocalizations and bending and rocking of the body that often suggest a parasomnia or waking behavior (28,68,69). The firm diagnosis is also complicated by the fact that the EEG is often normal and may only show epileptiform discharges during an actual nocturnal event (see Figure 5.7) (70). In one study carbamazepine abolished all seizures in 20%, with a significant reduction in seizure activity by at least 50% in another 48% of the patients treated (68).

CONCLUSIONS

Sleep comprises approximately half of the time spent in early childhood. Maturation of the neurological structures responsible for sleep normally leads to a fairly predictable progression of sleep patterns; nevertheless disruption of this process can lead to negative consequences. Sleep disorders in children can present as difficulties with sleep initiation and maintenance, inappropriate sleep, and undesired behaviors. The appropriate evaluation of pediatric sleep disorders requires a detailed pediatric sleep history, a focused physical examination, and in some cases PSG to assure accurate diagnosis and proper therapeutic intervention.

REFERENCES

1. Sheldon SH, Ferber R, Kryger M. Preface. In Sheldon SH, Ferber R, Kryger MH, eds. *Principles and Practice of Pediatric Sleep Medicine*. Philadelphia,PA: Elsevier Saunders; 2005:vii.
2. Mindell JA, Owens JA. *A clinical guide to pediatric sleep: diagnosis and management of sleep problems*. Philadelphia, PA: Lippincott, Williams & Wilkins;2003.
3. Drake C, Nickel C, Burduvali E, et al. The pediatric daytime sleepiness scale (PDSS): sleep habits and school outcomes in middle-school children. *Sleep*. 2003;26(4):455–458.
4. Kumar HV, Schroeder JW, Gang Z, Sheldon SH. Mallampati score and pediatric obstructive sleep apnea. *J Clin Sleep Med*. 2014;10(9):985–990.
5. Ballard CF. Adenoidal facies and mouth-breathing: a clinical analysis. *Med Press*, 1952;228(15): 347–351.
6. Chan W, Woldeyohannes M, Colman R, et al. Haemodynamic and structural correlates of the first and second heart sounds in pulmonary arterial hypertension: an acoustic cardiography cohort study. *BMJ Open*. 2013;3(4):1–10.
7. Sheldon SH. Polysomnography in infants and children. In: Sheldon SH, Ferber R, Kryger MH, eds. *Principles and Practice of Pediatric Sleep Medicine*. Philadelphia, PS: W.B. Saunders;2005:49–70.
8. Caton R. The electric currents of the brain. *Br Med J*. 1875;2:278.
9. Berger H. Uber das Elektrenkephalogramm des Menschen. *Arch of Psychiat*. 1929;87:527–570.
10. Brazier MAB. A History of the Electrical Activity of the Brain: The First Half-Century. London: Pitman Medical Publishing Co;1961.
11. Yamada T, Meng E. Chapter 1, Introduction: history and perspective of clinical neurophysiologic diagnostic tests. In: Yamada T, Meng E, eds. *Practical Guide for Clinical Neurophysiologic Testing– EEG*. Philadelphia, PA: Wolters Kluwer/Lippincott Williams & Wilkins;2010:1–4.
12. Loomis AL, Harvey N, Hobart GA. Cerebral states during sleep, as studied by human brain potentials. *J Exp Psychol*. 1937;21:127–144.
13. Aserinsky E, Kleitman N. Regularly occurring periods of eye motility, and concomitant phenomena, during sleep. *Science*. 1953;118:273–274.
14. Jouvet M. Neurophysiology of the states of sleep. *Physiol Rev*. 1967;47:117–177.
15. Rechtschaffen A, Kales A. *A manual of standardized terminology, techniques and scoring system for sleep stages in human subjects*. Washington, DC: US Government Printing Office;1968. (NIH Publication No. 204)

16. Berry RB, Brooks R, Gamaldo CE, et al. *American Academy of Sleep Medicine. The AASM manual for the scoring of sleep and associated events: rules, terminology and technical specifications, Version 2.0.* Darien, IL: American Academy of Sleep Medicine;2012. www.aasmnet.org
17. Anders T, Emde R, Parmalee A, eds. *A Manual of Standardized Terminology, Techniques and Criteria for Scoring of States of Sleep and Wakefulness in Newborn Infants.* Los Angeles: UCLA Brain Information Service, NINDS Neurological Information Network;1971.
18. American Academy of Sleep Medicine. International Classification of Sleep Disorders, 3rd ed. Darien, IL: American Academy of Sleep Medicine;2014.
19. Guilleminault C, van den Hoed J, Mitler M. Clinical overview of the sleep apnea syndromes. In: Guilleminault C, Dement WC, eds. *Sleep apnea syndromes.* New York, NY: Alan R Liss, Inc;1978:1–12.I
20. Iber C, Ancoli-Israel S, Chesson A, et al. *The AASM Manual for the Scoring of Sleep and Associated Events: Rules, Terminology and Technical Specifications*, 1st ed. Westchester, IL: American Academy of Sleep Medicine;2007.
21. Ruehland WR, Rochford PD, O'Donoghue FJ, et al. The new AASM criteria for scoring hypopneas: Impact on the apnea hypopnea index. *Sleep.* 2009;32(2):150–157.
22. Prasad M, Setty G, Ponnusamy A, et al. Cataplectic facies: clinical marker in the diagnosis of childhood narcolepsy-report of two cases. *Pediatr Neurol.* 2014;50(5):515–517.
23. Dyken ME, Yamada TY, Lin-Dyken DC, et al. Narcolepsy: unequivocal diagnosis after split-screen, video-polysomnographic analysis of a prolonged cataplectic attack. *Neurology.* 1994;44:760–761.
24. Dyken ME, Yamada T, Lin-Dyken DC, et al. Diagnosing narcolepsy through the simultaneous clinical and electrophysiologic analysis of cataplexy. *Arch Neurol.* 1996;53:456–460.
25. Krahn LE, Boeve BF, Olson EJ, et al. A standardized test for cataplexy. *Sleep Med.* 2000;1(2):125–130.
26. Saper CB, Fuller PM, Pedersen NP, et al. Sleep state switching. *Neuron.* 2010;68(6):1023–1042.
27. Dyken ME, Afifi AK, Lin-Dyken DC. Sleep-related problems in neurologic diseases. *Chest.* 2012;141(2):528–544.
28. Dyken ME, Yamada T, Lin-Dyken DC. Polysomnographic assessment of spells in sleep: nocturnal seizures versus parasomnias. *Semin Neurol.* 2001;21:377–390.
29. Dyken ME, Lin-Dyken DC. Parasomnias. In: Yamada T, Meng E, eds. *Practical Guide for clinical neurophysiologic testing: EP, LTM, IOM, PSG, and NCS.* Philadelphia, PA:Wolters Kluwer/Lippincott Williams & Wilkens;2011:260–277.
30. Berry RB. Fundamentals of Sleep Medicine. *Elsevier Health*, Kindle Edition. 2011:27849–27861.
31. American Academy of Sleep Medicine. *International Classification of Sleep Disorders:Diagnostic and Coding Manual.* 2nd ed. Westchester, IL: American Academy of Sleep Medicine;2005.
32. Roth B, Nevismalova S, Rechtschaffen A. Hypersomnia with "sleep drunkenness." *Arch Gen Psychiatry.* 1972;26:456–462.
33. Guilleminault C, Moscovitch A, Yuen K, Poyares D. Atypical sexual behavior during sleep. *Psychosom Med.* 2002;64:328–336.
34. Hublin C, Kaprio J, Partinen M, et al. Parasomnias: co-occurrence and genetics. *Psychiatr Genet.* 2001;11:65–70.
35. Reynolds C, Kupfer D, Sleep research in affective illness: state of the art circa 1987. *Sleep.* 1987;10:199–215.
36. Espa F, Ondze B, Deglise P, et al. Sleep architecture, slow wave activity, and sleep spindles in adult patients with sleepwalking and sleep terrors. *Clin Neurophysiol.* 2000;11:929–939.
37. Dyken ME, Lin-Dyken DC, Boyle J. Vignette 8; Sleep terrors, In: Chokroverty S, Thomas RJ, eds. *Atlas of Sleep Medicine.* 2nd ed. Philadelphia, PA: Elsevier Saunders;2014:386–387.
38. Schenck C, Mahowald M. On the reported association of psychopathology with sleep terrors in adults. *Sleep.* 2000;23:448–449.
39. Provini F, Tinuper P, Bisulli F, Lugaresi E. Arousal disorders. *Sleep Med.* 2011;12 Suppl 2:S22–S26.
40. Meltzer L, Mindell J. Sleep and sleep disorders in children and adolescents. *Sleep Med.* 2008;3(2):269–279.
41. Lask B. Sleep disorders. "Waking treatment" best for night terrors. *BMJ.* 1993;306(6890):1477.
42. Schenck CH, Bundlie SR, Mahowald MW. Human REM sleep chronic behavior disorders: a new category of parasomnia. *Sleep Res.* 1985;14:208.

43. Mahowald M, Schenck C, Basetti, et al. REM Sleep Behavior Disorder (Including Parasomnia Overlap Disorder and Status Dissociatus). In: American Academy of Sleep Medicine. *International classification of sleep disorders: Diagnostic and coding manual.* 2nd ed. Westchester, IL: American Academy of Sleep Medicine;2005:148–152.

44. Stores G. Rapid eye movement sleep behaviour disorder in children and adolescents. *Dev Med Child Neurol.* 2008:50:728–732.

45. Rye DB, Johnston LH, Watts RL, Bliwise DL. Juvenile Parkinson's disease with REM sleep behavior disorder, sleepiness, and daytime REM onset. *Neurology.* 1999;53:1868–1870.

46. Barros-Ferreira M, Chodkiewicz JP, Lairy GC, Salzarulo P. Disorganized relations of tonic and phasic events in REM sleep in a case of brain-stem tumour. *Electroenceph Clin Neurophysiol.* 1975;38:202–207.

47. Schenck CH, Bundlie SR, Smith SA, et al. REM behavior disorder in a 10 year old girl and aperiodic REM and NREM sleep movements in an 8 year old brother. *Sleep Res.* 1986;15:162.

48. Saper CB, Fuller PM, Pedersen NP, et al. Sleep state switching. *Neuron.* 2010;68(6):1023–1042.

49. Dyken ME, Afifi AK, Lin-Dyken DC. Sleep-related problems in neurologic diseases. *Chest.* 2012;141:528–544.

50. Boeve BF, Silber MH, Saper CB, et al. Pathophysiology of REM sleep behaviour disorder and relevance to neurodegenerative disease. *Brain.* 2007;130(pt 11):2770–2788.

51. Dyken ME, Lin-Dyken DC, Seaba P, et al. Violent sleep-related behavior leading to subdural hemorrhage. *Arch Neurol.* 1995;52:318–321.

52. Sheldon SH, Jacobson J. REM-sleep motor disorder in children. *J Child Neurol.* 1998;13:257–260.

53. Schenck CH, Mahowald MW. Polysomnographic, neurologic, psychiatric and clinical outcome report on 70 consecutive cases with REM sleep behavior disorder (RBD): sustained clonazepam efficacy in 89.5% of 57 treated patients. *Cleve Clin J Med.* 1990;57(Suppl):9–23.

54. Mahowald MW, Schenck CH. REM sleep Parasomnias. In: Kryger MH, Roth T, Dement WC, eds. *Principles and Practice of Sleep Medicine.* 4th ed. Philadelphia, PA: Elsevier Saunders;2005:897–916.

55. Dyken ME, Wenger EJ, Yamada T. REM alpha rhythm: diagnostic for narcolepsy? *J Clin Neurophysiol.* 2006;23:254–257.

56. Terrillon JC, Marques- Bonham, S. Does recurrent isolated sleep paralysis involve more than cognitive neurosciences? *J Sci Explor.* 2001;15:97–123.

57. Dyken ME, Lin-Dyken DC, Jerath N. Isolated sleep paralysis: an REM-"Sleep" polysomnographic phenomenon as documented with simultaneous clinical and electrophysiological assessment. In; Chokroverty S, Thomas RJ eds. *Atlas of Sleep Medicine;* 2nd ed. Philadelphia, PA; Elsevier Saunders;2014:375–377.

58. Cheyne JA, Rueffer SD, Newby-Clark IR. Hypnagogic and hypnopompic hallucinations during sleep paralysis: neurological and cultural construction of the night-mare. *Conscious Cogn.* 1999;8(3):319–337.

59. Walters AS, Rye DB. Review of the relationship of restless legs syndrome and periodic limb movements in sleep to hypertension, heart disease and stroke. *Sleep.* 2009;32(5):589–597.

60. Lee SJ, Kim JS, Song IU, et al. Poststroke restless legs syndrome and lesion location: anatomical considerations. *Mov Disord.* 2009;24(1):77–84.

61. Im KB, Strader S, Dyken ME. Management of sleep disorders in stroke. *Curr Treat Options Neurol.* 2010;12(5):379–395.

62. Littner MR, Kushida C, Anderson WM, et al. Practice parameters for the dopaminergic treatment of restless legs syndrome and periodic limb movement disorder. *Sleep.* 2004;27:557–559.

63. Ohayon M, Li K, Guilleminault C. Risk factors for sleep bruxism in the general population. *Chest.* 2001;119:53–61.

64. Rugh J, Harlan J. Nocturnal bruxism and temporomandibular disorders. *Adv Neurol.* 1988;49:329–341.

65. Ware J, Rugh J. Destructive bruxism: sleep stage relationship. *Sleep.* 1988;11:172–181.

66. Dyken ME, Lin-Dyken DC, Yamada T. Diagnosing rhythmic movement disorder with video-polysomnography. *Pediatr Neurol.* 1997;16:37–41.

67. Etzioni T, Katz N, Hering E, et al. Controlled sleep restriction for rhythmic movement disorder. *J Pediatr.* 2005;3:393–395.

68. Provini F, Plazzi G, Tinuper P, et al. Nocturnal frontal lobe epilepsy. A clinical and polygraphic overview of 100 consecutive cases. *Brain.* 1999;122:1017–1031.
69. Ryvlin P, Rheims S, Risse G. Nocturnal frontal lobe epilepsy. *Epilepsia.* 2006;47:83–86.
70. Dyken ME, Lin-Dyken DC. Seizure, parasomnia or behavioral disorder? In; Culebras A., ed. Case Studies in Sleep Neurology; Common and Uncommon Presentations. New York, NY: Cambridge University Press:2010;193–199.

Pediatric Muscular Dystrophies and Myopathies: The Role of Neurophysiology, Genetics, and Ancillary Testing

Russell J. Butterfield, MD, PhD
Mark B. Bromberg, MD, PhD

A traditional approach to diagnostic evaluation in neuromuscular disease centers on a thorough clinical history, physical examination, family history, and ancillary tests such as serum creatine kinase (CK) levels, neurophysiology, and muscle biopsy. The discovery of the *DMD* gene as the cause for Duchenne muscular dystrophy (DMD) in 1987 initiated the genetic era in neuromuscular disorders. The ever-increasing availability of genetic testing is challenging traditional approaches to diagnosis. Current paradigms for pediatric muscular dystrophies and myopathies continue to follow the traditional approach with respect to the clinical history, physical examination, and family history to narrow the differential diagnosis to one or a few disorders that can then be tested directly with a genetic test (1). For common disorders with distinctive phenotypes such as DMD, myotonic dystrophy, facioscapulohumeral dystrophy (FSHD), and spinal muscular atrophy (SMA), genetic testing has become a first-line test based on clinical history and examination.

The development of new, rapid, inexpensive, and expansive sequencing technology, termed next-generation sequencing (NGS) is further challenging traditional approaches and early use of sequencing is becoming more accepted (2). As the role of genetic testing becomes more prominent, the role played by ancillary testing has diminished. In this chapter, we review the role of ancillary testing and genetics in the evaluation of patients with suspected neuromuscular disease and discuss the changing paradigms presented by emerging genetic technologies.

CLINICAL EVALUATION/EXAMINATION

Evaluation of a child with a suspected myopathy or muscular dystrophy starts with a thorough history and physical examination. Differential diagnosis is shaped by clinical features, age at onset, and a dominant, recessive, or X-linked inheritance pattern (3). A number of different classification and diagnostic schemes have been proposed (4,5). These algorithms are complicated, however, by the ever increasing number of overlapping disorders.

Recognition of the relative frequency of disorders can guide the differential diagnosis by prioritizing more common diagnoses. DMD, FSHD, and myotonic dystrophy are substantially more common than any of the limb-girdle muscular dystrophies (LGMDs), congenital muscular dystrophies (CMDs), or congenital myopathy phenotypes in most populations (6). These more common diagnoses are often identifiable by clinical features, which prompt appropriate confirmatory genetic testing. Among CMDs, collagen VI–related muscular dystrophies (COL6-RDs) are most common except in Japanese populations where Fukuyama muscular dystrophy predominates due to a common founder mutation in the *FKTN* gene (7,8). COL6-RDs accounted for almost half of the genetically confirmed CMD patients in one study in the United Kingdom, with merosin-deficient CMD and alpha-dystroglycan-related CMD also relatively common, accounting for nearly 20% and 30% of the cases, respectively (8). *RYR1*-related central core myopathies are the most common congenital myopathies in the United Kingdom, accounting for half of the genetically confirmed cases, with *SEPN1* and *ACTA1* each accounting for 16% of the genetically confirmed congenital myopathies (9).

In the newborn period, patients with neuromuscular disorders typically present with muscle weakness, hypotonia, and joint contractures. Discrimination of neuromuscular vs. nonneuromuscular etiology in the hypotonic infant can be complex; however, infants with encephalopathy, seizure, or abnormal movements are suggestive of a central rather than peripheral etiology (10,11). Respiratory and feeding difficulties are common in both neuromuscular and nonneuromuscular disorders. A history of polyhydramnios and decreased fetal movements is common during pregnancy in patients with neuromuscular diseases. Normal cognitive functioning in the newborn period supports a neuromuscular diagnosis. Since it is common, evaluation of any hypotonic infant should include the consideration of congenital myotonic dystrophy. Examination of the mother for clinical features of myotonic dystrophy may assist in making a diagnosis in the child. It should be noted that the mother is often unaware of her diagnosis until the birth of an affected child.

Clinical features can assist in narrowing a differential diagnosis. Centronuclear myopathy or nemaline myopathy patients often have profound facial weakness in the neonatal period particularly in the lower face (5). Ptosis and ophthalmoparesis are also common features seen in severe congenital myopathies in the newborn period. Distal hyperlaxity and abnormal scar formation suggest a COL6-RD. Scoliosis and spinal rigidity are prominent features in myopathies related to *SEPN1*, *LAMA2*, *LMNA*, collagen VI, and *RYR1*. Cardiac involvement can be a clue to guide the differential diagnosis. Cardiac involvement is seen in some cases of *TTN*- and *MYH7*-related myopathies but is generally uncommon in most congenital myopathies (12,13). Cardiac findings are common in DMD, Emery-Dreifuss muscular dystrophy (EDMD), and myotonic dystrophy, but onset is usually in adolescence or adulthood, despite the onset of skeletal muscle weakness much earlier. Among CMD patients, *FKRP-* and *FKTN*-related muscular dystrophies are most commonly associated with cardiac problems.

ANCILLARY STUDIES

Creatine Kinase

Serum CK is often the first test performed for suspected neuromuscular disorder and can lead directly to specific genetic testing in the setting of typical presentations of common disorders, such as DMD. CK is an enzyme with wide expression in many tissues but is enriched in tissues specialized for rapid energy metabolism such as skeletal and cardiac muscle. An elevation in CK suggests disruption of the permeability of the sarcoplasmic membrane, allowing CK to leak from the cytoplasm. Disruption of the sarcoplasmic membrane is common in dystrophic disorders associated with mutations in the dystroglycan-associated complex (DAC) such as dystrophin, alpha-dystroglycan, merosin, and the sarcoglycans.

In DMD, CK elevations are often 10 to 100 times the upper limit of normal (ULN), and combined with a typical clinical presentation, leave little doubt of a neuromuscular diagnosis. CK elevations are present even in presymptomatic boys with DMD. Newborn screening based on CK elevations has been proposed to facilitate early diagnosis. In one large-scale trial, 37,000 newborns were screened for DMD based on elevated CK levels in routine blood spots. Six DMD cases and three LGMD cases were identified based on CK levels greater than 2,000 U/L (14). While newborn screening has not been systematically adopted, the development of gene-specific therapies such as nonsense read-through and exon skipping suggests the importance of early identification of these patients. In the absence of newborn screening, the first symptoms in patients with DMD can be identified as young as 2 years of age; however diagnosis is delayed until a mean of 4.7 years, a diagnostic delay that is unchanged in 25 years (15,16). Simple changes in practice such as early evaluation of the CK in patients with gross motor delay decreases the time to diagnosis in these patients.

CK elevation in asymptomatic and paucisymptomatic individuals is more complicated. Variations between individuals based on gender, race, and age are well established (17). Many factors unrelated to neuromuscular disease can cause elevations in CK (18). Systemic causes for CK elevation include viral illness, trauma, physical exertion, and endocrine disorders (especially thyroid and parathyroid). Medications such as HMG-CoA reductase inhibitors (statins) are a common cause of elevated CK. Other common medications that can cause CK elevation include fibrates, antiretrovirals, beta-blockers, and isotretinoin. Further, CK can be elevated as a secondary factor in patients with neurogenic disorders such as SMA or amyotrophic lateral sclerosis (ALS), particularly during periods of rapid denervation.

While reported normal ranges vary between laboratories, current evidence-based data suggests ULN of 97.5th percentile for serum CK. Patients with CK elevations greater than 1.5 times ULN based on age and race should be evaluated for a possible neuromuscular disorder (325 U/L for non-black females, 504 U/L for non-black males, 621 U/L for black females, and 1201 U/L for black males) (19).

Clinical Neurophysiology

Clinical neurophysiology or electrodiagnosis is often obtained early in the evaluation of children with suspected neuromuscular disorders and is considered an extension of the physical examination. Electrophysiology consists of three individual studies, nerve conduction studies (NCSs) assessing the integrity of sensory and motor nerves, repetitive stimulation assessing the integrity of the neuromuscular junction, and routine needle electromyography (EMG) to assess the integrity of muscle architecture. Technical aspects of these tests are detailed elsewhere in this volume and are especially important to consider when NCSs/EMGs are performed in infants (20). Of note, peripheral nerves structurally mature with age, with an increase in the number of large fibers from birth to 8 years and complete myelination by 5 years. Thus, nerve conduction values for amplitude and conduction velocities must be adjusted for age (21).

Routine needle EMGs/NCSs are associated with a degree of discomfort, and studies in children are usually limited to the extent of muscles studied, with the selection of those most likely to be diagnostic (proximal muscles in suspected myopathic disorders). The use of disposable smaller "facial electrodes" ensures a sharp point and small needle diameter. Topical anesthetic or light sedation can facilitate studies in poorly cooperative children. Routine studies require active contraction of muscles, and graded voluntary muscle activation is challenging in the pediatric population. Measurement of neuromuscular transmission jitter can be performed without patient cooperation by electrical stimulation of nerve branches (22). Repetitive nerve stimulation is usually performed when congenital myasthenia gravis is suspected. A more sensitive measurement of neuromuscular junction transmission is by the measurement of jitter by single-fiber EMG and its variations (23).

Children with low tone, weakness, gait abnormalities, or other symptoms and signs typical of neuromuscular disease are often referred for EMG/NCS as a first step in the evaluation. EMG/NCS primarily separates peripheral neuropathies or motor neuropathies from primary muscle disorders. In one review of 122 children under the age of 3 years with hypotonia and weakness, NCS and EMG were supportive of SMA in 48%, CMD in 16%, and neuropathy in 8% (24). In another large case series, 39% of the cases referred for pediatric EMG/NCS showed neurogenic findings and were ultimately diagnosed as primary neurogenic disorders (25). In that same series, muscle disorders were ultimately diagnosed in 10% of the cases and included congenital myopathies, CMDs, DMD, and others. A central nervous system (CNS) disorder was diagnosed in 26%, and 22% ultimately lacked a neurologic diagnosis. It should be noted that in many cases of myopathy, EMG findings may be normal or show neurogenic changes. In one series, mild-to-moderate neurogenic changes were the only EMG findings in 36% of the patients ultimately diagnosed with a myopathy (26).

For patients with suspected myopathic disorders, the utility of the EMG/NCS is primarily to exclude neuropathic conditions, provide objective evidence of myopathy, characterize the distribution (distal vs. proximal, and symmetry), and identify targets for muscle biopsy (27). While EMG findings can confirm the presence of a myopathic disorder, EMG cannot determine underlying pathologic processes, and a muscle biopsy or genetic testing is necessary to make a specific diagnosis, which is altered in many myopathies, by documenting changes in motor unit action potential waveforms. Abnormal spontaneous discharges include fibrillation potentials and positive sharp waves. These occur in both neuropathic and myopathic disorders and thus are not discriminating. The presence of myotonic discharges is traditionally associated with myotonic disorders (myotonic dystrophies, myotonia and paramyotonia congenital, and channelopathies), but they were also encountered in other forms of muscle disease (28). A 12-year review of 2,234 children revealed that 11 had myotonic discharges without other abnormalities on EMG that contributed to the diagnosis of myotonia congenital, paramyotonia congenital, congenital myopathy, and Pompe disease (29). Another group of eight patients had both myotonic discharges and myopathic motor units, which led to the diagnoses of congenital myopathy and non-Pompe glycogen storage diseases.

Characteristic findings in myopathic disorders include short-duration, polyphasic, and low-amplitude motor unit potentials (22). It is important to note that interpretation of motor unit waveforms in children younger than 2 years requires experience because muscle fibers are of lesser diameter, and normal motor units may appear myopathic (30). Fibrillation potentials, positive sharp waves, and myopathic motor units are observed in most muscular dystrophies and myopathies including LGMD, EDMD, FSHD, myotonic dystrophy, congenital myopathy, and, inflammatory myopathies (31). While NCSs are usually normal in primary muscle disease, some disorders such as merosin-deficient CMD may show slow motor conduction velocities without signs of denervation (32–34). Further, there may be a progression of motor nerve slowing over time in an individual patient (35). With myotonic dystrophy type 1, there is a mild and mostly subclinical neuropathy (36).

EMG can supplement other studies such as muscle biopsy. Among 17 children undergoing surgical procedures for the repair of clubfoot deformities without preoperative diagnoses, EMG combined with muscle biopsies at the time of surgery were helpful showing 70% with myopathic features (37). Data from a Mayo Clinic review of 72 children who had both an EMG study and a muscle biopsy showed that EMG was 91% sensitive and 67% specific in identifying myopathic disorders (28). Forty-six percent had an abnormal EMG study and a myopathic disorder (biopsy or genetic testing); 17% had an abnormal EMG but no pathologic or genetic testing evidence of a myopathic disorder; 4% had a normal EMG but a metabolic myopathic disorder; and 36% had normal studies. Congenital myopathies were the most commonly identified disorders in this review. All had abnormal EMG studies. While myotonic discharges are readily identified in adults with myotonic dystrophy, EMG findings in infants with congenital myotonic dystrophy may be absent months to years after birth, and the discharges may be sparse and atypical (ie, of shorter duration) (31).

Electrical Impedance Myography

Electrical impedance myography (EIM) is a noninvasive and painless procedure that assesses changes in muscle structure by passing low-intensity alternating current through one set of surface electrodes and recording the voltages with another set of surface electrodes (38). Changes in muscle composition including atrophy, edema, and fibrosis can be identified with EIM since these changes alter the underlying conductance of the muscle tissue. EIM has been used to characterize SMA and can successfully differentiate types 2 and 3 SMA (39). Furthermore, EIM has been proposed as a method to grade the severity and follow the progression of muscle disease and may become an important outcome for clinical trials. In this respect, EIM has been shown to distinguish boys with DMD from healthy subjects, and EIM measurements correlated with functional outcomes in boys with DMD (40).

Muscle Biopsy

A muscle biopsy is warranted in a child with weakness when CK elevation and/or myopathic features on EMG, imaging, or physical examination are present. Historically, most muscular dystrophies and myopathies were defined by features on the muscle biopsy, and muscle biopsy has been the mainstay of diagnostic testing (41). Muscle biopsy can be diagnostic of a specific disorder in many cases, including DMD, merosin-deficient CMD, sarcoglycanopathies, and dystroglycanopathies. Congenital myopathies such as central core myopathy, nemaline myopathy, and central nuclear myopathies are defined primarily by their histologic appearance and were considered distinct clinical entities until the identification of the genes underlying these disorders. Significant heterogeneity within myopathy subtypes and overlap between them has blurred the distinctions between disorders that were once thought to be distinct.

Selection of the muscle for biopsy should be guided by the distribution of weakness. A moderately affected muscle is preferred since very weak muscle shows severe changes that obliterate specific findings. Muscle imaging by ultrasound or MRI can direct selection of the biopsy site and avoid sampling of muscle that is either too severely affected or relatively unaffected (42). Muscle biopsy can be obtained through an open incision (43) or using a specialized needle (44). Needle biopsy procedures have the advantage of being less invasive and leaving a smaller scar but has the disadvantage of limited visualization of the sampling site and technical difficulty in very young children. Muscle biopsy samples should be taken immediately to the processing laboratory on saline-moistened gauze. Immersion of the sample or attempts to wash the sample can result in significant tissue artifacts.

Once in the laboratory, samples are split, with half fixed in formalin and half frozen to preserve enzymatic activity. Detailed handling procedures and utility of the different stains are outside the scope of this chapter but are well reviewed in the literature (45,46). Hematoxylin and eosin (H&E) and modified Gomori trichrome stains are routinely performed to evaluate overall tissue architecture and organization. Adenosine triphosphatase (ATPase) stains allow distinction of type 1 and type 2 fibers. Nicotinamide adenine dinucleotide tetrazolium reductase (NADH-TR), succinic dehydrogenase (SDH), and cytochrome oxidase (COX) are used to evaluate enzyme activity and distribution within the muscle fibers. Additional immunohistochemical stains are selected depending on the clinical question and include stains for sarcolemmal proteins such as dystrophin, sarcoglycans, dysferlin, caveolin, merosin, and others.

Normal muscle structure shows polygonal muscle fibers with peripherally located nuclei. Fibers are uniform in size and shape and surrounded by a thin layer of connective tissue (endomysium) (Figure 6.1). It should be noted that fiber size is dependent on age. An average fiber size of 15 μm is expected in neonates, gradually increasing to 50 μm in adolescent children and adults (41). Muscle biopsies in neonates are often deferred until after 6 months of age due to difficulty in interpretation because of the small fiber size. Discrete bundles of muscle fibers (fascicles) are surrounded by a connective tissue layer, the perimysium, which also contains nerve fibers and blood and lymphatic vessels. Fascicles are bundled together by a thick connective tissue layer, the epimysium, which is contiguous with the tendon sheath.

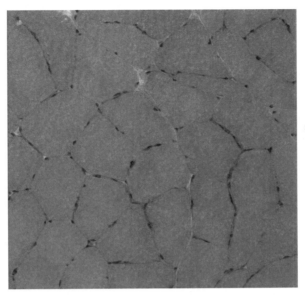

FIGURE 6.1 Normal muscle demonstrating polygonal fibers of uniform size with peripherally placed nuclei (hematoxylin and eosin [H&E] stain).

Histopathology in muscular dystrophies is generally distinct from myopathies by the prominence of dystrophic features such as fibrosis, fatty infiltration, and necrosis (Figure 6.2); however, severe, early-onset congenital myopathies may also have a dystrophic appearance (47,48). Myopathic features commonly seen in muscle biopsies include central displacement of nuclei,

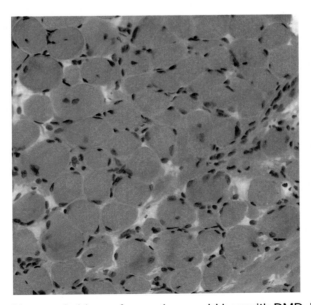

FIGURE 6.2 Dystrophic muscle biopsy from a 4-year-old boy with DMD. Note the marked variation in fiber size, hypertrophic fibers, necrotic fibers, and fibrosis (hematoxylin and eosin [H&E] stain).

atrophy or hypertrophy of fibers, degenerating/regenerating fibers, fibrosis, and fatty replacement. These features are somewhat nonspecific and can be seen in many different myopathic disorders. Congenital myopathies may have specific findings such as central cores, nemaline rods, or central nuclei (Figure 6.3). In many cases, congenital myopathies are defined by their histologic appearance, but genetic discoveries continue to blur distinctions between them. Specific histopathologic features are suggestive of more targeted diagnoses and can direct the selection of genetic tests.

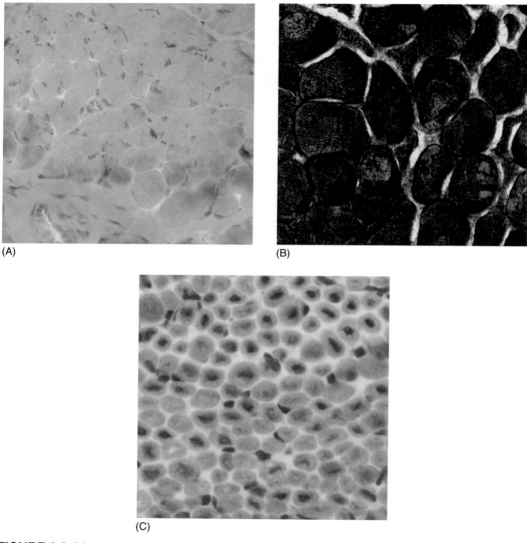

(A)

(B)

(C)

FIGURE 6.3 Muscle biopsy section from a patient with (A) nemaline myopathy demonstrating prominent cytoplasmic inclusions on Gomori trichrome stain, (B) central core myopathy demonstrating areas of central clearing in NADH-TR stain, and (C) centronuclear (myotubular) myopathy demonstrating immature fibers with predominantly centrally placed nuclei on hematoxylin and eosin (H&E) stain.

Muscle Imaging

Muscle imaging is an increasingly important tool in the evaluation of patients with suspected neuromuscular disorders. Imaging techniques including ultrasound (US), MRI, and CT have the advantage over neurophysiology and biopsy of being noninvasive and readily available at most centers. The use of muscle imaging in clinical settings is largely focused on the targeting of muscle biopsy and pattern recognition in the guidance of differential diagnosis. Research applications are advancing rapidly and are focused on the use of imaging markers of disease progression. In this regard, development of quantitative techniques has been an especially important area of investigation.

Ultrasound

Muscle US was first introduced in the 1980s and was promoted as a tool for a more accurate selection of muscle biopsy site (42,49,50). In recent years, US has been used increasingly as a tool for pattern recognition to aid in differential diagnosis (51). Normal muscle has low echodensity resulting in a black appearance on US. Underlying connective tissue appears bright, outlining the epimysial and perimysial architecture. In longitudinal orientation, the pennation pattern of individual muscles can be identified, and in the transverse plane, the muscle has a more speckled appearance. Bone, subcutaneous fat, and vascular structures can also be easily detected. Echodensity increases with age as muscle is replaced by fibrous connective tissue and fat.

In patients with suspected neuromuscular disorders, US can be used to assess both echogenicity (degree of fibrosis, fatty replacement, and overall degeneration of the muscle architecture) and size (atrophy/hypertrophy) of muscle. Specific features can be identified in some disorders, including a "central cloud" phenomenon in the rectus femoris in patients with COL6-RD and marked sparing of the rectus femoris in *RYR1*-related myopathies (Figure 6.4) (52,53).

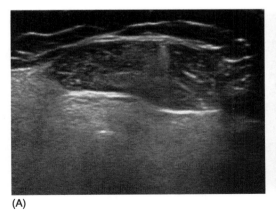 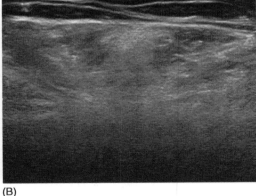

(A)   (B)

FIGURE 6.4 Ultrasound image of rectus femoris in patients with (A) RYR1-associated myopathy and (B) collagen VI–related muscular dystrophy (COL6-RD). Note the sparing of rectus femoris and marked increase in echogenicity in other muscle groups in the patient with RYR1-associated myopathy. In COL6-RD, the rectus is affected centrally and spared peripherally. The resulting "central cloud" phenomenon is pathognomic of COL6-RD. In both cases, the normal bone echo is obscured by the involved muscle.

Source: Image courtesy of Jahannaz Dastgir, MD, Columbia University.

Evaluation of deeper muscles in patients with severe disease may not be possible with US due to echogenicity of more superficial muscles. In very severely affected muscle, the underlying bone echo, which is very prominent in normal muscle US, can be completely obliterated. Prominence of the bone shadow has been used as a marker for grading the echodensity of the overlying muscle (50).

US has the advantage of portability, low cost, and immediate availability in the clinic setting. Serial evaluations can noninvasively identify progression. However interpretation is highly dependent on the skill of the examiner. In addition, technical differences related to equipment and different system settings complicate interrater reliability. US has the unique advantage of being a dynamic study, allowing the examiner to visualize movements in the muscle including fasciculations (54).

Computed Tomography

CT of muscle can be performed rapidly and can detect changes in muscle size and volume and structure. Myopathic changes in muscle tissue are characterized by fibrosis and fatty replacement and are easily identifiable on CT as areas of low attenuation. CT, however, has poor soft-tissue contrast to differentiate inflammatory changes (edema) (55). The main disadvantage of CT is the radiation exposure, which has led to a decline in its routine use (55).

Magnetic Resonance Imaging

MRI has largely replaced CT since it offers significantly better spatial resolution and requires no radiation exposure. While necessary sequences for MRI take longer to obtain compared with CT, most can be completed in a relatively short time frame. Typical MRI protocols for muscle imaging include T1-weighted, T2-weighted, and fat-suppressed (short tau inversion recovery [STIR]) images through hips, thighs, and calves. In most cases these studies can be done with little or no sedation in 15 to 30 minutes in children over 5 years old; however, sedation may be required for imaging in younger children.

Normal muscle is intermediate in signal intensity on all sequences. Evidence of muscle disease such as fatty replacement of muscle and fibrosis can be identified easily on T1- and T2-weighted scans as areas of increased signal. Edema, which can precede these more chronic changes, can be distinguished from fibrosis and fatty infiltration on fat-suppressed, STIR images as areas of increased signal. Standardized rating scales have been proposed but are not widely used clinically (56–58). Quantitative measures of fatty infiltration and fibrosis are active areas of investigation with an interest in developing reliable indicators of progression, but these are not used routinely in clinical setting (59–61).

From an imaging perspective, muscle can change in a limited number of ways (mass, shape, and signal intensity). Chronic myopathy results in fatty replacement without atrophy, while denervation results in atrophy. Since muscle changes in MRI are limited, a pattern recognition approach combining imaging characteristics and clinical features is most helpful. Changes in muscle can be described in four basic areas (62): (a) distribution and symmetry—focal vs. diffuse involvement, (b) morphology—size (atrophy, hypertrophy, pseudohypertrophy) and shape of muscle, (c) T1 changes—fatty replacement, usually diffuse in later stages and patchy in early stages of disease, and (d) T2 changes—largely due to edema suggesting inflammation.

Rapid advancement in the identification of genetic mutations associated with neuromuscular disease has led to the increasing complexity of differential diagnosis. Variability between patients even with the same disease makes pattern recognition difficult, and MRI is supplemental rather than diagnostic. To assist in differential diagnosis, pattern recognition algorithms have been developed to identify muscles or muscle groups that are affected or those that are spared in congenital myopathies (63), muscular dystrophies with rigidity of the spine (64), and LGMDs (65). While most imaging protocols involve only the hips, thighs, and calves, protocols have been introduced for upper limb-girdle and whole-body MRIs (66,67). These techniques are not widely available but may shed future light on pattern recognition when a more diverse group of muscles are imaged, including postural and facial muscles.

Imaging Findings in Specific Disorders

Duchenne and Becker Muscular Dystrophies

MRI of muscle in DMD and Becker muscular dystrophy (BMD) patients shows prominent involvement in the proximal leg, long head of biceps femoris, vastus lateralis, and rectus femoris. Biceps and gluteus maximus are less involved and progress more slowly over time (68). In the lower leg, there is greater involvement of posterior muscles (gastrocnemius greater than soleus) than anterior compartment muscles (anterior/posterior tibialis). Severity of MRI findings in DMD patients has been correlated with the severity and degree of fibroadipose tissue replacement in biopsy samples from extensor digitorum brevis muscle (69). MRI findings in BMD have been described and include prominent involvement of gluteal muscles, adductor magnus, long head of biceps femoris, semimembranosus, and the vasti; however, this pattern was not sufficiently distinct to clinically separate BMD from LGMD (70).

Congenital Myopathies/Muscular Dystrophies

Specific patterns have been identified for some CMD and congenital myopathy phenotypes. In some cases, imaging findings can directly inform confirmatory genetic testing and obviate the need for muscle biopsy.

Patients with myopathies due to *RYR1* mutations include a broad clinical spectrum from severely affected infants to mildly affected adults. Histopathologic findings are diverse and can include central core disease, multi-minicore disease, congenital fiber-type disproportion, and others. In contrast to the variability in clinical phenotypes, imaging characteristics are similar in most patients regardless of clinical and histopathologic findings (71). Imaging features include prominent involvement of the gluteal muscles, adductor magnus, sartorius, and vastus interomediolateralis and the sparing of rectus femoris and adductor longus (Figure 6.5) (72,73). These findings are easily identifiable by both US and MRI. There is some overlap with *SEPN1*-related myopathies, given severe involvement of the sartorius compared to gracilis, but sparing the posterior thigh muscles and vasti differentiates them (64). Patients with susceptibility to malignant hyperthermia due to *RYR1* mutations in the absence of other clinical features have normal imaging (73).

Atrophy of the sartorius with preservation of the rectus femoris is the hallmark of rigid spine muscular dystrophy type 1 (RSMD1) due to *SEPN1* mutations (73). Posterior thigh muscles and adductor magnus are also involved while other muscle groups are spared (64). Lower

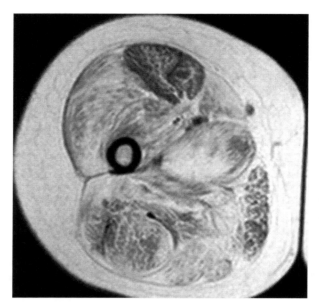

FIGURE 6.5 Transverse T1-weighted image through the thigh of a patient with RYR1-associated myopathy demonstrating sparing of the rectus femoris.

Source: Image courtesy of Jahannaz Dastgir, MD, Columbia University.

leg muscles are less severely affected, and on whole-body MRI, sternocleidomastoid muscles are severely affected, which may be a pathognomonic feature (66). In milder cases with *SEPN1* mutations, the sartorius may be the only significantly involved muscle by imaging features and may be difficult to identify due to severe atrophy. Overlapping clinical disorders such as CMD due to *LMNA* mutations are distinguished from *SEPN1*-related disorders by sparing of the sartorius.

Patients with COL6-RD such as Bethlem myopathy (BM) and Ullrich congenital muscular dystrophy (UCMD) show diffuse involvement of posterior and lateral thigh muscles with relative sparing of the sartorius, gracilis and adductor longus. COL6-RD patients have a characteristic rim of abnormal signal in the vastus lateralis and gastrocnemius with sparing of the central areas (52,74). Involvement of the rectus femoris is prominent centrally (Figure 6.6). This phenomenon, termed *central shadow* or *central cloud* in the rectus femoris is pathognomonic in COL6-RD patients and is identifiable on all imaging modalities. In nemaline myopathy patients with mutation in *NEB*, rectus femoris is the most affected, with significant involvement of the tibialis anterior (63). Involvement of the tibialis anterior may be out of proportion to clinical involvement (66).

Imaging characteristics of other congenital myopathy and muscular dystrophy phenotypes are less well characterized. Patients with *ACTA1* mutations have broad clinical phenotypes and no specific imaging pattern; however, involvement of the lower leg is less significant than that seen in patients with *NEB* mutations. EDMD due to a mutation in emerin is distinguished from EDMD due to a mutation in lamin A/C by disproportionate involvement of the medial head of gastrocnemius (75).

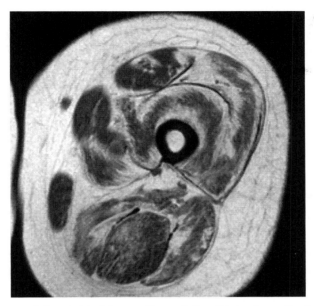

FIGURE 6.6 Transverse T1-weighted image through the thigh of a patient with Ullrich congenital muscular dystrophy demonstrating characteristic "central cloud" in the rectus femoris and rimming of vastus lateralis. Note also relative sparing of the sartorius and gracilis.

Source: Image courtesy of Jahannaz Dastgir, MD, Columbia University.

Limb-Girdle Muscular Dystrophy

LGMD is a genetically and clinically heterogeneous group of disorders characterized by weakness in the shoulder and hip flexors. Patterns of specific muscle involvement in LGMD identifiable by muscle imaging have been suggested (55,73); however, clinical, histological, and imaging findings are largely overlapping. Imaging characteristics are most distinctive early in the course of disease before motor impairment becomes severe (65).

Patients with LGMD2A due to mutations in *CAPN3* show early involvement of gluteal, posterior/medial thigh, adductors, and semimembranosus. With clinical progression, involvement is more diffuse but the vastus lateralis, sartorius, and gracilis are spared to some extent (76). LGMD2B due to *DYSF* mutations show a more diffuse pattern than LGMD2A. Patients with *DYSF* mutations can have either LGMD or a distal myopathy phenotype, Myoshi myopathy. In both cases, muscle involvement is diffuse, but the calf muscles are the earliest and most severely affected (73). LGMD2I due to mutations in *FKRP* is the most common LGMD in North American and European populations. Muscle involvement in the thigh is reminiscent of that seen in LGMD2A, but selective involvement of the medial gastrocnemius and soleus in the lower leg is seen in LGMD2A but is absent in LGMD2I (77). In contrast, sarcoglycanopathy (LGMD2C-2F) and dystrophinopathy patients showed early involvement of the anterior thigh and little involvement of the lower leg, differentiating them from other LGMDs (55,73).

GENETIC TESTING

Genetic testing in neuromuscular disease began with the discovery of mutations in the *DMD* gene as the cause for DMD in 1987 (78). Since then, the number of genes associated with neuromuscular phenotypes has grown rapidly. A comprehensive list of neuromuscular genes and phenotypes is maintained in the GeneTable of Neuromuscular Disorders (www.musclegenetable.fr) (79). The 2014 version of the GeneTable includes 685 different neuromuscular phenotypes associated with 360 different genes. New genes are identified regularly, with 27 new genes added in 2014. Application of genetic discoveries in the clinical setting was slow at first, but with the accelerating discovery of new genes and rapid improvement of the sequencing technology, genetic diagnosis has become an important part of the workup for any patient presenting with neuromuscular weakness.

Funding for genetic testing varies by country and by insurance coverage. Third-party payers and even many physicians have been hesitant to pursue genetic testing since specific treatments for most neuromuscular disorders are not available. Coverage often is dependent on a demonstration of clinical utility. Given the increasing complexity of genetic testing, inclusion of a genetic counselor early in the diagnostic evaluation can often facilitate education for families, insurance preauthorization, and identification of appropriate genetic tests.

In most cases, genetic testing is sent to specialized laboratories. Laboratories vary widely in cost and quality, even for the same test, and care must be taken to select both the lab and the genetic test appropriately. Sequencing panels are emerging using both traditional and NGS approaches. These panels can be helpful for disorders with significant heterogeneity but can be wasteful if clinical and diagnostic features suggest a more specific diagnosis. Selection of the appropriate genetic test and appropriate laboratory for testing can be facilitated by a number of online resources including the Genetic Testing Registry at the National Institute of Health and www.genetests.org.

From a diagnostic standpoint, genetic testing offers a definitive diagnosis. The clinical utility of a definitive diagnosis for patients and families in the midst of a prolonged diagnostic odyssey is difficult to understate. An accurate genetic diagnosis facilitates genetic counseling and estimation of recurrence risk, guides appropriate surveillance, and avoids unnecessary and costly testing. Clinical utility is demonstrated by a significant impact on both survival and quality of life for patients with disease-specific surveillance facilitated by accurate genetic diagnosis (80,81). Furthermore, development of specific treatments depends on having well-characterized, genetically distinct groups of participants. Participation in most clinical trials requires a genetic diagnosis. The benefits of genetic testing must be balanced with the costs, which can be high, especially if multiple genetic tests are required. The rapid evolution of NGS technologies and rapid drop in cost of sequencing will ultimately change this balance in favor of early genetic testing.

As early as the year 2000, genetic testing was recommended as a first-line test, before either EMG/NCS or muscle biopsy in cases of suspected DMD/BMD, EDMD, FSHD, myotonic dystrophy, and congenital myotonias (31). Standards of care have been developed in recent years for DMD, congenital myopathies, CMDs, myotonic dystrophy, and others. Appropriate application of these standards depends on accurate and specific genetic diagnosis, even when a diagnosis is already made by biopsy or other means (80,82–84). Genetic testing as a first-line test is the current standard for DMD, myotonic dystrophy type 1, and SMA in patients with typical clinical presentations (82–85).

Disorders such as COL6-RD have distinctive clinical features. These findings, which are easily recognizable in the clinic include weakness in the presence of proximal contractures and distal joint laxity and skin changes, and should prompt appropriate genetic testing (86). Genetic testing early in the evaluation speeds the diagnosis and avoids more invasive diagnostic tests such as EMG/NCS and muscle biopsy.

Selection of genetic tests may depend on regional factors. In Japan, Fukuyama-type CMD (FCMD) is the most common CMD, accounting for almost half of the cases (7,87,88). The high number of FCMD patients in Japanese populations has been traced to the insertion of a 3-kb retrotransposon in the *FKTN* gene in a founder 102 generations ago (88). The high prevalence of this founder mutation in Japanese populations (1/188 individuals) suggests that molecular testing should be performed early in the evaluation of CMD patients in Japanese populations but should be a later consideration in other populations where *FKTN* mutations are more rare.

Complications of Genetic Testing in Neuromuscular Disorders

Genetic testing is complicated by the large size of many of the genes involved in neuromuscular disorders. These include some of the largest genes in the human genome including *TTN*, *DMD*, *NEB*, and *RYR1*. Sequencing of these genes by traditional methods (Sanger sequencing) is time-consuming and very expensive. Initial efforts at molecular diagnosis identified mutational hot spots where disease-causing mutations clustered, ie, exons 44 to 51 in the *DMD* gene for DMD and the C-terminal transmembrane domain of the *RYR1* gene for central core myopathy (78,89).

To save costs, many clinically available tests for these large genes screen only mutational hot spots, and failure to identify a mutation does not rule out a disorder associated with one of these genes. Technological improvements have made comprehensive analysis of these genes possible and have led to the identification of significant mutations throughout these very large genes (90–92). Titin, encoded by the *TTN* gene, the largest gene in the human genome, encompassing 364 exons in a 100-kb-long transcript was first associated with tibial muscular dystrophy, due to mutations in the M-line domain (93). For some time, sequencing of the *TTN* gene focused primarily on this region of the gene. With newer technologies that allow sequencing of the entire gene, a variety of skeletal muscle and cardiac phenotypes have been associated with mutations throughout the *TTN* gene, but no clear genotype-phenotype association has emerged (92).

Genetic and Phenotypic Heterogeneity

In many cases, patients with suspected neuromuscular disorders have few distinguishing features and a large number of potential genetic etiologies. Genetic diagnosis in these cases is complicated by high levels of clinical and genetic heterogeneity. Rather than simplifying the diagnostic approach, the rapid discovery of new genes in these disorders has only added to the known heterogeneity and blurred what appeared to be specific genetic associations in early genetic studies. Among the genes causing LGMD phenotypes, for example, the 2014 GeneTable lists 8 autosomal dominant and 21 autosomal recessive genes. A dominant, recessive, or X-linked family history may guide a differential; however, in some cases such as COL6-RD, inheritance may follow a dominant or recessive pattern depending on the specific mutation (94).

Increasingly, disorders such as COL6-RD that were thought to be specific phenotypes show a broad spectrum of involvement. UCMD was first described in the 1930s as a syndrome with weakness from early infancy and a mix of proximal joint contracture and distal joint hyperlaxity (95). Forty years later, BM was described as a slowly progressive congenital myopathy presenting with contracture in the elbows, ankles, and long finger flexors and onset in later childhood or adolescence (96). It was not until the genetic era that mutations in collagen VI were identified as the cause for both disorders (97,98). With increasing experience in genotype-phenotype correlations, a spectrum of clinical phenotypes is now recognized that spans from severe UCMD to mild BM cases, with most cases intermediate between the classically described phenotypes (99).

A striking example of the phenotypic variability from a single gene comes from mutations in the nuclear envelope protein lamin A/C encoded by the *LMNA* gene (OMIM 150330). Mutations in *LMNA* cause a diverse set of neuromuscular and nonneuromuscular phenotypes including EDMD, LGMD1B, a severe CMD with dropped head, Charcot-Marie-Tooth type 2B1 (CMT2B1), dilated cardiomyopathy 1A (CMD1A), familial partial lipodystrophy, Dunnigan type 2 (FPLD2), and Hutchinson-Gilford progeria syndrome (100). In turn, EDMD, a fairly specific clinical entity characterized by progressive weakness in a scapulo-peroneal-humeral distribution, early contractures in ankles and elbows, and cardiomyopathy can be caused by as many as three different genes, *EMD*, *FHL1*, and *LMNA* (101). In each case, the clinical phenotype is identical. Family history can help to narrow the search for the causative gene, but inheritance can be difficult to assess in small families and may not be completely informative since both *EMD* and *FHL1* are X-linked and *LMNA* can be either autosomal dominant or recessive.

Duchenne and Becker Muscular Dystrophy

Soon after the identification of the *DMD* gene in 1987 (78), clinical genetic tests quickly became available; however, this testing was technically challenging and costly. Due to the large size of the *DMD* gene, clinically available tests did not include a comprehensive analysis of the entire gene but focused on mutational hot spots where deletions were common. With the development of newer sequencing strategies, genetic diagnosis for DMD became widely available from the early 2000s (90). As genetic testing has become more readily available in the clinic, genetic testing for DMD has become a standard part of the workup for most cases. For DMD, the current standard for genetic testing consists of stepwise analysis for deletion/duplication mutations followed by direct sequencing of all 79 exons in cases where a deletion or duplication is not identified (84). Genetic testing is usually sent early in the evaluation of boys with appropriate clinical presentation and elevation in CK and obviates the need for muscle biopsy or other diagnostic tests.

Using current technology, a genetic diagnosis can be made in more than 95% of the cases where clinical history and elevated CK suggest a diagnosis of DMD (90,102). Deletion or duplication mutations in the *DMD* gene are the most common and are identified in 72% of the cases, while nonsense mutations are identified in 17% patients (103). Generally speaking, BMD and DMD can be differentiated based on the reading frame rule. Nonsense mutations and deletions or duplications that disrupt the reading frame result in a DMD phenotype. Missense mutations and deletion or duplication mutations that leave the reading frame intact result in BMD.

Genetic testing for DMD is readily available in most developed countries and genetic testing has become the standard of care in patients with appropriate clinical presentation (84). Muscle biopsy and other testing should be limited to unusual cases or cases where genetic testing fails to identify a mutation. Even in cases where muscle biopsy has been done and suggests DMD due to absent dystrophin expression, current care guidelines suggest that genetic diagnosis is mandatory (84). Given the development of mutation-dependent therapies such as nonsense read-through and exon skipping, the importance of an accurate and early genetic diagnosis is becoming even more critical (104,105).

Mutations in the *DMD* gene are de novo in one-third of affected boys with the remaining two-third inheriting their mutation from their carrier mothers (106). Once a mutation has been identified in an affected boy, carrier testing for the mother is critical. With a high recurrence risk (50% for sons of carrier mothers), and many mothers still of childbearing age at the initial diagnosis, appropriate genetic counseling can give important guidance to family planning decisions. As with any genetic test, a normal finding on carrier testing does not exclude the possibility that an individual might pass the mutation to future offspring due to the possibility of germ-line mosaicism. In DMD, the risk that an individual with negative carrier testing has the mutation in the germ line has been estimated at 8.6%, resulting in a 4.3% chance that she will pass the mutant allele to future offspring (107). Technologies such as preimplantation diagnosis are available to families where carrier status has been confirmed. Daughters of carrier mothers are at 50% risk for carrier status and should be appropriately counseled about recurrence risk. Carrier testing should be offered when potential carriers are of appropriate age to consent to testing.

It should also be noted that female carriers of DMD mutations can have a variety of manifestations of disease, including a full DMD phenotype (108). In most cases clinical features are mild and include myalgias and fatigability, but progressive cardiomyopathy has been described (109). Since carriers can have some manifestations of disease, especially cardiac, establishment of recurrence risk and identification of carrier status can inform medical decision making and surveillance for carriers (110).

Congenital Myopathies

Diagnosis in the congenital myopathies has traditionally centered on findings in the muscle biopsy. Histopathologic classes including nemaline myopathies, core myopathies, centronuclear myopathies, and myopathies with congenital fiber-type disproportion have been well described (5). In each case, multiple genes have been identified with each histopathologic group (Table 6.1). Nemaline myopathy is caused by mutations in nebulin (*NEB*) in up to half of the cases and *ACTA1* in 20% to 25% of the cases; however, as many as six other genes can cause a myopathy with nemaline rods (5). Since these disorders lack clinical or histopathologic features to differentiate them, genetic sequencing is necessary to make a specific diagnosis. Clinical features can sometimes narrow the differential diagnosis to a smaller group of genes. The presence of ophthalmoplegia in a patient with centronuclear myopathy on biopsy suggests a mutation in *MTM1*, *RYR1*, or *DNM2*. Cardiac involvement in a patient with otherwise nonspecific myopathy suggests a *TTN* or *MYH7* mutation. Sequencing of many of these genes is

TABLE 6.1 Overview of Genes Associated With Congenital Myopathies

GENE	PROTEIN	INHERITANCE	BIOPSY	UNIQUE FEATURES
NEMALINE MYOPATHIES				
ACTA1	Alpha actin, skeletal muscle	AD, AR	NR, C, CFTD	20–25% of nemaline myopathy; 50% of severe neonatal cases
KBTBD13	Kelch repeat and BTB (POZ) domain containing 13	AD	NR, C	Rare; slow voluntary movements; spares face
CFL2	Cofilin 2 (muscle)	AR	NR	Rare; only 3 families reported
KLHL40	Kelch-like family member 40	AR	NR	Severe neonatal, often lethal
NEB	Nebulin	AR	NR	Most common nemaline myopathy; 50% of cases
TNNT1	Slow troponin T	AR	NR	Only reported in Amish families
TPM2	Tropomyosin 2 (beta)	AD	NR, CFTD	Also seen in congenital arthrogryposis, pterygia
TPM3	Tropomyosin 3	AD, AR	NR, CFTD	Common cause of CFTD without nemaline rods
CORE MYOPATHIES				
RYR1	Ryanodine receptor 1 (skeletal)	AD, AR	C, CFTD	Most common core myopathy; usually AD; associated with susceptibility to malignant hyperthermia
MYH7	Myosin, heavy polypeptide 7, cardiac muscle, beta	AD	CN	May have cardiac involvement
SEPN1	Selenoprotein N1	AR	CN, CFTD	Multi-minicore; axial weakness and respiratory involvement out of proportion to weakness
TTN	Titin	AR	CN	May have cardiac involvement
CENTRONUCLEAR MYOPATHIES				
BIN1	Amphiphysin	AR	CN	
DNM2	Dynamin 2	AD	CN	

(continued)

TABLE 6.1 Overview of Genes Associated With Congenital Myopathies (*continued*)

GENE	PROTEIN	INHERITANCE	BIOPSY	UNIQUE FEATURES
CENTRONUCLEAR MYOPATHIES				
MTM1	Myotubularin	X-linked	CN	Myotubular myopathy. Prominent central nuclei is the characteristic feature histologically. Similar features are seen in patients with congenital myotonic dystrophy. Clinical features and family history usually differentiate the two disorders.

Abbreviations: AD, autosomal dominant; AR, autosomal recessive; C, cores or multi-minicores; CFTD, congenital fiber-type disproportion; CN, central nuclei; NR, nemaline rods.

complicated by the large size of the genes, which can make genetic testing cost-prohibitive. Nebulin is especially notable in this respect, with 183 exons.

Congenital Muscular Dystrophies

CMD includes a group of disorders that vary widely in clinical features but share dystrophic features on muscle biopsy (Table 6.2). A combination of clinical features and ancillary testing such as muscle imaging and biopsy can direct specific genetic testing. COL6-RDs are the most common CMDs and present with distal joint hyperlaxity and proximal joint contractures. The presence of skin changes such as keloid scars and hyperkeratosis pilaris with distal laxity should prompt the consideration of a COL6-RD, even without biopsy or imaging tests. Patients with merosin-deficient CMD are not easily distinguished from other CMDs clinically but are readily identified by the absence of merosin on muscle immunohistochemistry. In these cases, genetic testing targeted to the *LAMA 2* gene is readily available and confirms the diagnosis at a molecular level. The most genetically diverse group of CMDs is due to defects in the glycosylation of alpha-dystroglycan. These disorders include a spectrum from very severe in the Walker-Warburg and muscle-eye-brain phenotypes to the relatively mild LGMD phenotypes. While a disruption of glycoslylation of alpha-dystroglycan can be readily identified on muscle biopsy samples, distinction between the 12 or more genes identified to date including *FKTN, POMT1, POMT2, FKRP, POMGNT1, ISPD, GTDC2, B3GNT1, GMPPB, LARGE, DPM1, DPM2, ALG13, B3GALNT2,* and *TMEM5* is only accomplished by sequencing each of the genes.

Next-Generation Sequencing

Given the increasing complexity of genetic diagnosis including the increasing number of genes per phenotype and increasing numbers or phenotypes per gene and the inherent difficulty of sequencing many of the very large genes associated with neuromuscular disorders, selection of an appropriate genetic test can be very difficult. The dramatic expansion of sequencing

TABLE 6.2 Overview of Genes Associated With Congenital Muscular Dystrophies

SUBTYPE	GENE(S)	INHERITANCE	CLINICAL FEATURES
Merosin	*LAMA2*	AR	Most never achieve independent ambulation. Peripheral neuropathy in later childhood. Normal intelligence despite abnormality in white matter on brain MRI. 30% with seizures. Milder phenotypes possible with partial deficiency.
Collagen VI	*COL6A1, COL6A2, COL6A3*	AD, AR	Milder BM and severe UCMD phenotypes, but most patients intermediate. Distinguishing features are marked distal hyperlaxity with proximal contractures. Skin changes include keloid formation, hyperkeratosis pilaris, and soft palms and soles. CK may be normal to mildly elevated.
Alpha-dystroglycan	*FKTN, POMT1, POMT2, FKRP, POMGNT1, ISPD, GTDC2, B3GNT1, GMPPB, LARGE, DPM1, DPM2, ALG13, B3GALNT2, TMEM5*	AR	Defect in glycosylation of alpha-dystroglycan. Broad spectrum of clinical phenotypes from very severe Walker-Warburg syndrome and muscle-eye-brain disease to milder limb-girdle MD phenotypes. CNS involvement can be profound in severe cases and includes cobblestone lissencephaly, severe mental retardation, and seizures. Fukuyama subtype due to FKTN mutation is common in Japan because of ancestral mutation. FKRP most common in other populations.
Rigid spine	*SEPN1*	AR	Broad spectrum of severity including overlap with congenital myopathy phenotypes. CMD phenotype with early spinal rigidity and weakness in neck, postural muscles. Early respiratory compromise is typical and precedes loss of ambulation.
RYR1	*RYR1*	AR/AD	On spectrum with congenital myopathy phenotypes caused by RYR1 including central core, multiminicore, and congenital fiber-type proportion. May present with early scoliosis and loss of ambulation.

(continued)

TABLE 6.2 Overview of Genes Associated With Congenital Muscular Dystrophies (*continued*)

SUBTYPE	GENE(S)	INHERITANCE	CLINICAL FEATURES
Laminopathy	*LMNA*	AR	CMD phenotype includes neonatal onset of severe weakness for neck/postural muscles (dropped head syndrome) with early loss of ambulation. Other phenotypes include EDMD, FPL, LGMD, dilated cardiomyopathy, CMT disease, and Hutchinson-Gilford progeria syndrome.

Abbreviations: AD, autosomal dominant; AR, autosomal recessive; BM, Bethlem myopathy; CK, creatine kinase; CMD, congenital muscular dystrophy; CMT, Charcot-Marie-Tooth; CNS, central nervous system; EDMD, Emery-Dreifuss muscular dystrophy; FPL, familial partial lipodystrophy; LGMD, limb-girdle muscular dystrophy; MD, muscular dystrophy; UCMD, Ullrich congenital muscular dystrophy.

capacity afforded by NGS techniques will likely result in a shift in traditional diagnostic paradigms, since many genes (or all genes) can be sequenced simultaneously at a relatively low cost.

The Human Genome Project was launched in 1990, just 3 years after the discovery of the *DMD* gene, with a goal to sequence the entire human genome. Sequencing for the Human Genome Project started with traditional Sanger sequencing methods and ended by taking advantage of increasing computing power and high-throughput "parallel" sequencing techniques. Using these techniques, sequencing the first full human genome cost an estimated $300 million and involved the efforts of many hundreds of scientists. The completed sequence was published in 2004 (111).

Taking advantage of lessons learned in sequencing the first human genome, new technologies emerged to greatly amplify the efficiency and parallelization of the sequencing. These advances in sequencing technology, broadly termed *next-generation sequencing* have allowed a dramatic decrease in the cost per base for sequence generation and has led to a rapid acceleration in the development of sequencing applications (112,113). A variety of technologies have emerged but all take advantage of the ability to rapidly sequence millions of short fragments of DNA (or cDNA) in a parallel fashion. Among the first to use NGS technologies, Lupski et al. identified a variant in the *SH3TC2* gene in a family with CMT neuropathy by whole genome sequencing at an estimated cost of $50,000 per genome (114). Continued rapid development of these technologies has been promoted by the *National Institutes of Health* (NIH) and others with a goal toward providing a complete genome sequence for under $1,000 (115). Realization of these goals is anticipated to result in dramatic changes in the utilization of DNA sequencing in both clinical and research applications. While the issues of obtaining sequence data have been largely addressed, issues of data analysis including data storage, patient privacy, insurability, and handling of incidental findings remain significant (116–118).

Targeted Gene and Exome Sequencing
While NGS technology has made sequencing of the whole genome feasible, targeted NGS approaches have simplified some of the complex data analysis issues and allowed a more

straightforward application for clinical use. Using this approach, samples of interest are subjected to an enrichment step during sample preparation that restricts the sequenced DNA to only those areas of interest. For exome sequencing, the targeted sequences are the exons of all genes. The exome sequence covers 30 million bases in 180,000 exons from 23,000 genes or about 1% of the total human sequence. Within that 1% of the genomic sequence is an estimated 85% of the pathogenic mutations. Thus exome sequencing can significantly limit the search space and at the same time identify mutations in almost every gene without a priori knowledge of the phenotype.

A number of different exon capture technologies are available. All have gaps in coverage, and analysis of the resulting sequence data should acknowledge the possibility that some genes or exons may not be well covered (119). With current exome capture technologies, most leave 10% of exomes poorly covered and 3% of exons not targeted at all. Gaps in exome coverage are somewhat systematic and reflect difficulties in hybridization due to high guanine-cytosine (GC) content and other factors in the primary sequence. Rapid development in these areas is expected to improve coverage; however, gaps are likely to remain.

Beyond exome sequencing, strategies have been developed to target different disorders by limiting the number of exons in the enrichment step to a relatively small number of genes of interest. Targeted gene panels such as this take advantage of the capacity of the sequencing technology to cover a large number of genes and yet limit the search for mutations to those genes with a relationship to the phenotype of interest (120). In one study, 267 genes selected from the Muscle GeneTable were selected for sequencing in eight myopathy patients with known molecular diagnoses and eight patients with neuromuscular disorders but without a molecular diagnosis (121). Pathogenic mutations were identified in 13 of the 16 patients with a variety of neuromuscular disorders.

For disorders where genetic and phenotypic heterogeneity is the rule, genetic testing using panels of neuromuscular genes will likely change the diagnostic approach. This approach is likely to include genetic testing at a much earlier point, perhaps even before the use of ancillary tests such as EMG/NCS, imaging, and muscle biopsy, especially as costs for sequencing by exome or by targeted sequencing drop below those of traditional tests. Clinical use of targeted sequencing panels is rapidly evolving and targeted NGS panels for neuromuscular disorders are currently available from a number of commercial labs. Selection of the appropriate panel requires careful review of the genes included on the panel and assessment of clinical phenotype. A panel for 8 to 10 genes associated with nemaline myopathy, for example, may be sufficient if nemaline rods are identified on muscle biopsy. However, if the clinical phenotype and ancillary tests are less specific, a larger, more diverse panel may be more appropriate.

Difficulties of NGS

Despite its enormous potential, there are pitfalls in using NGS. Sequencing using these technologies is inherently less precise on a per-base level than traditional Sanger sequencing. Analytical tools such as those to assess the quality of the base calls and repeated sequencing of the same base in different reads (read depth) can help to overcome this imprecision, but there can be systematic errors. These errors can usually be handled by a detailed look at the primary data and by validation of identified mutations by Sanger sequencing. NGS can miss some mutations due to technical reasons inherent in the technology. Expansions of triplet repeats such as the ones causing myotonic dystrophy, for example, are not identifiable using NGS due to the repetitive nature of the sequence and difficulties in aligning short reads to a repetitive sequence. Further, chromosomal rearrangements and large deletions can be difficult to identify using NGS.

Interpretation of variants of unknown significance (VUSs) is a problem for any genetic sequencing technology but is a particular problem when using NGS due to the sheer magnitude of the sequencing. In an exome sequencing study, an individual may have as many as 20,000 to 30,000 variants from the reference sequence. Filtering rare but benign variants from potentially pathogenic variants is difficult. A number of bioinformatic analyses are available to assess pathogenicity of variants. Locus-specific databases such as the Leiden Muscular Dystrophy pages highlight variants with known pathogenicity (www.dmd.nl). Tools such as the Single Nucleotide Polymorphism database (dbSNP), the Exome Variant Server, and 1000 Genomes Project can help to identify rare variants that have been previously identified in other populations (122–124). Analytic tools including SIFT (sorting intolerant from tolerant) and PolyPhen2 (polymorphism phenotyping) use conservation of the locus and biochemical disruption of the altered amino acid to the peptide to predict pathogenicity of a particular variant (125,126). Inclusion of DNA from parents and other family members can help to characterize the variant as benign, VUS, or pathogenic, based on segregation of the variant with the phenotype. Most commercial NGS tests include this type of segregation analysis. Taken together, these tools can be used to filter and classify variants identified in an individual or family and narrow the search for a potentially pathogenic mutation.

Given the complexity of the analysis, there are a number of cases where whole genome or exome sequencing has failed to identify a mutation when it was indeed present. In these cases, the bioinformatic tools failed to properly classify a variant as pathogenic. In one recently published case, a family with clinical symptoms typical of BM presented after obtaining their own whole genome sequencing (127). Several variants were identified in genes associated with neuromuscular disorders, but none fully explained the phenotype. Reassessment of the clinical phenotype including imaging gave additional weight to the possibility of a collagen VI mutation. Traditional Sanger sequencing was performed and a pathogenic mutation in *COL6A3*, typical of BM was identified. In this case, the whole genome data was reanalyzed, given the known mutation in *COL6A3*, and it was determined that the variant was indeed present in the whole genome sequence but was misclassified by bioinformatics analysis. The authors concluded that the sequence data must be matched with careful phenotypic analysis and understanding of clinical aspects of the suspected disorder in order to come to an appropriate interpretation of the data.

CONCLUSION

Current approaches to the diagnosis of neuromuscular disorders focus on careful clinical examination and application of ancillary tests to define probable disorders that are then confirmed by genetic testing. The role of clinical neurophysiology is limited primarily to distinguishing muscle disorders from nerve disorders. In the process, certain abnormalities, such as the presence of myotonic discharges can support a limited range of potential diagnoses. In recent years, the number of genetic tests has markedly increased. However, there remain disorders not diagnosed by commonly available tests. The rapid evolution of sequencing technology that allows sequencing of the entire genome or exome at a relatively low cost is likely to change diagnostic strategies in these situations. Rapid discovery of new genes involved with neuromuscular disease and broad overlap of phenotypes will prompt earlier application of broad sequencing strategies such as exome sequencing or sequencing of large targeted gene panels. While the importance of ancillary tests such as neurophysiology, muscle biopsy, and imaging will likely be diminished in diagnostic application, they will likely become increasingly important in treatment and monitoring applications. Recent advances in EIM and imaging for muscle disorders have focused on quantitative measures, which will have great application in the monitoring of treatments and progression of these disorders.

REFERENCES

1. Arnold WD, Flanigan KM. A practical approach to molecular diagnostic testing in neuromuscular diseases. *Phys Med Rehabil Clin N Am.* 2012;23:589–608.
2. Vasli N, Laporte J. Impacts of massively parallel sequencing for genetic diagnosis of neuromuscular disorders. *Acta Neuropathol.* 2013;125:173–185.
3. Fardeau M, Desguerre I. Diagnostic workup for neuromuscular diseases. *Handb Clin Neurol.* 2013;113:1291–1297.
4. Bonnemann CG, Wang CH, Quijano-Roy S, et al. Diagnostic approach to the congenital muscular dystrophies. *Neuromuscul Disord.* 2014;24:289–311.
5. North KN, Wang CH, Clarke N, et al. Approach to the diagnosis of congenital myopathies. *Neuromuscul Disord.* 2014;24:97–116.
6. Norwood FL, Harling C, Chinnery PF, et al. Prevalence of genetic muscle disease in Northern England: in-depth analysis of a muscle clinic population. *Brain.* 2009;132:3175–3186.
7. Okada M, Kawahara G, Noguchi S, et al. Primary collagen VI deficiency is the second most common congenital muscular dystrophy in Japan. *Neurology.* 2007;69:1035–1042.
8. Clement EM, Feng L, Mein R, et al. Relative frequency of congenital muscular dystrophy subtypes: Analysis of the UK diagnostic service 2001–2008. *Neuromuscul Disord.* 2012;22:522–527.
9. Maggi L, Scoto M, Cirak S, et al. Congenital myopathies—clinical features and frequency of individual subtypes diagnosed over a 5-year period in the United Kingdom. *Neuromuscul Disord.* 2013;23:195–205.
10. Richer LP, Shevell MI, Miller SP. Diagnostic profile of neonatal hypotonia: an 11-year study. *Pediatr Neurol.* 2001;25:32–37.
11. Vasta I, Kinali M, Messina S, et al. Can clinical signs identify newborns with neuromuscular disorders? *J Pediatr.* 2005;146:73–79.
12. Carmignac V, Salih MA, Quijano-Roy S, et al. C-terminal titin deletions cause a novel early-onset myopathy with fatal cardiomyopathy. *Ann Neurol.* 2007;61:340–351.
13. Overeem S, Schelhaas HJ, Blijham PJ, et al. Symptomatic distal myopathy with cardiomyopathy due to a MYH7 mutation. *Neuromuscul Disord.* 2007;17:490–493.
14. Mendell JR, Shilling C, Leslie ND, et al. Evidence-based path to newborn screening for Duchenne muscular dystrophy. *Ann Neurol.* 2012;71:304–313.
15. Ciafaloni E, Fox DJ, Pandya S, et al. Delayed diagnosis in duchenne muscular dystrophy: data from the Muscular Dystrophy Surveillance, Tracking, and Research Network (MD STARnet). *J Pediatr.* 2009;155:380–385.
16. Crisp DE, Ziter FA, Bray PF. Diagnostic delay in Duchenne's muscular dystrophy. *JAMA.* 1982;247:478–480.
17. Wong ET, Cobb C, Umehara MK, et al. Heterogeneity of serum creatine kinase activity among racial and gender groups of the population. *Am J Clin Pathol.* 1983;79:582–586.
18. Silvestri NJ, Wolfe GI. Asymptomatic/pauci-symptomatic creatine kinase elevations (hyperckemia). *Muscle Nerve.* 2013;47:805–815.
19. Kyriakides T, Angelini C, Schaefer J, et al. EFNS guidelines on the diagnostic approach to pauci- or asymptomatic hyperCKemia. *Eur J Neurol.* 2010;17:767–773.

20. Jones HR, Harmon RL, Harper CM, Bolton DF. An approach to pediatric electromyography. In: Bolton DF, Harper CM, eds. *Pediatric Clinical Electromyography.* Phildelphia, PA: Lippincott-Raven;1996:1–36.
21. Oh SJ. Pediatric Nerve Conduction Studies. In: Oh SJ, eds. *Clinical Electromyography: Nerve Conduction Studies.* Phildalphia, PA: Lippincott Williams & Wilkins; 2003: 107–135.
22. Pitt M. Paediatric electromyography in the modern world: a personal view. *Dev Med Child Neurol.* 2011;53:120–124.
23. Pitt M. Update in electromyography. *Curr Opin Pediatr.* 2013;25:676–681.
24. Bady B, Vila A, Boulliat G, et al. [Value of electromyography in the child. Apropos of 1,624 examinations performed over a 3 year period]. *Rev Electroencephalogr Neurophysiol Clin.* 1983;13:282–288.
25. Hellmann M, von Kleist-Retzow JC, Haupt WF, et al. Diagnostic value of electromyography in children and adolescents. *J Clin Neurophysiol.* 2005;22:43–48.
26. Rabie M, Jossiphov J, Nevo Y. Electromyography (EMG) accuracy compared to muscle biopsy in childhood. *J Child Neurol.* 2007;22:803–808.
27. Paganoni S, Amato A. Electrodiagnostic evaluation of myopathies. *Phys Med Rehabil Clin N Am.* 2013;24:193–207.
28. Ghosh PS, Sorenson EJ. Diagnostic Yield of Electromyography in Children With Myopathic Disorders. *Pediatr Neurol.* 2014; 51(2):215–219.
29. Shah DU, Darras BT, Markowitz JA, et al. The spectrum of myotonic and myopathic disorders in a pediatric electromyography laboratory over 12 years. *Pediatr Neurol.* 2012;47:97–100.
30. Pitt MC. Nerve conduction studies and needle EMG in very small children. *Eur J Paediatr Neurol.* 2012;16:285–291.
31. Darras BT, Jones HR. Diagnosis of pediatric neuromuscular disorders in the era of DNA analysis. *Pediatr Neurol.* 2000;23:289–300.
32. Shorer Z, Philpot J, Muntoni F, et al. Demyelinating peripheral neuropathy in merosin-deficient congenital muscular dystrophy. *J Child Neurol.* 1995;10:472–475.
33. Mercuri E, Pennock J, Goodwin F, et al. Sequential study of central and peripheral nervous system involvement in an infant with merosin-deficient congenital muscular dystrophy. *Neuromuscul Disord.* 1996;6:425–429.
34. Quijano-Roy S, Renault F, Romero N, et al. EMG and nerve conduction studies in children with congenital muscular dystrophy. *Muscle Nerve.* 2004;29:292–299.
35. Fujii Y, Sugiura C, Fukuda C, et al. Sequential neuroradiological and neurophysiological studies in a Japanese girl with merosin-deficient congenital muscular dystrophy. *Brain Dev.* 2011;33:140–144.
36. Peric S, Stojanovic VR, Nikolic A, et al. Peripheral neuropathy in patients with myotonic dystrophy type 1. *Neurol Res.* 2013;35:331–335.
37. Zanette G, Manani G, Pittoni G, et al. Prevalence of unsuspected myopathy in infants presenting for clubfoot surgery. *Paediatr Anaesth.* 1995;5:165–170.
38. Rutkove SB. Electrical impedance myography: Background, current state, and future directions. *Muscle Nerve.* 2009;40:936–946.
39. Rutkove SB, Shefner JM, Gregas M, et al. Characterizing spinal muscular atrophy with electrical impedance myography. *Muscle Nerve.* 2010;42:915–921.
40. Rutkove SB, Darras BT. Electrical impedance myography for the assessment of children with muscular dystrophy: a preliminary study. *J Phys Conf Ser.* 2013;434.
41. Dubowitz V, Sewry CA. Muscle biopsy: a practical approach. 3rd ed. Philadelphia, PA: Saunders/Elsevier; 2007.
42. Heckmatt JZ, Dubowitz V. Ultrasound imaging and directed needle biopsy in the diagnosis of selective involvement in muscle disease. *J Child Neurol.* 1987;2:205–213.
43. Joyce NC, Oskarsson B, Jin LW. Muscle biopsy evaluation in neuromuscular disorders. *Phys Med Rehabil Clin N Am.* 2012;23:609–631.
44. Tarnopolsky MA, Pearce E, Smith K, Lach B. Suction-modified Bergstrom muscle biopsy technique: experience with 13,500 procedures. *Muscle Nerve.* 2011;43:717–725.
45. Jaradeh SS, Ho H. Muscle, nerve, and skin biopsy. *Neurol Clin.* 2004;22:539–561
46. Meola G, Bugiardini E, Cardani R. Muscle biopsy. *J Neurol.* 2012;259:601–610.

47. Romero NB, Monnier N, Viollet L, et al. Dominant and recessive central core disease associated with RYR1 mutations and fetal akinesia. *Brain*. 2003;126:2341–2349.
48. Wallefeld W, Krause S, Nowak KJ, et al. Severe nemaline myopathy caused by mutations of the stop codon of the skeletal muscle alpha actin gene (ACTA1). *Neuromuscul Disord*. 2006;16:541–547.
49. Heckmatt JZ, Dubowitz V, Leeman S. Detection of pathological change in dystrophic muscle with B- scan ultrasound imaging. *Lancet*. 1980;1:1389–1390.
50. Heckmatt JZ, Leeman S, Dubowitz V. Ultrasound imaging in the diagnosis of muscle disease. *J Pediatr*. 1982;101:656–660.
51. Pillen S, Arts IM, Zwarts MJ. Muscle ultrasound in neuromuscular disorders. *Muscle Nerve*. 2008;37:679–693.
52. Bonnemann CG, Brockmann K, Hanefeld F. Muscle ultrasound in Bethlem myopathy. *Neuropediatrics*. 2003;34:335–336.
53. Bharucha-Goebel DX, Santi M, Medne L, et al. Severe congenital RYR1-associated myopathy: the expanding clinicopathologic and genetic spectrum. *Neurology*. 2013;80:1584–1589.
54. Pillen S, van Alfen N. Skeletal muscle ultrasound. *Neurol Res*. 2011;33:1016–1024.
55. Wattjes MP, Kley RA, Fischer D. Neuromuscular imaging in inherited muscle diseases. *Eur Radiol*. 2010;20:2447–2460.
56. Mercuri E, Talim B, Moghadaszadeh B, et al. Clinical and imaging findings in six cases of congenital muscular dystrophy with rigid spine syndrome linked to chromosome 1p (RSMD1). *Neuromuscul Disord*. 2002;12:631–638.
57. Kornblum C, Lutterbey G, Bogdanow M, et al. Distinct neuromuscular phenotypes in myotonic dystrophy types 1 and 2: a whole body highfield MRI study. *J Neurol*. 2006;253:753–761.
58. Fischer D, Kley RA, Strach K, et al. Distinct muscle imaging patterns in myofibrillar myopathies. *Neurology*. 2008;71:758–765.
59. Fischmann A, Hafner P, Gloor M, et al. Quantitative MRI and loss of free ambulation in Duchenne muscular dystrophy. *J Neurol*. 2013;260:969–974.
60. Willis TA, Hollingsworth KG, Coombs A, et al. Quantitative muscle MRI as an assessment tool for monitoring disease progression in LGMD2I: a multicentre longitudinal study. *PLoS One*. 2013;8:e70993.
61. Arpan I, Willcocks RJ, Forbes SC, et al. Examination of effects of corticosteroids on skeletal muscles of boys with DMD using MRI and MRS. *Neurology*. 2014;83:974–980.
62. Costa AF, Di Primio GA, Schweitzer ME. Magnetic resonance imaging of muscle disease: a pattern- based approach. *Muscle Nerve*. 2012;46:465–481.
63. Quijano-Roy S, Carlier RY, Fischer D. Muscle imaging in congenital myopathies. *Semin Pediatr Neurol*. 2011;18:221–229.
64. Mercuri E, Clements E, Offiah A, et al. Muscle magnetic resonance imaging involvement in muscular dystrophies with rigidity of the spine. *Ann Neurol*. 2010;67:201–208.
65. ten Dam L, van der Kooi AJ, van Wattingen M, et al. Reliability and accuracy of skeletal muscle imaging in limb-girdle muscular dystrophies. *Neurology*. 2012;79:1716–1723.
66. Quijano-Roy S, Avila-Smirnow D, Carlier RY. Whole body muscle MRI protocol: pattern recognition in early onset NM disorders. *Neuromuscul Disord*. 2012;22 Suppl 2:S68–S84.
67. Tasca G, Monforte M, Iannaccone E, et al. Upper girdle imaging in facioscapulohumeral muscular dystrophy. *PLoS One*. 2014;9:e100292.
68. Hollingsworth KG, Garrood P, Eagle M, Bushby K, Straub V. Magnetic resonance imaging in Duchenne muscular dystrophy: longitudinal assessment of natural history over 18 months. *Muscle Nerve*. 2013;48:586–588.
69. Kinali M, Arechavala-Gomeza V, Cirak S, et al. Muscle histology vs MRI in Duchenne muscular dystrophy. *Neurology*. 2011;76:346–353.
70. Tasca G, Iannaccone E, Monforte M, et al. Muscle MRI in Becker muscular dystrophy. *Neuromuscul Disord*. 2012;22 Suppl 2:S100–S106.
71. Jungbluth H, Davis MR, Muller C, et al. Magnetic resonance imaging of muscle in congenital myopathies associated with RYR1 mutations. *Neuromuscul Disord*. 2004;14:785–790.
72. Fischer D, Herasse M, Ferreiro A, et al. Muscle imaging in dominant core myopathies linked or unlinked to the ryanodine receptor 1 gene. *Neurology*. 2006;67:2217–2220.

73. Straub V, Carlier PG, Mercuri E. TREAT-NMD workshop: pattern recognition in genetic muscle diseases using muscle MRI: 25–26 February 2011, Rome, Italy. *Neuromuscul Disord.* 2012;22 Suppl 2:S42–S53.
74. Mercuri E, Lampe A, Allsop J, et al. Muscle MRI in Ullrich congenital muscular dystrophy and Bethlem myopathy. *Neuromuscul Disord.* 2005;15:303–310.
75. Lovitt S, Moore SL, Marden FA. The use of MRI in the evaluation of myopathy. *Clin Neurophysiol.* 2006;117:486–495.
76. Mercuri E, Bushby K, Ricci E, et al. Muscle MRI findings in patients with limb girdle muscular dystrophy with calpain 3 deficiency (LGMD2A) and early contractures. *Neuromuscul Disord.* 2005;15:164–171.
77. Fischer D, Walter MC, Kesper K, et al. Diagnostic value of muscle MRI in differentiating LGMD2I from other LGMDs. *J Neurol.* 2005;252:538–547.
78. Koenig M, Hoffman EP, Bertelson CJ, et al. Complete cloning of the Duchenne muscular dystrophy (DMD) cDNA and preliminary genomic organization of the DMD gene in normal and affected individuals. *Cell.* 1987;50:509–517.
79. Kaplan JC, Hamroun D. The 2014 version of the gene table of monogenic neuromuscular disorders (nuclear genome). *Neuromuscul Disord.* 2013;23:1081–1111.
80. Wang CH, Dowling JJ, North K, et al. Consensus statement on standard of care for congenital myopathies. *J Child Neurol.* 2012;27:363–382.
81. Moxley RT, 3rd, Pandya S, Ciafaloni E, et al. Change in natural history of Duchenne muscular dystrophy with long-term corticosteroid treatment: implications for management. *J Child Neurol.* 2010;25:1116–1129.
82. Gagnon C, Chouinard MC, Laberge L, et al. Health supervision and anticipatory guidance in adult myotonic dystrophy type 1. *Neuromuscul Disord.* 2010;20:847–851.
83. Wang CH, Finkel RS, Bertini ES, et al. Consensus statement for standard of care in spinal muscular atrophy. *J Child Neurol.* 2007;22:1027–1049.
84. Bushby K, Finkel R, Birnkrant DJ, et al. Diagnosis and management of Duchenne muscular dystrophy, part 1: diagnosis, and pharmacological and psychosocial management. *Lancet Neurol.* 2010;9:77–93.
85. Turner C, Hilton-Jones D. The myotonic dystrophies: diagnosis and management. *J Neurol Neurosurg Psychiatry.* 2010;81:358–367.
86. Bonnemann CG. The collagen VI-related myopathies: muscle meets its matrix. *Nat Rev Neurol.* 2011;7:379–390.
87. Toda T, Kobayashi K, Kondo-Iida E, Sasaki J, Nakamura Y. The Fukuyama congenital muscular dystrophy story. *Neuromuscul Disord.* 2000;10:153–159.
88. Watanabe M, Kobayashi K, Jin F, et al. Founder SVA retrotransposal insertion in Fukuyama-type congenital muscular dystrophy and its origin in Japanese and Northeast Asian populations. *Am J Med Genet A.* 2005;138:344–348.
89. Davis MR, Haan E, Jungbluth H, et al. Principal mutation hotspot for central core disease and related myopathies in the C-terminal transmembrane region of the RYR1 gene. *Neuromuscul Disord.* 2003;13:151–157.
90. Flanigan KM, von Niederhausern A, Dunn DM, et al. Rapid direct sequence analysis of the dystrophin gene. *Am J Hum Genet.* 2003;72:931–939.
91. Klein A, Lillis S, Munteanu I, et al. Clinical and genetic findings in a large cohort of patients with ryanodine receptor 1 gene-associated myopathies. *Hum Mutat.* 2012;33:981–988.
92. Chauveau C, Rowell J, Ferreiro A. A Rising Titan: TTN Review and Mutation Update. *Hum Mutat.* 2014; 35(9):1046–1059.
93. Hackman P, Vihola A, Haravuori H, et al. Tibial muscular dystrophy is a titinopathy caused by mutations in TTN, the gene encoding the giant skeletal-muscle protein titin. *Am J Hum Genet.* 2002;71:492–500.
94. Jimenez-Mallebrera C, Maioli MA, Kim J, et al. A comparative analysis of collagen VI production in muscle, skin and fibroblasts from 14 Ullrich congenital muscular dystrophy patients with dominant and recessive COL6A mutations. *Neuromuscul Disord.* 2006;16:571–582.

95. Ullrich O. Kongenitale, atonisch-sklerotische Muskeldysrophie, ein weiterer typus der heredono-degenerativen Erkankungen des neuromuskularen Systems. *Z Gestamte Neurol Psychiat.* 1930;126:171–201.

96. Bethlem J, Wijngaarden GK. Benign myopathy, with autosomal dominant inheritance. A report on three pedigrees. *Brain.* 1976;99:91–100.

97. Jobsis GJ, Keizers H, Vreijling JP, et al. Type VI collagen mutations in Bethlem myopathy, an autosomal dominant myopathy with contractures. *Nat Genet.* 1996;14:113–115.

98. Camacho Vanegas O, Bertini E, Zhang RZ, et al. Ullrich scleroatonic muscular dystrophy is caused by recessive mutations in collagen type VI. *Proc Natl Acad Sci U S A.* 2001;98:7516–7521.

99. Butterfield RJ, Foley AR, Dastgir J, et al. Position of glycine substitutions in the triple helix of COL6A1, COL6A2, and COL6A3 is correlated with severity and mode of inheritance in collagen VI myopathies. *Hum Mutat.* 2013;34:1558–1567.

100. Bonne G, Quijano-Roy S. Emery-Dreifuss muscular dystrophy, laminopathies, and other nuclear envelopathies. *Handb Clin Neurol.* 2013;113:1367–1376.

101. Bonne G, Leturcq F, Ben Yaou R. Emery-Dreifuss Muscular Dystrophy. In: Pagon RA, Adam MP, Ardinger HH, et al., eds. GeneReviews [Intermet]. Seattle, WA: Univeristy of Washington; 2013.

102. Flanigan KM, Dunn DM, von Niederhausern A, et al. Mutational spectrum of DMD mutations in dystrophinopathy patients: application of modern diagnostic techniques to a large cohort. *Hum Mutat.* 2009;30:1657–1666.

103. Dent KM, Dunn DM, von Niederhausern AC, et al. Improved molecular diagnosis of dystrophinopathies in an unselected clinical cohort. *Am J Med Genet A.* 2005;134:295–298.

104. Bushby K, Finkel R, Wong B, et al. Ataluren treatment of patients with nonsense mutation dystrophinopathy. *Muscle Nerve.* 2014; 50(4):477–487.

105. Mendell JR, Rodino-Klapac LR, Sahenk Z, et al. Eteplirsen for the treatment of Duchenne muscular dystrophy. *Ann Neurol.* 2013;74:637–647.

106. Lee T, Takeshima Y, Kusunoki N, et al. Differences in carrier frequency between mothers of Duchenne and Becker muscular dystrophy patients. *J Hum Genet.* 2014;59:46–50.

107. Helderman-van den Enden AT, de Jong R, den Dunnen JT, et al. Recurrence risk due to germ line mosaicism: Duchenne and Becker muscular dystrophy. *Clin Genet.* 2009;75:465–472.

108. Soltanzadeh P, Friez MJ, Dunn D, et al. Clinical and genetic characterization of manifesting carriers of DMD mutations. *Neuromuscul Disord.* 2010;20:499–504.

109. Schade van Westrum SM, Hoogerwaard EM, Dekker L, et al. Cardiac abnormalities in a follow-up study on carriers of Duchenne and Becker muscular dystrophy. *Neurology.* 2011;77:62–66.

110. Bushby K, Muntoni F, Bourke JP. 107th ENMC international workshop: the management of cardiac involvement in muscular dystrophy and myotonic dystrophy. 7th–9th June 2002, Naarden, the Netherlands. *Neuromuscul Disord.* 2003;13:166–172.

111. Consortium IHGS. Finishing the euchromatic sequence of the human genome. *Nature.* 2004;431:931–945.

112. Wetterstrand KA. DNA Sequencing Costs: Data from the NHGRI Genome Sequencing Program (GSP). www.genome.gov/sequencingcosts. Accessed August 2014.

113. Metzker ML. Sequencing technologies - the next generation. *Nat Rev Genet.* 2010;11:31–46.

114. Lupski JR, Reid JG, Gonzaga-Jauregui C, et al. Whole-genome sequencing in a patient with Charcot-Marie-Tooth neuropathy. *N Engl J Med.* 2010;362:1181–1191.

115. Hayden EC. Technology: The $1,000 genome. *Nature.* 2014;507:294–295.

116. Mardis ER. The $1,000 genome, the $100,000 analysis? *Genome Med.* 2010;2:84.

117. Green RC, Berg JS, Grody WW, et al. ACMG recommendations for reporting of incidental findings in clinical exome and genome sequencing. *Genet Med.* 2013;15:565–574.

118. Bamshad MJ, Ng SB, Bigham AW, et al. Exome sequencing as a tool for Mendelian disease gene discovery. *Nat Rev Genet.* 2011;12:745–755.

119. Chilamakuri CS, Lorenz S, Madoui MA, et al. Performance comparison of four exome capture systems for deep sequencing. *BMC Genomics.* 2014;15:449.

120. Nigro V, Piluso G. Next generation sequencing (NGS) strategies for the genetic testing of myopathies. *Acta Myol.* 2012;31:196–200.

121. Vasli N, Bohm J, Le Gras S, et al. Next generation sequencing for molecular diagnosis of neuromuscular diseases. *Acta Neuropathol.* 2012;124:273–283.

122. Sherry ST, Ward MH, Kholodov M, et al. dbSNP: the NCBI database of genetic variation. *Nucleic Acids Res.* 2001;29:308–311.
123. Abecasis GR, Altshuler D, Auton A, et al. A map of human genome variation from population-scale sequencing. *Nature.* 2010;467:1061–1073.
124. Exome Variant Server. In. 2014 ed: *NHLBI GO Exome Sequencing Project* (ESP). Seattle, WA; 2014.
125. Ng PC, Henikoff S. Accounting for human polymorphisms predicted to affect protein function. *Genome Res.* 2002;12:436–446.
126. Adzhubei IA, Schmidt S, Peshkin L, et al. A method and server for predicting damaging missense mutations. *Nat Methods.* 2010;7:248–249.
127. Foley AR, Pitceathly RD, He J, et al. Whole-genome sequencing and the clinician: a tale of two cities. *J Neurol Neurosurg Psychiatry.* 2014;85:1012–1015.

Clinical Evaluation in Pediatric Peripheral Neuropathies

Zarife Sahenk, MD, PhD, FAAN

In comparison to adults, peripheral neuropathies in the pediatric age group are a highly heterogeneous group of disorders. These disorders, however, share similarities with the adult patient in that a pattern recognition approach is required, based on pathobiological considerations ultimately leading to diagnosis and appropriate management. The diagnostic approach will rely heavily on careful history taking, skillful physical exam including detailed family history supplemented by electrodiagnostic studies as well as molecular and metabolic analysis, and occasionally sural nerve biopsy. Compared to the adult population, while peripheral neuropathy is less common, the inherited forms represent a much larger proportion of childhood neuropathies including various types of Charcot-Marie-Tooth (CMT) neuropathies (30%–70%) (1,2).

Neuropathological studies of experimental toxic neuropathies from the 1970s were essential to understanding the evolution of "distal axonopathy" and set the foundation for formulating a classification of peripheral nerve disorders according to the anatomical site most altered (3–6). This morphologic classification approach, based on experimental evidence, has been endorsed widely since then and has proven clinically useful (7,8). Based on the anatomical site of involvement, disorders of peripheral nerve include those that affect the neuron's cell body or neuronopathies and those affecting the peripheral process or peripheral neuropathies. The peripheral neuropathies can largely be subdivided into axonopathies and myelinopathies. A length-dependent distal axonal disease or "dying back neuropathy" is the most common presentation of neuropathic disorders. Regardless of the underlying cause, the final common path, distal axonal degeneration occurs in a fairly stereotypic manner. As in the adult population, most axonal diseases present with distal axonopathy resulting from pathologic changes first occurring in a multifocal manner in the distal portions of long and large-diameter axons. It is important to recognize that this pattern is valid for many genetic conditions affecting peripheral as well as central nervous system (CNS) axons. Moreover, most CMT patients including those with primary Schwann cell genetic defects present with a clinical phenotype of length-dependent axonal disease. The so-called secondary axonal pathology in hereditary myelinopathies, thought to result from impaired Schwann cell support of axons is now well recognized, representing an important feature that directly correlates with the clinical disability (9–13). Another less common pattern of distal axonal degeneration is central–peripheral distal axonopathy found in spinocerebellar degenerations such as Friedreich's ataxia, the best-studied example of an inherited system degeneration (6). Some forms of hereditary spastic paraplegia that again are characterized by a distal axonal degeneration are confined predominantly to the CNS, representing the central distal axonopathy (14). Each of these disorders has distinct clinical features that enable neurologists to recognize the various patterns of the disease process. Once a particular pattern is established, further laboratory studies can be performed to confirm the clinical impression. Detailed history, exam, and electrophysiological studies should assist the clinician in determining the differential diagnosis and appropriate direction for investigation. This review only focuses on the diagnostic approach based on clinical presentation of the most common infantile and childhood polyneuropathies and comments on those rare ones with simple clinical clues.

CLINICAL APPROACH

During history taking and clinical examination of a child with suspected neuropathy, the clinician should follow a framework to extract information that will establish the pattern of an ongoing disease process. This could be achieved with the following approach:

Which Systems and Nerve Fiber Size Are Involved?

The aim of the clinician should be to determine if the child's symptoms and signs are most compatible with predominant dysfunction of motor, sensory, or both, pure sensory, autonomic, or some combination of these. Motor fibers are composed of heavily myelinated large-diameter Aα axons. Sensory modalities on the other hand are transmitted by two sets of axons, referred to as "small fibers "and "large fibers" based on their diameters. Pain, temperature, and light touch modalities are carried by the small-diameter and unmyelinated C-type axons and thinly myelinated Aδ-type fibers, while vibration and position sense are carried by the large-diameter sensory afferents. Predominantly, large-fiber distal axonopathy is the most common type of disease process and presents as length-dependent distal motor fiber involvement along with significant large-fiber sensory deficits leading to impaired or absent sensory nerve action potentials, or SNAPs. The prototype of such a pattern is seen in CMT disease, referred to as classic CMT. It should be noted, however, that although large fiber sensory deficit predominates, the disease process does affect small fibers to a lesser extent, giving rise to a pan-modality sensory dysfunction involving large fibers to a greater extent than small fibers.

Pure motor neuropathies are uncommon in childhood. Progressive muscle weakness without sensory symptoms should suggest a disease of motor neurons such as spinal muscular atrophy (SMA), an autosomal recessive (AR) motor neuronopathy of childhood (15). Patients with pure motor distal weakness with a clinical phenotype of axonal CMT neuropathy with no discernible sensory involvement are now classified as distal hereditary motor neuropathies (dHMNs) and distal spinal muscular atrophies (dSMAs) (16,17). Diagnosing these conditions depends on the associated upper motor neuron findings, age of onset of symptoms, and family history. dHMNs represent about 10% of all inherited neuropathies and cover a spectrum of clinically and genetically heterogeneous diseases characterized by the selective involvement of motor neurons. The disease usually begins in childhood or adolescence with weakness and wasting of distal muscles of the anterior tibial and peroneal compartments. Subsequently, weakness and atrophy of the proximal muscles of the lower limbs and/or of the distal upper limbs may ensue.

While some peripheral neuropathies may present with only motor symptoms, the clinician can usually find evidence of sensory involvement on neurologic examination, or the patients themselves may report paresthesias or pain. The best examples of this scenario include acquired autoimmune neuropathies, Guillain-Barré syndrome (GBS), and chronic inflammatory demyelinating polyneuropathy (CIDP). In these disorders, information obtained from the pattern of distribution and temporal evolution of the weakness are crucial for directing the diagnostic workup as discussed further in this chapter. Multifocal motor neuropathy as a variant of CIDP appears to be a very rare condition in childhood, reported to occur with a similar pattern of asymmetric distal upper extremity weakness and conduction block as seen in adults (18,19).

Sensory prominent neuropathies may impair small-fiber or large-fiber functional modalities or both. Assessment of sensory dysfunction can be challenging and unreliable early in life; therefore, confirmational evidence by clinical history from the parents is critical. Sensory examination in the cooperative older age group will require careful inquiry to differentiate diminished or lack of sensation (numbness) from altered sensation (tingling/paresthesia) or pain. Neuropathic pain can be described as burning, dull and poorly localized, presumably transmitted by C nociceptor fibers, or a sharp and lancinating type, relayed by Aδ fibers. If severe pain is a prominent feature of presentation, painful peripheral neuropathies due to peripheral nerve vasculitis or GBS must be considered because these disorders are potentially treatable. Vasculitic neuropathies are very rare in children, but have been reported in adolescents with Wegener granulomatosis, systemic lupus, and Henoch-Schonlein purpura (20–23). The pain in vasculitic neuropathy is generally distal and asymmetric in the most severely involved extremity. It is important to determine the pattern of peripheral nerve involvement as mononeuropathy in which the sensory and/or motor deficit is confined to a single nerve distribution versus mononeuritis multiplex, defined by sensory and motor symptoms involving two or more nerves, and developing acutely or subacutely. In general, entrapment neuropathies such as those occurring in hereditary neuropathy with a predisposition to pressure palsies (HNPPs) are typically painless in the pediatric age group. This is in contrast to adults in whom one-third report the development of neuropathic pain several years after the initial onset of painless neuropathic symptoms (24). Children with GBS commonly present with severe back pain associated with symmetric numbness and paresthesias in the extremities. A well-established genetic condition associated with neuropathic pain is Fabry disease (25). Episodic crises of severe hand or foot pain in males with Fabry disease typically present in early childhood, whereas the disease in female carriers often presents in late adolescence or adulthood. Other conditions associated with severe neuropathic pain include situations where nerve damage has occurred, eg, posttraumatic pain, phantom limb pain, postchemotherapy pain, some chronic conditions or infections such as HIV/AIDS, and complex regional pain syndrome (26,27).

Although neuropathic pain is a relatively common feature of diabetic neuropathy in adults, among children with diabetes, the complications do not progress to the point that painful neuropathy would be of concern. On the other hand, recent studies have shown that almost half of the children with type 1 diabetes have subclinical large- and small-fiber neuropathies (28). Overt autonomic neuropathy is rare in childhood and adolescence, while subclinical signs of autonomic dysfunction in cardiovascular nerve function testing and pupillometry are common and can be found soon after diabetes diagnosis (29). Duration of diabetes, poor glycemic control, and the presence of aldose reductase gene polymorphisms constitute risk factors for autonomic neuropathy in young people (30). Puberty may accelerate autonomic dysfunction.

Most *inherited sensory neuropathies* present with reduced or absent sensation. History may provide examples of the child having had painless hand or foot lacerations, blisters, or cellulitis. This is the typical presentation of the rare forms of hereditary sensory neuropathies or hereditary sensory autonomic neuropathies (HSNs/HSANs). In extreme cases, children may present with self-inflicted injury or limb mutilation. Clinicians should be aware of this since electrophysiology will fail to detect neuropathy due to predominantly small-fiber involvement.

HSANs comprise the rarest subgroup within the hereditary neuropathies and are clinically and genetically heterogeneous. Although by definition, HSANs impact the development, survival, function, and migration of sensory autonomic nerves, in some autosomal dominant (AD) forms that present in the second and third decades, clear distal weakness may be present, giving rise to the classical CMT phenotype. This group designated as HSAN I includes *SPTLC1* (encoding serine palmitoyl transferase long-chain base subunit 1) and *RAB7* (encoding RAS-associated protein RAB7) mutations presenting with a prominent sensory, minimal autonomic, and variable motor involvement (31). Interestingly, neuropathic pain can be a distinguishing clinical feature in that patients with *SPTLC1* mutations often have neuropathic pain, while those with *RAB7* mutations do not (32,33). In contrast, the AR forms usually have an early or congenital onset and commonly present with striking sensory and autonomic abnormalities or in some rare cases as pure autonomic disorders. Well-characterized recessive forms include HSAN II, an early-onset ulcero-mutilating sensory neuropathy (34); HSAN III, Riley-Day syndrome or familial dysautonomia presenting as a predominantly autonomic disorder with congenital onset, (35); and HSAN IV, congenital insensitivity to pain with anhidrosis (CIPA), with characteristic features of recurrent episodic fevers due to anhidrosis, absence of reaction to painful stimuli, self-mutilating behavior, and mental retardation (36). A very rare entity designated as HSAN V is caused by mutations in nerve growth factor beta and presents with a phenotype closely related to CIPA, but in contrast, patients do not display prominent mental retardation, and the disease onset is in childhood.

The other important sensory abnormality that significantly narrows the differential diagnosis is severe proprioceptive loss. The prototype example is Friedreich's ataxia, a central peripheral distal axonopathy classically presenting with increasing clumsiness, gait ataxia, or tremor in early adolescence. The ataxia results from distally prominent progressive degeneration of the long tracts in the CNS (spinocerebellar and corticospinal) as well as central and peripheral projections of dorsal root ganglia neurons. During the course of the disease, sensory nerve action potentials and nerve conduction velocities (NCVs) may become undetectable due to predominately large myelinated fiber degeneration.

Sensorimotor polyneuropathies comprise the largest group of childhood neuropathies encompassing the most common hereditary and treatable acquired autoimmune demyelinating neuropathies. The distribution of the patient's weakness and the temporal evolution of disease are crucial for an accurate diagnosis as delineated in the following text.

What Is the Distribution of Motor Weakness?

The crucial task for the examiner is to extract the relevant information and localize the weakness as (a) only involving the distal extremities or (b) involving both proximal and distal extremities and assessing if the weakness is focal/asymmetric or symmetric. The finding of *weakness in both proximal and distal muscle groups in a symmetrical fashion* is the hallmark for acquired immune demyelinating polyneuropathies, both the acute form (GBS) and the chronic form (CIDP). This clinical presentation is in perfect line with the histopathological site of involvement since in these entities (acquired myelinopathy), segmental demyelination occurs randomly all along the peripheral nerves including the nerve roots with innervation of proximal limb muscles. Good recovery from an acquired monophasic myelinopathy is common, and patients are usually left with little or no residual weakness. In contrast, in cases of CIDP characterized by a relapsing remitting course, partially treated or refractory cases can occur and in these cases, secondary axonal loss is common. This axonal loss may result in distally prominent residual weakness in a length-dependent manner. The examiner should consider this possibility in children with a long-standing history of distal greater than proximal muscle weakness that is more pronounced in the lower extremities.

Focal or asymmetric weakness is also a feature that helps to narrow the diagnostic possibilities. Traumatic injury or nerve compressions are common causes of mononeuropathies. HNPPs or familial brachial plexus neuropathies can present with focal, asymmetric leg or arm weakness, or with multifocal nerve involvement, but they rarely occur in childhood. The presence of unilateral motor and sensory signs confined to one extremity is much more likely to be due to a simple entrapment, compressive neuropathy, or radiculopathy (37,38).

Predominant lower extremity symmetrical distal weakness is the most common distribution pattern of weakness seen in hereditary neuropathies. If a patient presents with both symmetrical sensory and motor findings involving the distal lower extremities first, with or without associated distal weakness in the upper extremities, the disorder generally reflects a length-dependent distal axonopathy. The recognition of this classic CMT phenotype cannot be overemphasized because it occurs in both the so-called "demyelinating" forms, CMT1 where axonal loss is secondary and in CMT2 forms with primary axonopathy.

Exceptions to the classic CMT phenotypic presentation are rare. Among the rare types of AD CMT2, *BSCL2*/seipin mutations are known to present with predominant upper limb involvement (39). Distal atrophy in the upper extremities and spastic legs are notable features of Silver syndrome; in 33% of the cases, presentation is that of atrophy in the upper limbs only (40). So far, the second gene known to cause predominant involvement of the small hand muscles is the *GARS* gene responsible for synthesizing glycyl tRNA synthetase. *GARS* mutations cause CMT2D, also called distal spinal muscular atrophy type V (dSMA-V) characterized by atrophy and weakness of hand muscles, which can be asymmetric (41).

Is There Evidence for Upper Motor Neuron Involvement and/or Other Associated Clinical Features?

Upper motor neuron signs and other associated clinical features may help narrow the differential diagnosis. Among them, the mitofusin 2(*MFN2*) gene is an important one with mutations causing the most common form of axonal CMT, CMT2A and representing currently about 20% of all AD CMT2 cases (42). Patients with *MFN2* mutations commonly present with an early childhood onset and severe CMT phenotype; classical CMT phenotype in a later age group is less common. Unique mutations in *MFN2* were described initially in six families (also designated as hereditary motor and sensory neuropathy, HMSN VI with optic atrophy) presenting with early childhood onset and severe symptoms including proximal weakness and vocal cord paralysis (43). Optic atrophy usually presents subacutely and may improve. Several publications expanded the CMT2A phenotype to include cases with spasticity (44), cognitive impairment and mitochondrial dysfunction (45), severe early-onset axonal neuropathy with compound heterozygous *MFN2* mutations (46), and severe neuropathy with fatal encephalopathy (47).

In addition to *MFN2* mutations, other rare CMT2 neuropathies with AD gene defects in *GDAP1,* and *NEFL*, are known to have pyramidal features. Recessive cases of *GDAP1* mutations represent the most common CMT4 with greater than 40 mutations usually associated with a severe clinical phenotype with early onset (neonatal or infancy) and disabling hand and foot deformities occurring toward the end of the first decade. Loss of autonomy occurs in the second decade with the development of proximal muscle weakness. Hoarse voice and vocal cord paralysis may be part of the phenotype in some cases (48). *TRPV4* is another gene, recently recognized to present with a wide range of features including vocal cord and respiratory involvement, congenital dSMA, and scapuloperoneal spinal muscle atrophy (49).

Finally, the overall investigation of a child presenting with a peripheral neuropathy is incomplete without a careful search for evidence of CNS involvement. A history of seizures, visual impairment, developmental delay, regression of motor milestones, cognitive impairment, especially language, intellectual acquisition, or behavioral changes including increasing irritability or hyperactivity provide important clues that must heighten suspicion for a metabolic disorder concomitantly affecting the CNS and peripheral nervous system. Poor weight gain and loss of developmental milestones, and multisystem disease (cardiac, renal and liver) should alert the clinician for possible mitochondrial disease. Other well-recognized clues include orange-colored tonsils for Tangier disease, tendinous xanthomas for cerebrotendinous xanthomatosis, kinky hair for giant axonal neuropathy (GAN), angiokeratomas for Fabry disease, and hyper-pigmentation of the buccal mucosa or axilla for adrenoleukodystrophy.

What Is the Age of Onset and Temporal Evolution?

Of obvious importance is the age of onset, duration, and evolution of symptoms and signs. Polyneuropathies in the neonatal group are exceedingly rare. However, when faced with a newborn with extreme hypotonia and weakness, congenital hypomyelinating neuropathy (CHN) is usually included in the differential diagnosis. Molecular testing is recommended to rule out SMA first, and if the electrophysiologic studies suggest a peripheral neuropathy, a nerve biopsy may be required to establish the diagnosis. In the pregenetic era of HMSN classi-fication, severely affected children with early-onset demyelinating polyneuropathy of infancy were classified as having HMSNIII, also called CHN or Dejerine-Sottas disease (DSD), and in some current classifications, this group is referred to as CMT3. This group, originally pre-dicted to be mainly AR now includes patients with de novo AD mutations in the genes that commonly cause AD CMT1 (*PMP22*, myelin protein zero [*MPZ*], and early growth response 2 [*EGR2*]). It is now advocated to refer to these patients as having severe CMT1 although this is not universally agreed upon and the terms CMT3, CHN, and DSD are still commonly used. It should also be kept in mind that several lysosomal storage disorders can present with an infant-onset polyneuropathy and concomitant profound CNS symptoms; these include globoid cell leukodystrophy (GCL), metachromatic leukodystrophy (MLD), and peroxisomal disor-ders such as infantile Refsum disease.

The temporal evolution is important for determining genetic versus acquired disease pro-cess. Does the disease have an acute (days–4 wks), subacute (4–8 wks), or chronic (>8 wks) course? Is the course monophasic, progressive, or relapsing? In general, these sets of questions apply to both adult and pediatric populations. A subacute initial course is more common for CIDP in children than adults.

GBS is the most common acute-onset rapidly evolving weakness in childhood and gen-erally referred to as acute inflammatory demyelinating polyradiculoneuropathy (AIDP). The Miller Fisher variant presents with ophthalmoplegia, ataxia, and areflexia. Another subtype is referred to as acute motor axonal neuropathy (AMAN), characterized by acute paralysis and loss of reflexes without sensory loss caused by an antibody- and complement-mediated attack on the axolemma of motor fibers in contrast to AIDP in which the antigenic target is myelin proteins. AMAN patients in most cases have antecedent infection with *Campylobacter jejuni* and usually have a poor outcome compared with patients with GBS (50). In the majority of children with GBS, symptoms typically develop over several days and may include back and/or extremity pain and paresthesias. Respiratory failure and autonomic symptoms are less common compared to adults with GBS. CIDP differs from GBS by its more chronic progression evolving over at least 1 to 2 months (51). Children with CIDP may demonstrate either a progressive or a relapsing course. Although many patients exhibit a slow insidious onset of weakness and sen-sory loss, it is not unusual for an acute-onset presentation that clinically mimics GBS in about one-fifth of the cases (52,53). Unlike GBS, paresthesia may be more common in children with CIDP, while back pain, autonomic symptoms, or respiratory failure are rare.

The most common CMT forms, CMT1A and CMTX, generally present in early adolescence with symptoms of distal muscle weakness (foot drop) and atrophy and evolve slowly over years.

Is There Evidence for Hereditary Neuropathy?

In patients with a chronic, very slowly progressive distal weakness over many years, with very little in the way of sensory symptoms, the first step is to determine whether the patient has a genetic neuropathy. A history of delayed motor milestones, toe walking, ankle-twisting episodes, and poor performance in sports compared to peers may be clues to an underlying slowly progressive CMT/hereditary neuropathy. Particular attention to the family history should be made to inquire about foot deformities and entrapment neuropathies in immediate relatives. On examining the patient, the clinician must look carefully at the feet for arch and toe abnormalities (high or flat arches, hammertoes, overlapping toes, inability to spread the toes) and look at the spine for scoliosis. In suspicious cases, it may be necessary to perform both neurologic and electrophysiologic studies on family members. A genetic neuropathy diagnosis can be straightforward when there are an affected parent and child, making either AD or X-linked (if there is no definite male-to-male transmission) inheritance more likely or when there are multiple affected siblings from a consanguineous marriage, making AR inheritance likely. X-linked inheritance should always be kept in mind unless there is unequivocal evidence of male-to-male transmission. Even if there is no family history, families are small, or extensive family histories are not available, it is important not to rule out an inherited neuropathy if the clinical features raise the possibility. It should be kept in mind that these apparently sporadic patients may have mutations in the common AD genes (including in some cases, de novo dominant mutations) and less commonly in the AR genes.

Is the Neuropathic Process Superimposed on a Preexisting Asymptomatic Hereditary Neuropathy?

In rare cases, clinicians may face a challenge with the diagnosis and management of children who develop an autoimmune demyelinating polyneuropathy or a rapidly evolving severe chemotherapy-induced toxic neuropathy superimposed on a preexisting asymptomatic CMT. A history of distal greater than proximal weakness and distal sensory symptoms that are more pronounced in the lower extremities and that evolve over 1 to 2 months is characteristic of atypical CIDP superimposed on a preexisting asymptomatic distal axonopathy, which in most cases has a genetic basis. The clinician should consider this possibility especially in the presence of minor/obvious foot deformities and conduct further diagnostic studies as outlined in the illustrative case report.

Length-dependent distal axonopathies secondary to chemotherapy have a dose-dependent onset and stereotypic evolution with well-recognized cumulative effects of dosing and concomitant agents. A rapidly evolving distal weakness with paresthesias predominating in lower extremities outside the range of the expected neurotoxicity profile of a chemotherapeutic drug

ILLUSTRATIVE CASE REPORT

Clinical History: A 14-year-old male with high arches and hammertoes first noticed changes in his feet and some difficulties with running approximately 5 years prior to presentation. One year prior, he had a gastrointestinal illness associated with weight loss, proteinuria, and an elevated C-reactive protein (CRP). Subsequently he had progressive gait difficulties to the point of losing his balance, and generalized weakness. His mother reported more recent loss of functional abilities, difficulties getting up from the floor, frequent falls due to foot drop, and muscle loss and weakness.

Examination Highlights: His manual muscle testing using Medical Research Council (MRC) scale revealed grade 4 proximal weakness in the upper and lower extremities and ankle dorsiflexor strength of 3-. He was areflexic throughout. Sensory exam revealed significantly decreased vibration and position sense loss and less prominent pin appreciation at the toes. Electrophysiological studies revealed evidence of a chronic, length-dependent, sensorimotor demyelinating polyneuropathy with secondary axonal features. The findings were relatively symmetric, with evidence of temporal dispersion and conduction block suggesting an acquired condition. His cerebrospinal fluid (CSF) protein was elevated at 129 mg/dL with no white blood cells (WBCs).

Sural nerve biopsy revealed severe nerve fiber loss and the presence of widespread onion bulb formations, typical of an underlying Charcot-Marie-Tooth type I. In addition, there were many medium-to-large-diameter axons, which either lacked compacted myelin or contained a very thin layer of myelin indicative of recently occurring demyelination/remyelination events. In this clinical setting, these findings are compatible with an acquired chronic demyelinating neuropathy superimposed on a preexisting hereditary neuropathy. He responded to intravenous immunoglobulin (IVIG) and steroids within 3 weeks, with muscle strength returning to normal in 3 to 4 months.

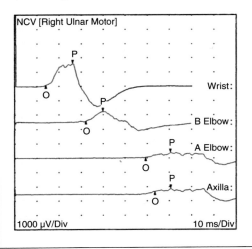

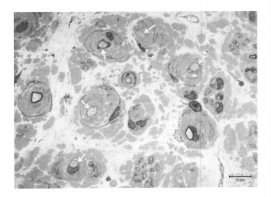

should alert the clinician for the possibility of underlying neuropathy. Typically, continuation or further worsening of symptoms can occur for some weeks after cessation of the offending drug. Amongst them, vincristine, a chemotherapeutic agent used for the treatment of leukemia, lymphoma, and solid tumors is extremely toxic for patients with either demyelinating or axonal forms of CMT (54–56). Therefore, it is not unusual for a patient with no past history of CMT to develop a severe polyneuropathy after a few doses of vincristine; if evidence of underlying CMT is suspected, vincristine should be discontinued to avoid additive damage. Routinely, neurologists should consider all concomitant and previously used medications when investigating a child with an underlying neuropathy.

ELECTRODIAGNOSTIC TESTING

Nerve conduction study (NCS) and needle electromyogram (EMG) are important in order to obtain objective information regarding the specific peripheral nerve fibers involved (sensory, motor, or mixed), the type of injury (demyelinating, axonal, or combined), and the severity of the neuropathy. Demyelinating features include prolongation of distal latencies and slowing of NCV less than 38 m/s in the upper extremity motor nerves. Conduction velocity slowing may be uniform, implying that the myelin abnormalities are similar along the length of the axon as the typical feature of primary demyelinating disorders that develop due to Schwann cell genetic defects. Nonuniform slowing is more commonly seen in acquired demyelinating disorders such as GBS or CIDP in which the myelinopathy is secondary to an autoimmune attack. Conduction block, considered a sign of secondary myelinopathy, can also be seen with HNPP and toxin exposure (57,58).

Needle EMG, performed in children under sedation or when awake is important in defining motor unit changes suggesting a possible neurogenic disease (large amplitude rapidly firing) or a possible myopathic lesion (smaller amplitude and polyphasic). The electromyographer needs to use judgment in obtaining the most necessary information, limiting testing to specific sites most likely to provide an accurate diagnosis and avoiding excessive study that does not provide further information.

NERVE BIOPSY

With recent advances in molecular testing, nerve biopsy is rarely required as a diagnostic test and is only performed in children if histopathologic examination of nerve tissue should provide important and useful information. If the patient is suspected to have a vasculitic neuropathy, it is imperative to obtain tissue diagnosis before initiating immunosuppressant therapy. Other circumstances in which the information from nerve biopsy may be important in formulating a management plan include cases of possible atypical CIDP superimposed on subclinical CMT. In rare cases of AR, early-onset CMT nerve biopsy may offer information directing the clinician toward a genetic diagnosis, such as focally folded myelin sheaths that are unique features of CMT4B caused by gene mutations in myotubularin 2 and 13 (*MTMR2, MTMR13*) (59,60).

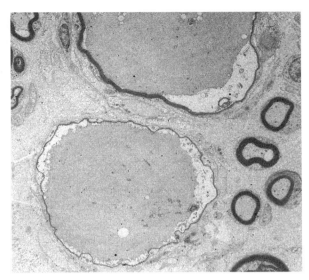

FIGURE 7.1 Electron micrograph of a sural nerve from a 5-year-old Indian girl with a history of difficulty running and proximal weakness since the age of 1 year. She was born with pas planus and "kinky hair" and walked around 14 to 15 months of age. Exam revealed normal cognition, slow running, and areflexia. She was unable to toe walk and had markedly diminished muscle bulk in her legs, particularly the posterior compartment. Nerve biopsy demonstrated no significant fiber loss but several abnormally enlarged "giant axons" with diameter up to 25 µm packed with neurofilaments. GAN diagnosis was confirmed with identification of R242X homozygous mutation in exon 4 of gigaxonin gene. She later developed predominant large-fiber sensory loss, bilateral foot drop, ataxic gait, and dysmetria consistent with central peripheral distal axonopathy. Nerve biopsy remains a useful diagnostic test in centers without access to genetic testing for GAN and in children with ataxia, neurodegeneration and neuropathy without kinky hair.

Until whole genome sequencing becomes readily available at a low cost, it is justifiable to perform nerve biopsy in selected cases in which the information can be diagnostic. The rare condition, GAN, which presents with a clinical phenotype of central peripheral distal axonopathy, is one of those conditions (Figure 7.1) with a unique histopathological feature showing neurofilament-packed swollen (giant) axons. It needs to be emphasized that the clinicians requesting the procedure should be aware of the highly specialized requirements for surgical removal, fixation, and the processing of nerve biopsy specimens in order to ensure its diagnostic yield and freedom from handling artifacts. Therefore, it is recommended that nerve biopsies be carried out at centers with the experience and expertise to appropriately process and provide a diagnostic service.

Early and late childhood–onset and adolescent pediatric peripheral neuropathies are grouped according to temporal evolution of symptoms, pathological site and pattern of involvement, and key clinical and genetic features in Tables 7.1 and 7.2.

TABLE 7.1 Early Childhood–Onset Pediatric Peripheral Neuropathies

TEMPORAL EVOLUTION OF SYMPTOMS	DISORDERS	PATHOLOGICAL SITE/ PATTERN OF INVOLVEMENT	KEY CLINICAL/ DIFFERENTIATING FEATURES	GENETIC DEFECT/PROTEIN BIOLOGICAL FUNCTION
Acute/ subacute onset	Guillain-Barré syndrome	Acquired/autoimmune myelinopathy (large fiber predominant; motor sensory)	Symmetric proximal and distal weakness with sensory loss	
	Mitochondrial (Leigh syndrome/ -NARP)	Predominant myelopathy (caused by SURF1 mutations); sensory and motor, CNS > PNS	Progressive psychomotor retardation, hypotonia, weakness, ataxia, optic atrophy, ophthalmoplegia, nystagmus, dystonia, evidence of brainstem dysfunction, lactic acidosis, pes cavus, absent ankle jerks	Different mitochondrial and nuclear gene mutations have been reported in Leigh syndrome (SURF1, the most common nuclear gene involved; MTATP6, the most common mitochondrial gene involved)
		Predominantly central-peripheral distal axonopathy (caused by MTATP6 mutations)		
	CMT3(DSD/CHN)	Distal axonopathy secondary to hereditary myelinopathy (large fiber predominant; sensory < motor)	Severe CMT1 phenotype usually presents as floppy infant at or shortly after birth	de novo AD mutations in the genes that commonly cause AD CMT1 (PMP22, MPZ, and EGR2; rare AR cases)
Insidious onset/slow progression	CMT4	Myelinopathy and axonopathy length dependent, motor sensory	Earlier onset and much severe than other CMTs; demyelinating and axonal phenotypes	AR, comprises 5%–10% of all CMT cases
	CMT4A		Usually early onset and severe vocal cord and diaphragm paralysis	GDAP1 mutations (25% of all CMT4 cases)
	CMT2A	Length-dependent distal axonopathy, sensory and motor	Onset before age 5, often in infancy, with rapidly progressive weakness throughout childhood. Severe distal weakness and atrophy below knees and elbows; early proximal weakness; planus foot deformity; optic atrophy up to 20% of cases	AD, MFN2 mutations (comprises 30% of CMT2 cases, 3% of infantile neuropathies)

(continued)

TABLE 7.1 Early Childhood–Onset Pediatric Peripheral Neuropathies *(continued)*

TEMPORAL EVOLUTION OF SYMPTOMS	DISORDERS	PATHOLOGICAL SITE/ PATTERN OF INVOLVEMENT	KEY CLINICAL/ DIFFERENTIATING FEATURES	GENETIC DEFECT/PROTEIN BIOLOGICAL FUNCTION
	HSAN IIA	Reduction in sensory neurons	Inability to feel pain, temperature, and touch sensations and autonomic disturbances	AR, caused by mutations in the *WNK1* gene
	HSAN IIB	Loss of nociceptive neurons by apoptosis	Impairment of the autonomic function. Chronic ulcerations and multiple injuries to fingers and feet, autoamputation	AR, caused by mutations in the *FAM134B* gene
Insidious onset/slow progression	HSAN III (RDS)	Progressive sympathetic and sensory neuron loss	Onset at birth, prominent dysautonomic features	Germline point mutation in *ILP1/IKBKAP* gene causing impairment of postmigratory sensory and sympathetic neuron survival and target tissue innervation
	HSAN IV (CIPA)	Absence or deficiency of C and Aδ fibers in the epidermis, absent or hypoplastic dermal sweat glands without innervation	Onset at infancy, lack of pain, self-mutilation, anhidrosis, and mild intellectual disability	AR, mutation of NTRK1 accounts for all cases of properly classified CIPA
	HSAN V	Absence of nociceptive sensory innervation; selective absence of small myelinated fibers	Onset at birth or early infancy, loss of deep pain, heat, and cold. Repeated severe injuries, normal intelligence	AR, mutations in the NGFβ gene leading to production of an abnormal protein, cannot bind to receptor

(continued)

TABLE 7.1 Early Childhood–Onset Pediatric Peripheral Neuropathies *(continued)*

TEMPORAL EVOLUTION OF SYMPTOMS	DISORDERS	PATHOLOGICAL SITE/PATTERN OF INVOLVEMENT	KEY CLINICAL/DIFFERENTIATING FEATURES	GENETIC DEFECT/PROTEIN BIOLOGICAL FUNCTION
	Krabbe disease	CNS > PNS myelinopathy, myelin-independent axonopathy—due to toxic psychosine accumulation	Infantile phenotype (onset > 6 months—95% of known cases); hyperirritability, episodic fever, marked hypertonicity. Late infantile (onset 6 mos–3 yrs), irritability, psychomotor regression, stiffness, ataxia, and loss of vision	AR, mutations in *galc* gene resulting in beta-galactosylceramidase deficiency, impaired degradation of some lipids
Insidious onset/slow progression	Metachromatic leukodystrophy	CNS > PNS myelinopathy, neuronopathy—due to sulfatide storage causing functional impairment	Late infantile (onset < 3 years of age), most common form includes abnormal movement patterns, gait disturbances, developmental regression	AR, lysosomal sphingolipid storage disorder, caused by a deficiency of arylsulfatase A
	Giant axonal neuropathy	Central peripheral distal axonopathy (large fiber predominant; motor sensory; cerebellar tracts involvement)	Onset < 7 yrs; delayed early milestones, distal lower limb prominent progressive weakness, impaired position, vibration; Babinski sign, ataxia, nystagmus, dysarthria, small stature, kinky hair	AR, mutations in gigaxonin gene lead to slowdown in ubiquitin-mediated protein degradation. Interaction between gigaxonin and intermediate filament degradation is proposed

Abbreviations: AR, autosomal recessive; CIPA, congenital insensitivity to pain with anhidrosis; CMT, Charcot-Marie-Tooth disease; CNS, central nervous system; DSD/CHN, Dejerine-Sottas disease/congenital hypomyelination neuropathy; EGR2, early growth response 2; FAM134B, Family with sequence similarity 134, member B; SURF1, surfeit locus protein 1; GDAP1, ganglioside-induced differentiation-associated protein 1; HSAN, hereditary sensory autonomic neuropathy; ILP1/IKBKAP, inhibitor of kappa light polypeptide gene enhancer in beta cells, kinase complex-associated protein; MPZ, myelin protein zero; MFN2, mitofusin 2; MTATP6, mitochondrial ATP synthase 6; NGFβ, nerve growth factor β; NTRK1, neurotrophic tyrosine kinase, receptor type 1; PMP22, peripheral myelin protein 22; PNS, peripheral nervous system; RDS, Riley-Day Syndrome; WNK1, WNK lysine deficient protein kinase 1.

TABLE 7.2 Late Childhood-to-Adolescent-Onset Pediatric Peripheral Neuropathies

TEMPORAL EVOLUTION OF SYMPTOMS	DISORDERS	PATHOLOGICAL SITE/PATTERN OF INVOLVEMENT	KEY CLINICAL/DIFFERENTIATING FEATURES	GENETIC DEFECT/PROTEIN BIOLOGICAL FUNCTION
	Guillain–Barré syndrome	Acquired/autoimmune myelinopathy (large fiber predominant; motor sensory)	Symmetric proximal and distal weakness with sensory loss	
	HNPP	Hereditary myelinopathy	Early adulthood presentation with painless mononeuropathy commonly involving peroneal or ulnar nerve; less commonly with recurrent paresthesia, painless brachial plexopathy or polyneuropathy	AD, *PMP22* deletion
Acute/subacute onset	Vasculitic neuropathy	Acquired/autoimmune vasculopathy causing segmental ischemic insult, Wallerian degeneration	Distal weakness with sensory loss; asymmetric, neuropathic pain at onset	
	Porphyria	Motor-predominant axonopathy	Childhood porphyrias typically with photosensitivity and unique skin lesions	AD, defects in the heme biosynthetic pathway. Subtypes include acute intermittent porphyria, hereditary coproporphyria, and variegate porphyria
	CIDP	Acquired/autoimmune myelinopathy (large fiber predominant; motor sensory)	Symmetric proximal and distal weakness with sensory loss	

(continued)

TABLE 7.2 Late Childhood-to-Adolescent-Onset Pediatric Peripheral Neuropathies (continued)

TEMPORAL EVOLUTION OF SYMPTOMS	DISORDERS	PATHOLOGICAL SITE/PATTERN OF INVOLVEMENT	KEY CLINICAL/DIFFERENTIATING FEATURES	GENETIC DEFECT/ PROTEIN BIOLOGICAL FUNCTION
	CMT1	Length-dependent distal axonopathy secondary to hereditary myelinopathy (large fiber predominant; sensory < motor)	Classic CMT phenotype with demyelinating-range NCVs	
	CMT1A			AD, *PMP22* duplication (70% of CMT1 cases)
	CMT1B			AD, *MPZ* mutations (5%– 10% of CMT1 cases)
	CMT2	Length-dependent distal axonopathy (large fiber predominant; sensory < motor)	Classic CMT phenotype with axonal-range NCVs	AD, comprises 20% of all CMT cases
	CMTX	Length-dependent distal axonopathy secondary to hereditary myelinopathy (large fiber predominant; sensory < motor)	Classic CMT phenotype with mutation-dependent variable severity and demyelinating-range NCVs in males; milder phenotype in females with intermediate-range NCVs	X-linked, 15%–20% of al CMT cases
	CMTX1			*GJB1* mutations (90% of all CMTX cases)
Insidious onset/slow progression	dHMN	Predominantly motor length-dependent distal axonopathy	Symmetric distal weakness without sensory loss—rare in childhood	AD forms (*HSPB1, HSPB8, BSCL2* mutations)
	Friedreich ataxia	Central-peripheral distal axonopathy (large fiber predominant; sensory < motor)	Limb and truncal ataxia and absent tendon reflexes in the legs present within 5 yrs of presentation; dysarthria, signs of pyramidal tract eventually occur. Cardiomyopathy, diabetes may develop in later life	AR, loss of function due to GAA trinucleotide repeat expansion in *FXN* gene encoding a small mitochondrial protein, involved in iron-sulfur clusters, iron chaperoning, and storage, and control of iron-mediated oxidative damage

TABLE 7.2 Late Childhood-to-Adolescent-Onset Pediatric Peripheral Neuropathies (continued)

TEMPORAL EVOLUTION OF SYMPTOMS	DISORDERS	PATHOLOGICAL SITE/PATTERN OF INVOLVEMENT	KEY CLINICAL/DIFFERENTIATING FEATURES	GENETIC DEFECT/ PROTEIN BIOLOGICAL FUNCTION
Insidious onset/slow progression	Fabry disease	Small-fiber distal axonopathy	Onset between ages 3 and 10 yrs, with boys affected earlier and more severely. Presenting features: burning pain, hypohidrosis/hyperhidrosis, strokes, angiokeratoma, proteinuria, or cardiomyopathy. Loss of temperature sensation in the hands and feet, and reduced tolerance to cold; episodic painful crises or chronic pain starting distally in extremities exacerbated by exercise and heat; autonomic neuropathy symptoms	X-linked; glycosphingolipidosis caused by deficiency of a lysosomal hydrolase, alpha-galactosidase A, required for the degradation of globotriaosylceramide in multiple cell types resulting in a multisystem disorder. Pathophysiology not fully understood: Gb3 deposition in neurons of DRG vs chronic nerve ischemia secondary to Gb3 deposition within the endothelial cells of the blood vessels supplying nerve fibers

Abbreviations: AD, autosomal dominant; AR, autosomal recessive; BSCL2, Bernardinelli-Seip congenital lipodystrophy type 2; CIDP, chronic inflammatory demyelinating polyneuropathy; CMT, Charcot-Marie-Tooth disease; CMTX, X-linked CMT; dHMN, distal hereditary motor neuropathy; DRG, dorsal root ganglia; FXN, frataxin; GAA, guanine adenine adenine; GJB1, gap junction Beta 1; HNPP, hereditary neuropathy with liability to pressure palsies; HSPB1, heat shock 27-kDa protein 1; HSPB8, heat shock 22-kDa protein 8; MPZ, myelin protein zero; NCV, nerve conduction velocity; PMP22, peripheral myelin protein 22.

REFERENCES

1. Evans OB. Polyneuropathy in childhood. *Pediatrics.* 1979;64(1):96–105.
2. Ouvrier RA, McLeod JG. Chronic peripheral neuropathy in childhood: an overview. *Aust Paediatr J.* 1988;24(suppl 1):80–82.
3. Schaumburg HH, Spencer PS. Toxic Neuropathies: clinical review. *Neurology.* 1979;29:429–431.
4. Schaumburg HH, Wieniewski HM, Spencer PS. Ultrastructural studies of the dying-back process: I. Peripheral nerve terminal and axonal degeneration in systemic acrylamide intoxication. *J Neuropathol Exp Neurol,* 1974;33:260–284.
5. Spencer PS, Schaumburg HH. Ultrastructural studies of the dying-back process: III. The evolution of experimental peripheral giant axonal degeneration. *J Neuropathol Exp Neurol.* 1977;36:276–299.
6. Spencer PS, Schaumburg HH. Central-peripheral distal axonopathy: The pathology of dying-back neuropathies. In: Zimmerman H, ed. *Progress in Neuropathology.* Vol 3. New York, NY: Grune & Stratton, Inc; 1977:253–295.
7. Overell, JR. Peripheral neuropathy: pattern recognition approach for the pragmatist. *Pract Neurol.* 2011;11:62–70.
8. Barohn RJ, Amato, AA. Pattern recognition approach to neuropathy and neuronopathy. *Neurol Clin.* 2013;31(2):343–361.
9. Dyck, PJ, Lais, AC, Offord, KP. The nature of myelinated nerve fiber degeneration in dominantly inherited hypertrophic neuropathy. *Mayo Clin Proc.* 1974;49:34–39.
10. Sahenk, Z, Chen, L. Abnormalities in the axonal cytoskeleton induced by a connexin32 mutation in nerve xenografts. *J Neurosci Res.* 1998;51:174–184.
11. Sahenk, Z, Chen, L, Mendell, JR. Effects of PMP22 duplication and deletions on the axonal cytoskeleton. *Ann Neurol.* 1999;45:16–24.
12. Sahenk, Z. Abnormal Schwann cell-axon interactions in CMT neuropathies. The effects of mutant Schwann cells on the axonal cytoskeleton and regeneration-associated myelination. *Ann N Y Acad Sci.* 1999;883:415–426.
13. Krajewski, KM, Lewis RA, Fuerst DR, et al. Neurological dysfunction and axonal degeneration in Charcot-Marie-Tooth disease type 1A. *Brain.* 2000;123(7):1516–1527.
14. Thomas PK, Schaumburg HH, Spencer PD, et al. Central Distal Axonopathy Syndromes: Newly Recognized Models of Naturally Occurring Human Degenerative Disease. *Ann Neurol.* 1984;15(4):313–315.
15. Iannaccone ST, Burghes A. Spinal muscular atrophies. *Adv Neurol.* 2002;88:83–98.
16. Irobi J, Dierick I, Jordanova A, Claeys KG et al. Unraveling the genetics of distal hereditary motor neuronopathies. *Neuromolecular Med.* 2006;8(1–2):131–146.
17. Dierick I, Baets J, Irobi J, et al. Relative contribution of mutations in genes for autosomal dominant distal hereditary motor neuropathies: a genotype-phenotype correlation study. *Brain.* 2008;131(Pt 5):1217–1227.
18. Moroni I, Bugiani M, Ciano C, et al. Childhood-onset multifocal motor neuropathy with conduction blocks. *Neurology.* 2006;66:922–924.
19. Wakamoto H, Chisaka A, Inoue N, et al. Childhood multifocal acquired demyelinating sensory and motor neuropathy. *Muscle Nerve.* 2008;37(6):790–795.
20. Ryan MM, Tilton A, De Girola mi UD, et al. Paediatric mononeuritis multiplex: a report of three cases and review of the literature. *Neuromuscul Disord.* 2003;13(9):751–756.
21. Orlowski JP, Clough JD, Dyment PG. Wegener's granulomatosis in the pediatric age group. *Pediatrics.* 1978;61(1):83–90.
22. Wang SJ, Yang YH, Lin YT, et al. Child hood Churg Strauss syndrome: report of a case. *J Microbiol lmmunol Infect.* 2000;33(4):263–266.
23. Belman AL, Leicher CR, Moshe SL, et al. Neurological manifestations of Schoenlein-Henoch purpura: report of three cases and review of the literature. *Pediatrics.* 1985;75(4):687–692.
24. Yilmaz U, Bird TT, Carter GT et al. Pain in hereditary neuropathy with liability to pressure palsy: an association with fibromyalgia syndrome?. *Muscle Nerve.* 2015;51(3):385–390.
25. Laney DA, Atherton AM, Manwaring LP et al. Fabry disease in infancy and early childhood: a systematic literature review. *Genet Med.* 2014. doi: 10.1038/gim.2014.120.
26. Walco GA, Dworkin RH, Krane EJ, et al. Neuropathic pain in children: Special considerations. *Mayo Clin Proc.* 2010;85(3 Suppl):S33–S41.

27. Howard RF, Wiener S, Walker SM. Neuropathic pain in children. *Arch Dis Child.* 2014;99:84–89.
28. M. Blankenburg M, Kraemer N, Hirschfeld G et al. Childhood diabetic neuropathy: functional impairment and non-invasive screening assessment. *Diabet Med.* 2012;29(11):1425–1432.
29. Cho YH, Craig ME, Hing S et al. Microvascular complications assessment in adolescents with 2- to 5-yr duration of type 1 diabetes from 1990 to 2006.[Erratum appears in *Pediatr Diabetes.* 2012 Feb;13(1):135]. *Pediatr Diabetes.* 2011;12:682–689.
30. Tang M, Donaghue KC, Cho YH, Craig ME. Autonomic neuropathy in young people with type 1 diabetes: a systematic review. *Pediatric Diabetes.* 2013;14:239–248.
31. Auer-Grumbach M. Hereditary sensory and autonomic neuropathies. In: Said G, Krarup C, eds. *Handbook of Clinical Neurology* (Vol 115). Amsterdam: Elsevier B.V, 2013;893–906.
32. Houlden H, King R, Blake J, et al. Clinical, pathological and genetic characterization of hereditary sensory and autonomic neuropathy type 1 (HSAN I). *Brain.* 2006;129:411–425.
33. Verhoeven K, De Jonghe P, Coen K, et al. Mutations in the small GTP-ase late endosomal protein RAB7 cause Charcot-Marie-Tooth type 2B neuropathy. *Am J Hum Genet.* 2003;72(3):722–727.
34. Lafreniere RG, MacDonald ML, Dube MP, et al. Identification of a novel gene (HSN2) causing hereditary sensory and autonomic neuropathy type II through the Study of Canadian Genetic Isolates. *Am J Hum Genet.* 2004;74(5):1064–1073.
35. Slaugenhaupt SA, Blumenfeld A, Gill SP et al. Tissue-specific expression of a splicing mutation in the IKBKAP gene causes familial dysautonomia. *Am J Hum Genet.* 2001;68:598–605.
36. Axelrod FB, Gold-von Simson G. Hereditary sensory and autonomic neuropathies: types II, III, and IV. *Orphanet J Rare Dis.* 2007;2:39.
37. Antonini G, Luchetti A, Mastrangelo M, et al. Early-onset hereditary neuropathy with liability to pressure palsy. *Neuropediatrics.* 2007;38:50–54.
38. Bayrak AO, Battaloglu E, Turker H, et al. Hereditary neuropathy with liability to pressure palsy (HNPP) in childhood: a case study emphasizing the relevance of detailed electrophysiological examination for suspected HNPP in the first decade. *Brain Dev.* 2009;31(6):445–448.
39. Rohkamm B, Reilly MM, Lochmuller H, et al. Further evidence for genetic heterogeneity of distal HMN type V, CMT2 with predominant hand involvement and Silver syndrome. *J Neurol Sci.* 2007;263:100–106.
40. Auer-Grumbach M, Schlotter-Weigel B, Lochmuller H, et al. Phenotypes of the N88S Berardinelli-Seip congenital lipodystrophy 2 mutation. *Ann Neurol.* 2005;57:415–424.
41. Antonellis A, Ellsworth RE, Sambuughin N, et al. Glycyl tRNA synthetase mutations in Charcot-Marie-Tooth disease type 2D and distal spinal muscular atrophy type V. *Am J Hum Genet.* 2003;72:1293–1299.
42. Zuchner S, Mersiyanova IV, Muglia M, et al. Mutations in the mitochondrial GTPase mitofusin 2 cause Charcot-Marie-Tooth neuropathy type 2A. *Nat Genet.* 2004;36:449–451.
43. Zuchner S, De Jonghe P, Jordanova A, et al. Axonal neuropathy with optic atrophy is caused by mutations in mitofusin 2. *Ann Neurol.* 2006;59:276–281.
44. Zhu D, Kennerson ML, Walizada G, Züchner S, et al. Charcot-Marie-Tooth with pyramidal signs is genetically heterogeneous: families with and without MFN2 mutations. *Neurology.* 2005;65(3):496–497.
45. Del Bo R, Moggio M, Rango M, et al. Mutated mitofusin 2 presents with intrafamilial variability and brain mitochondrial dysfunction. *Neurology.* 2008;71(24):1959–1966.
46. Nicholson GA, Magdelaine C, Zhu D, et al. Severe early-onset axonal neuropathy with homozygous and compound heterozygous MFN2 mutations. *Neurology.* 2008;70(19):1678–1681.
47. Boaretto F, Vettori A, Casarin A, et al. Severe CMT type 2 with fatal encephalopathy associated with MFN2 splicing mutation. *Neurology.* 2010;74(23):1919–1921.
48. Parman Y, Battaloglu E. Recessively transmitted predominantly motor neuropathies. In: Said G, Krarup C, eds. *Handbook of Clinical Neurology*(Vol. 115). Amsterdam: Elsevier B.V;2013:847–861.
49. Zimon M, Baets J, Auer-Grumbach M, et al. Dominant mutations in the cation channel gene transient receptor potential vanilloid 4 cause an unusual spectrum of neuropathies. *Brain.* 2010;133: 1798–1809.
50. Reisin RC, Cersosimo R, Garcia Alvarez M, et al. Acute "axonal" Guillain-Barré syndrome in childhood. *Muscle Nerve.* 1993;16(12):1310–1316.

51. American Academy Neurology AIDS Task Force. Research criteria for diagnosis of chronic inflammatory demyelinating polyneuropathy (CIDP). *Neurology.* 1991;41(5):617–618.
52. McCombe PA, Pollard JD, McLeod JG. Chronic inflammatory demyelinating polyradiculoneuropathy: a clinical and electrophysiological study of 92 cases. *Brain.* 1987;110(6):1617–1630.
53. Rabie M, Nevo Y. Childhood acute and chronic immune-mediated polyradiculoneuropathies.*Eur J Paediatr Neurol.* 2009;13(3):209–218.
54. Chauvenet AR, Shashi V, Selsky C, et al. Vincristine-induced neuropathy as the initial presentation of Charcot-Marie-Tooth disease in acute lymphoblastic leukemia: a Pediatric Oncology Group study. *J Pediatr Hematol Oncol.* 2003;25(4):316–320.
55. Cil T, Altintas A, Tamam Y, et al. Low dose vincristine-induced severe polyneuropathy in a Hodgkin lymphoma patient: a case report (vincristine-induced severe polyneuropathy). *J Pediatr Hematol Oncol.* 2009;31(10):787–789.
56. Nishikawa T, Kawakami K, Kumamoto T, et al. Severe neurotoxicities in a case of Charcot-Marie-Tooth disease type 2 caused by vincristine for acute lymphoblastic leukemia. *J Pediatr Hematol Oncol.* 2008;30(7):519–521.
57. Uncini A, Di Guglielmo G, Di Muzio A, et al. Differential electrophysiological features of neuropathies associated with 17p11.2 deletion and duplication. *Muscle Nerve.* 1995;18(6):628–635.
58. Pratt RW, Weimer LH. Medication and Toxin-Induced Peripheral Neuropathy. *Semin Neurol.* 2005;25(2) 204–216.
59. Gambardella A, Bolino A, Muglia M, et al. Genetic heterogeneity in autosomal recessive hereditary motor and sensory neuropathy with focally folded myelin sheaths (CMT4B). *Neurology.* 1998;50(3):799–801.
60. Senderek J, Bergmann C, Weber S, et al. Mutation of the SBF2 gene, encoding a novel member of the myotubularin family, in Charcot-Marie-Tooth neuropathy type 4B2/11p15. *Hum Mol Genet.* 2003;12(3):349–356.

EMG Considerations in the Pediatric Patient

Gloria M. Galloway, MD, FAAN

FEAR AND DISCOMFORT

Performing electrodiagnostic procedures in pediatric patients can be challenging in part because the test can be uncomfortable but more importantly because the young child will be fearful of a new procedure and not understand what will be involved. Therefore having a realistic expectation of the patient's (and parents') level of cooperation is necessary. In some cases, electrodiagnostic evaluations in young children and infants may be limited due to limits on patient and parent tolerance. This is particularly true in very small children and infants.

MYOPATHIC DISORDERS

One situation in particular where electrodiagnostic testing can be difficult in a small child is in the workup of suspected myopathic disorders. In these studies, much patience in obtaining motor unit analysis is needed and can be more time-consuming than a young child (or parent) can tolerate. Several studies have evaluated the role and accuracy of an electromyogram (EMG) in the diagnosis of neuromuscular disorders in children and infants. EMG has also been compared to muscle biopsy in diagnostic specificity and sensitivity of the procedures. In a majority of these studies, the accuracy of diagnosis with EMG improves in older children compared to the very young, likely mainly due to the level of tolerance of the procedure. However, EMG remains most difficult in the case of myopathic disorders in infants and very young children (1).

Ghosh and colleagues evaluated over a several-year period the diagnostic sensitivity of EMG in pediatric patients between the ages of 6 months and 18 years who underwent both EMG and muscle biopsy evaluations in cases of suspected myopathic disorders. A myopathic EMG was defined as having motor potentials that are of short duration, low amplitude, and polyphasic along with rapid recruitment. In their population, the most common diagnoses in decreasing order of frequency were congenital myopathy, metabolic myopathy, muscular dystrophy, genetically confirmed myopathy, myopathy undefined, and inflammatory myopathy. The authors concluded from their experience and comparisons that pediatric electromyography was 91% sensitive and 67% specific in diagnosing myopathic disorders with metabolic myopathies most commonly missed using EMG in this patient population (2).

THE ROLE OF GENETIC TESTING

One would expect the use of genetic testing in the diagnosis of muscular disorders to correspond to a decrease in the use of EMG in the pediatric population. However, this may not always be the case. In a study at Boston Children's Hospital (3) over a 10-year period from 2001 to 2011, a total of 2,100 studies were evaluated. In their review, the volume of studies actually increased from approximately 160 to 250 studies/year, with a trend toward studying older children. Referral for EMG was predominately from neurologists, including neuromuscular specialists. One reason for this is that with the possibility of genetic diagnosis, an EMG may be considered more useful in its ability to allow screening when these disorders are suspected. This screening may mitigate the expense of genetic testing to those disorders in which there is greater likelihood of a valid genetic diagnosis, a change to a health care plan of action, or a family's decision to have additional children. Also important in this process is that in many cases, genetic testing may not be reimbursed by a patient's health insurance plan. In this way, genetic testing along with EMG used to screen for myopathy in these patients may allow additional options available for the patient and family. In this Boston Children's Hospital study, polyneuropathies and mononeuropathies were the most common reason for referral. They found that 57% of the studies were normal, but EMG was able to provide diagnostically useful information in 94% of the cases.

EMG IN CLINICAL TRIALS

Using EMG parameters to follow a patient's response to treatment or course of disease is being used increasingly in clinical trials. In pediatric multicenter clinical trials in spinal muscular atrophy (SMA), using the maximum ulnar compound muscle action potential (CMAP) amplitude and area has been shown to provide a valid and reliable outcome measure that significantly correlates with clinical motor function. CMAP amplitude and area therefore have potential value as measures to evaluate and follow disease status in the trials of pediatric patients (4).

USE OF SEDATION

Adding to the challenge of performing these procedures in young children and infants is the fact that frequent pain assessments and the need for adequate pain control are often stipulated by the facility or institution and can be the subject of health performance survey data as part of the patient satisfaction score known as HCHAPS (Hospital Consumer Assessment of Healthcare Providers and Systems) (5). These surveys are increasingly used to judge the performance of a facility and are accessible to the public for review and scrutiny. Therefore, an incentive exists for each health care facility to merit a high score on survey data of patient satisfaction. Health care providers are encouraged to provide a "pain-free environment" and this may be at odds with the ability to perform complete and adequate electrodiagnostic evaluations in young children. The use of sedation can interfere with the complete evaluation of interference patterns, and depending on the level of sedation, motor unit analysis can be significantly impacted. More so than in studies in adult patients, preparation of the environment along with an honest discussion about expectations with the parents and child is needed in order to accomplish an appropriate study. Importantly it should be communicated to the parent and child that some level of discomfort should be expected. Since voluntary movements can interfere with the ability to adequately evaluate spontaneous resting activity, successful evaluation can only be obtained in a calm child. The use of conscious sedation during electrodiagnostic procedures in infants and children requires additional staffing to meet most regulatory requirements. This includes a provider skilled (and certified) in sedation procedures to be present for monitoring oxygen and vitals throughout the procedure and for a period thereafter. Additionally this provider needs to not be the provider performing the electrodiagnostic procedure. Although the use of conscious sedation is possible while obtaining nerve conduction studies, the child would need to be awake for the EMG component of the study. In general, the use of sedation significantly prolongs the total test time. Once the sedation wears off, it can be frightening for a young child to awaken and find an uncomfortable procedure about to begin, making cooperation often even less likely. In these cases, a realistic expectation would be that only limited information will be possible from the study. Motor unit analysis can be possible only with patience, a knowledgeable sedating team, informed parents, and a cooperative child (6).

DISEASE ETIOLOGIES

In some instances, neuromuscular disorders compare similarly in children and adults with little variation. One example of this is in the case of critical illness myopathy or critical illness polyneuropathy. Critical illness polyneuropathy and critical illness myopathy are associated with generalized weakness along with respiratory compromise and difficulty in weaning from mechanical ventilation. This has been reported in approximately 30% of the patients hospitalized for more than 3 days with a life-threatening illness (7). Since clinically and electrophysiologically polyneuropathic and myopathic features can be seen in the same patient, the disorder is often referred to as critical illness polyneuropathy and myopathy (CIPNM) (8).

In contrast, in many cases, the underlying etiological factors underlying a disorder vary significantly in infants and children compared to the adult population. An example of this is seen prominently with mononeuropathies. Mononeuropathies represent one of the most common sources of referrals for electrodiagnostic evaluation in the adult population but are less common in pediatrics. In children when carpal tunnel syndrome is seen in association with trigger finger and joint stiffness, a suspicion for mucopolysaccharidoses should be raised. Mucopolysaccharidoses are associated with joint stiffness and swelling and can also be associated with contractures (9).

Additionally, the more common sites for mononeuropathies are different in young children. Carpal tunnel and ulnar neuropathy make up the majority of adult mononeuropathy referrals in the outpatient setting with early presentation of paresthesias and progression to motor weakness. In contrast, in pediatric patients, sciatic mononeuropathy may account for 25% of all such cases (10). In the majority of these cases, the presentation is that of motor weakness. The underlying etiology of sciatic mononeuropathy may include trauma and injury from surgical causes and less commonly vascular or neoplastic processes. Other etiologies include prolonged extrinsic compression and immobilization. As in adults, the prognosis for recovery depends on the electrodiagnostic findings and degree of severity. Idiopathic etiologies may result from orthopedic surgeries or after prolonged compression with a cast. In most of these cases, peroneal followed by tibial nerve–innervated muscles are involved. Use of intraoperative EMG monitoring during surgical procedures in which the sciatic nerve is at risk of injury may reduce the risk of nerve-related injury. The severity can be evaluated both clinically and electrodiagnostically. The presence of reinnervation is a good prognostic sign as is the presence of normal-amplitude nerve action potentials (NAPS). Other rare causes of sciatic mononeuropathy include intraneural perineurioma of the sciatic nerve, which is treatable and has an indolent course. Electrodiagnosis and imaging with MRI in the appropriate clinical setting of intraneural perineurioma provide the correct diagnosis (11). Vascular etiologies are uncommonly seen as the cause of sciatic neuropathies in children but when present, may be due to vasculitis, embolization, or infectious etiologies (12).

Carpal tunnel syndrome or median neuropathy at the wrist is the most common mononeuropathy of adulthood but uncommon in children. It is characterized by paresthesias in the hand overlying the first three digits and can be associated with hand weakness and wrist pain. Electrophysiological findings include slowing of nerve conduction velocity at the palm-to-wrist segment along with latency prolongation at the wrist. In adults most often, this disorder is due to repetitive use of the hands and can be seen commonly in those with diabetes, other endocrine conditions, connective tissue disorders, and in pregnancy. In children however, in mucopolysaccharidoses and mucolipidoses, trauma to the median nerve, malformations of the wrist, brachial plexopathy, obesity, and inherited susceptibility to pressure palsies (PMP 22 gene deletion) are all possible as etiologies. In addition, family history of median neuropathy at the wrist is commonly seen (13).

Another example of different underlying etiologies for the same clinical condition in children compared to adults is in the case of acute axonal peripheral polyneuropathy. Toxic etiologies account for more than 50% of cases of acute axonal peripheral polyneuropathies in children, a larger percentage than in adults. In the case of purely sensory peripheral neuropathy, diabetes is responsible for most cases in children, whereas in adults, a purely sensory peripheral neuropathy necessitates a thorough diagnostic investigation for other etiologies including paraneoplastic disorders. Autoantibodies to gangliosides GM1, GM1b, GD1a, GD1a, or galNac-GD1a may be present is some children with acute motor axonal neuropathy and their clinical presentations are similar to those seen in adult patients (14). When these ganglioside markers are present in children, recovery from the neuropathy may be prolonged. In contrast to axonal neuropathies, pediatric cases of childhood multifocal acquired demyelinating sensory and motor neuropathy have been reported with and without conduction block on electrophysiological studies. These cases may respond to intravenous immunoglobulin (IVIG) therapy with more favorable long-term outcomes.

CLINICAL COURSE, ELECTRODIAGNOSIS, AND OUTCOME

Another consideration when interpreting EMG findings in children is that the same clinical condition may have very different presentations, electrodiagnostic findings, and outcomes. An example of this is with pediatric thoracic outlet syndrome. In these cases, vascular compromise is much more common than in adults. There is significant clinical and electrodiagnostic involvement and surgical rib resection is likely to result. In addition, a significant number of these cases are due to hypercoagulable disorders (15). Another example of the variability seen in children is in children with Guillain-Barré syndrome, the presentation may be that of leg pain and gait disturbance, but prognosis for complete recovery with IVIG is good (16). In the newborn and infant age group, often the presentation is that of muscle weakness or of a floppy infant. In this scenario, the differential diagnosis is wide and includes spinal muscular atrophy type 1, poliomyelitis (not so often in developed nations), as well as hereditary myopathies, infantile botulism, and Guillain-Barré syndrome.

Another potentially devastating disorder with a different clinical course in children is that of chronic inflammatory demyelinating polyneuropathy (CIDP). CIDP is characterized by clinical weakness, increased cerebrospinal fluid protein, and electrophysiological evidence of demyelination with varying degrees of axonal involvement. It is much less common in children than in adults, and in general, children tend to have a more severe and rapidly progressive course. Children, however, often show a more rapid improvement after therapy and ultimately have a more favorable overall outcome. Favorable response to IVIG or plasmapheresis is typical. However, in those patients who are not responsive to IVIG or plasmapheresis, a more prolonged course of recovery is found and variable responsiveness to other immune modulating treatments is also seen (17).

Neuromuscular junction disorders in children generally have a more severe clinical presentation than that seen in adults. Clinical presentations include floppy infant and apnea episodes leading to a broad differential diagnosis and can delay diagnosis and treatment (18). The genetic abnormalities involved in these disorders are numerous, so genetic screening without EMG confirmation is impractical. Neuromuscular junction disorders in children include the congenital myasthenic syndromes and autoimmune myasthenia gravis, which are uncommon. Stimulated single-fiber electromyography (stim SFEMG) of a proximal muscle such as the orbicularis oculi has a high sensitivity and specificity for diagnosis and although technically more difficult to do, at least in older children it may be very well tolerated.

Understandably, EMG in pediatric patients can be more challenging than in adults due to limitations in tolerance. Having an understanding of the limitations of the study in each case and maximizing the ability to obtain as much information as possible can be realized with informed parents and a sedating team when sedation is needed or required. Engaging both the parents and the sedating team in furthering the cooperation of the child is optimum and a key to the successful completion of EMG studies in these patients.

REFERENCES

1. Rabie M, Jossiphov J, Nevo Y. Electromyography (EMG) accuracy compared to muscle biopsy in childhood. *J Child Neurol.* 2007;22(7):803–808.
2. Ghosh PS, Sorensen EJ. Diagnostic yield of electromyography in children with myopathic disorders. *Pediatr Neurol.* 2014;51(2):215–221.

3. Karakis I, Liew W, Darras BT, et al. Referral and diagnostic trends in pediatric electromyography in the molecular era. *Muscle Nerve.* 2014;50(2):244–249.
4. Lewelt A, Krosschell KJ, Scott C, et al. Compound muscle action potential and motor function in children with spinal muscular atrophy. *Muscle Nerve.* 2010;42(5):703–708.
5. http://www.hcahpsonline.org. Centers for Medicare & Medicaid Services. Baltimore, MD 2015
6. Galloway G. The preoperative assessment. In: Galloway G, Nuwer M, Lopez J, Zamel K. eds. *Intraoperative Neurophysiologic monitoring.* New York, NY: Cambridge University Press;2010:10–18.
7. Jones, HR, Darras, BT. Acute care pediatric electromyography. *Muscle Nerve Suppl.* 2000;9:S53–S62.
8. Williams S, Horrocks A, Ouvrier RA, et al. Critical illness polyneuropathy and myopathy in pediatric intensive care: A review. *Pediatr Crit Care Med.* 2007;8(1):18–22.
9. Cimaz R, La Torre F. Mucopolysaccharidoses. *Curr Rheumatol Rep.* 2014;16:389.
10. Srinivasan J, Ryan MM., Escolar DM, et al. Pediatric sciatic neuropathies: a 30 year prospective study. *Neurology.* 2011;76:976–980.
11. Ostergaard JR, Smith T, Stausbol-Gron B. Intraneural perineurioma of the sciatic nerve in early childhood. *Pediatr Neurol.* 2009;41(1):68–70.
12. Srinivasan J, Escolar D, Ryan M. et al. pediatric sciatic neuropathies due to unusal vascular casuses. *J Child Neurol.* 2008;23(7):738–741.
13. Davis L, Vedanarayanan V. Carpal tunnel syndrome in children. *Pediatr Neurol.* 2014;50(1):57–59.
14. Nishimoto Y, Susuki K, Yuki N. Serologic marker of acute motor axonal neuropathy in childhood. *Pediatr Neurol.* 2008;39(1):67–70.
15. Arthur LG, Teich S, Hogan M. et al Pediatric thoracic outlet syndrome: a disorder with serious vascular complications. *J Pediatr Surg.* 2008;43(6):1089–1094.
16. Devos D, Magot A, Perrier-Boeswillwald J, et al. GB syndrome during childhood: particular clinical and electrophysiological features. *Muscle Nerve.* 2013;48(2):247–251.
17. Riekhoff AG, Jadoul C, Mercelis R, et al. Childhood chronic inflammatory demyelinating polyneuroradiculopathy—three cases and a review of the literature. *Eur J Paediatr Neurol.* 2012;16(4):315–31.
18. Wakamotor H, Chisaka A, Inoue N, Nakano N. Childhood multifocal acquired demyelinating sensory and motor neuropathy. *Muscle Nerve.* 2008;37(6):790–795.

Clinical Neurophysiology in Pediatric Peripheral Neuropathy

Gloria M. Galloway, MD, FAAN

This chapter provides descriptions of the electrophysiology involved in a variety of inherited and acquired peripheral neuropathies in the pediatric population. Although not meant to be an exhaustive list, it provides a review of the electrophysiology involved and although clinical features are included here to complete the discussion, the clinical aspects should be reviewed in greater detail in Chapter 7. A summary of inherited and acquired peripheral polyneuropathies is included in Table 9.1.

Peripheral neuropathy can present in a variety of ways in children. Symptoms can include sensory paresthesias and distal weakness, and when severe or chronic, distal atrophy can also be present. Sensory paresthesias often begin in the distal extremities, particularly the lower extremities first. These sensations can be described as burning, shooting, or throbbing in nature. In some patients, these sensations can be evoked or worsened by a physical stimulus such as touching the affected extremity or the touch of a blanket, and in some patients there is a hypersensitivity to cold or heat, referred to as allodynia or hyperalgesia. The paresthesias and the distal weakness can cause functional loss and disability. In general, many peripheral neuropathies progress over time and greater involvement can occur over more proximal regions of the body. Peripheral neuropathies may be chronic or acute in onset and therefore the progression differs, depending on the etiology involved. Many etiologies are shared with adult forms of the disease; however, clinical features, electrophysiology, treatment, and outcomes can differ significantly from the adult forms. Pain in pediatric peripheral neuropathy may in some cases be undertreated (1). This may be due to a lack of familiarity with this condition in children resulting in a delay in referral for specialty evaluation and hesitancy in medication treatment.

TABLE 9.1 Electrophysiology Summary Table

NEUROPATHY		ELECTROPHYSIOLOGY
HMSN		Slow nerve conduction velocities and prolonged latency. On EMG, increased polyphasic motor unit activity and variable abnormal spontaneous activity.
	HNPP	Slow nerve conduction velocities in sensory and motor nerves; significant latency prolongation; mild to no amplitude loss. Nerve conduction slowing is more pronounced across typical compression sites. Motor units are long duration with increased polyphasia.
	CMT	Significantly slow nerve conduction velocities; prolonged distal latency in motor and sensory nerves. In many cases, sensory nerve responses cannot be obtained at all. Amplitude loss. Distal abnormal spontaneous activity can be variably seen.
HSAN		Significant symmetric sensory amplitude loss; loss of sensory responses; sensory velocities may be normal. Normal motor conductions.
	Subtype 4	Normal or mild reductions in sensory amplitude; mild prolongation of distal latencies. QST will demonstrate markedly abnormal temperature thresholds.
	Spinal muscular atrophies	Motor axon loss without significant conduction slowing or latency changes; generally sparing of sensory nerves. Fasciculations and findings in several myotomes help to support the diagnosis.
	Mitochondrial deficiency	Amplitude loss; mild slowing of nerve conduction velocity.
	Lysosomal and glycogen storage disorder	Amplitude loss in motor and sensory nerves without abnormal findings. Muscle fiber irritability is on needle EMG particularly in proximal muscles.
	Giant axonal neuropathy	Significantly reduced motor amplitudes with mild-to-normal conduction velocities and absent sensory responses.
	Sickle cell disease	Abnormalities on QST; in general, normal nerve conduction studies.
GBS		Latency prolongation; nerve conduction slowing; amplitude loss. Often F responses are prolonged or absent. Muscle fiber irritability can be seen but may be missed if the study is done before 10 to 14 days after the onset.
Nutritional and malabsorption		Amplitude loss in motor nerves.
Chemotherapy		Motor amplitude loss.
DPN		Slowing of nerve conduction velocities involving motor and sensory nerves along with latency prolongations, and when severe, amplitude loss can be seen as well.

Abbreviations: DPN, diabetic peripheral neuropathy; EMG, electromyogram; GBS, Guillain-Barré syndrome; HMSN, hereditary motor and sensory neuropathy; HNPP, hereditary neuropathy with liability to pressure palsy; HSAN, hereditary sensory autonomic neuropathy; QST, quantitative sensory testing.

INHERITED PERIPHERAL NEUROPATHIES

Peripheral polyneuropathies presenting in children may be hereditary in nature due to genetic mutations in one or more peripheral nerve proteins. When expressed in the infant or early neonatal period, these may be part of a developmental syndrome and the congenital neuropathy may be one of many abnormalities present in that patient. In other cases, the peripheral neuropathy is expressed as the presenting symptom in later childhood with weakness, sensory loss, frequent falls, pain, or recurrent palsies. These later forms of peripheral neuropathy are discussed here.

Hereditary Motor and Sensory Neuropathies

In hereditary motor and sensory neuropathies (HMSNs), either demyelination or axonal loss can predominate. With demyelination, Schwann cell loss (see Chapter 7) results in segmental demyelination pathologically. Electrophysiology findings include slowing of nerve conduction velocities with prolongation of latency measures on electrophysiological testing. Electromyography (EMG) will demonstrate increased polyphasic motor unit activity due to the chronic nature of the disorder over time. As the name "polyphasic" implies, these motor units are the ones with multiple phases of long duration but generally ongoing abnormal spontaneous activity is not characteristic. There are multiple known subtypes of HMSNs linked to mutations at the peripheral myelin protein 22 (PMP22) on chromosome 17p.

Hereditary Neuropathy With Liability to Pressure Palsy

Hereditary neuropathy with liability to pressure palsy or HNPP is one subtype and is associated with a deletion on chromosome 17p11.2-12. It is an autosomal dominant disorder. Nerve conduction studies show slowing of nerve conduction velocities in sensory and motor nerves along with significant latency prolongation with mild to no amplitude loss. There is more pronounced slowing noted over areas where focal nerve compression can occur such as over the peroneal nerve across the fibula head. Early in the disease process, abnormal spontaneous activity may be seen. Motor unit changes can include long duration and increased polyphasia. Pathologically, one sees demyelination of nerves, and the affected nerves are described as *tomaculous* or sausage-shaped figures due to focal irregularities of the myelin sheath.

Charcot-Marie-Tooth Disease

Charcot-Marie-Tooth disease (CMT) is a form of HMSN and is the most common hereditary peripheral polyneuropathy with an incidence of 1/2,500. CMT has several different subtypes with characteristic associated features. CMT is associated with the clinical onset of distal sensory loss, weakness, hyporeflexia or areflexia, and pes cavus foot deformities. It is also associated in the majority of pediatric patients with pain and can effect quality-of-life measures (2). It varies in severity from mild functional impairment to significant disability. CMT1A is the most common form of CMT disease and is responsible for an estimated 50% of CMT cases. It is due to the overexpression of the *PMP22* gene. Electrophysiologic testing reveals significant slowing of nerve conduction velocities even in young children, and prolongation of distal latency is seen in motor and sensory nerves. In many cases, sensory nerve responses cannot be obtained at all. Over the first two decades, amplitude loss occurs as well with axonal involvement. The axon loss will be associated with more involved motor weakness. Distal abnormal spontaneous activity can be variably seen.

The second most common form of CMT is X-linked Charcot-Marie-Tooth (CMTX) and is responsible for approximately 10% of all CMT cases. It is associated with mutations in the gap junction protein beta 1 gene (GJB1 encoding for connexin-32.2 protein). Current research is aimed at evaluating the benefit of neurotrophic factors in CMT disorders on the progression of disease (3).

Hereditary Sensory and Autonomic Neuropathies

Hereditary sensory and autonomic neuropathies (HSANs) are of five subtypes, all characterized by impairment in sensation due to loss of unmyelinated and small myelinated peripheral nerve fibers. Autonomic involvement can be seen as well. Electrophysiologic testing can reveal significant symmetric amplitude loss in sensory nerves distally (sural), and when severe, there is loss of sensory nerve responses but nerve conduction velocities may be normal. Motor conductions are typically normal. Subtype IV is associated with pain insensitivity. This condition can be associated with injuries due to loss of sensation to pain, oral mutilation, fractures, and anhidrosis. This condition can be very functionally debilitating, and delay in diagnosis can cause severe morbidity (4). The intradermal histamine test demonstrates lack of a normal axon flare response and is consistent with a diagnosis of HSAN. Since large myelinated fibers are generally not impacted significantly, electrophysiology testing may be normal or reveal mild reductions in sensory amplitude and mild prolongation of distal latencies. Quantitative sensory testing will be markedly abnormal for temperature thresholds.

Spinal Muscular Atrophies

The most common forms are autosomal recessive and are due to homozygous deletion of exon 7 in the *SMN1* gene. The *SMN* gene produces an SMN protein involved in mRNA synthesis affecting motor neurons of the spine and peripheral nervous system. The severity of the disorder depends on the extent of involvement of other exons on the *SMN1* gene and the number of copies of SMN2 present. If more than two copies of SMN2 are present, it mitigates the severity of the disorder. Involvement in infancy (SMA1) is usually the most severe form of the disease with respiratory compromise and early death. SMA2 typically has onset after 6 months of age and severity is variable, with some patients continuing into adulthood. The mildest form is SMA3 with onset in adolescence typically with motor weakness and slower overall progression of disease. Electrophysiological findings in these forms include motor axon loss without significant conduction slowing or latency changes and generally sparing of sensory nerves. The presence electrophysiologically of fasciculations and the presence of findings in several myotomes help to support the diagnosis.

Mitochondrial Deficiency Neuropathies

Mitochondrial deficiency neuropathies are due to abnormalities in the mitochondrial DNA. These usually reveal significant amplitude loss on electrophysiological testing, with mild slowing of nerve conduction parameters seen. These usually present in later childhood and are progressive. They may also present with ophthalmoplegia. These can present uncommonly in infancy and depending on the number and type of mutations, can include more systemic features including lactic acidosis, stroke symptoms, and encephalopathy (MELAS), ataxia, and external ophthalmoplegia.

Lysosomal and Glycogen Storage Disorders

Although classically described as a muscle disorder, Pompe's disease is a glycogen storage disease type II disorder also known as acid maltase deficiency (5). It is called acid maltase deficiency because it encompasses mutations in the gene encoding the lysosomal enzyme acid alpha glucosidase or GAA and is inherited in an autosomal recessive pattern. As a result of this mutation, an abnormal accumulation of glycogen of normal structure occurs within the lysosomes of various organs and in particular in skeletal, hepatic, and cardiac muscle in infants. The storage of glycogen occurs also in the central and peripheral nervous systems. Electrophysiologic findings typically involve motor nerves with amplitude loss, while sensory nerves do not typically show abnormal findings. Muscle fiber irritability is seen on needle EMG, particularly in proximal muscles (6).

Giant Axonal Neuropathy

Giant axonal neuropathy (GAN) is a rare pediatric neurodegenerative disease characterized by "giant" axons pathologically. These giant axons are caused by accumulations of intermediate filaments. GAN is associated with severe and chronic progression. Onset of disease clinically is by age 3 years, with progressive systemic involvement and respiratory compromise typically by the third decade. Central nervous system (CNS) involvement includes ataxia, oculomotor apraxia, and dysmetria. Patients may also have dysarthria and hearing loss (7). This disorder is an autosomal recessive disease with mutations in the *GAN* gene, which encodes for a protein called gigaxonin, involved in cytoskeleton support. Nerve conduction testing reveals significantly reduced motor amplitudes with mild-to-normal conduction velocities and absent sensory responses.

Sickle Cell Disease

Sickle cell disease is an autosomal recessive disorder in which pain is known to occur during crisis. However, reports of neuropathic pain symptoms are described in approximately 40% of sickle cell patients, independent of sickle cell crisis. Symptoms increase in intensity with longer disease duration. The pain is described as thermal hyperalgesia and can be seen in adolescent patients along with abnormalities on quantitative sensory testing. Electrophysiology reveals the presence of a small fiber neuropathy (8).

ACQUIRED PERIPHERAL NEUROPATHIES

Guillain-Barré Syndrome

In contrast to inherited peripheral nerve disorders, Guillain-Barré Syndrome (GBS) is the most common acquired cause of acute flaccid paralysis in children, with the potential for delay in diagnosis, given the variable presentation. It typically presents after a gastrointestinal or respiratory infection in more than half of all patients, and weakness is symmetric and ascending in onset. Distal pain and paresthesias may more prominently accompany the weakness in children.

Areflexia and cranial nerve involvement is typical. Ataxia in children is a common feature. The Miller Fisher variant of ophthalmoplegia, areflexia, and ataxia may be seen as well. Other pediatric variants include a presentation with acute respiratory failure; quadriparesis with respiratory compromise; more prominent proximal weakness at onset; preserved peripheral tendon reflexes; acute inflammatory purely motor neuropathy (AMAN); and a presentation of severe autonomic involvement including hypertension and headache. GBS is thought to arise from a variety of infectious agents resulting in B-cell and T-cell activation and production of antibodies directed at peripheral nerve antigenic proteins (9). The electrophysiologic findings mimic the clinical findings with involvement of sensory and motor nerves. Variable degrees of axonal along with demyelinative characteristics are seen with latency prolongation, nerve conduction slowing, and amplitude loss. Often F responses are prolonged or absent, suggesting proximal nerve involvement. Muscle fiber irritability can be seen but may be missed if the study is done before 10 to 14 days after the onset. Elevated protein levels in cerebrospinal fluid (CSF) and enhancement of peripheral nerve roots and cauda on MRI may be seen. Treatment involves respiratory monitoring and treatment as needed and attention to autonomic parameters including pulse, blood pressure and orthostatic hypotension as significant autonomic impairment can occur. Treatment with intravenous immunoglobulin (total of 2 g/kg given over 2–4 days) or plasmapheresis is the mainstay of therapy resulting in a decrease in circulating autoantibodies and speedier rate of recovery. GBS in children may progress more rapidly than in adults, but generally have a good prognosis for full recovery within several months after onset.

Nutritional and Malabsorption Syndromes

Nutritional and vitamin deficiencies including B12, folate, and thiamine can be associated with a peripheral neuropathy, often axonal in nature. These deficiencies may happen due to gastrointestinal diseases such as Crohn's, malnutrition, or alcohol use. In adolescents, these vitamin deficiencies can be seen with anorexia nervosa, an eating disorder characterized by starvation, vomiting, and severe weight loss (10). Vitamin E deficiency can be associated with a distal motor neuropathy and mutation in the alpha-tocopherol transfer protein gene. Electrophysiologic findings include neurogenic motor units and low-amplitude to absent motor responses on nerve conduction testing (11). Vitamin E deficiency and peripheral neuropathy have also been shown to occur in patients with cystic fibrosis. Cystic fibrosis is an autosomal recessive multisystem disorder affecting 1/3,200 live births. The peripheral neuropathy is responsive to vitamin E supplementation.

Chemotherapy-Induced Peripheral Neuropathy

With improvements in pediatric cancer, chemotherapeutic agents have been more widely used in pediatric patients. These patients report the development of neuropathic symptoms. An example is that of vincristine-induced neuropathy in the treatment of acute lymphoblastic leukemia (ALL). ALL is the most common pediatric cancer responsible for 30% of all cases under the age of 14 years. Clinically, patients typically present 2+ years after chemotherapy and may have paresthetic complaints and loss of ankle reflexes on clinical exam (12). Electrophysiologic findings include predominately motor amplitude loss.

Diabetic Peripheral Neuropathy

As in adults, the most common form of peripheral neuropathy due to diabetes in children is a distal symmetric sensory-motor form. Most pediatric patients with diabetic peripheral neuropathy (DPN) are asymptomatic but have subclinical disease based on clinical examination and electrophysiology studies. There is increased risk with type 1 diabetes more than 5 years or with post-pubertal type 2 diabetics. Nerve conduction testing reveals slowing of nerve conduction velocities involving motor and sensory nerves along with latency prolongations, and severe amplitude loss can be seen as well (13).

Peripheral neuropathies in pediatric patients have a variety of clinical and electrophysiologic presentations. In some cases, these presentations are similar to those found in adults. In other cases, the pediatric presentation is unique. Determining whether the underlying process is inherited or acquired can be done based on clinical and family history. Electrophysiology can support the clinical diagnosis and help guide the determination of etiologic factors. In some cases, EMG can be used to monitor treatment outcomes or progression of disease.

REFERENCES

1. Kachko L, Ami S, Lieberman A, et al. Neuropathic pain other than CRPS in children and adolescents: incidence, referral, clinical characteristics, management, and clinical outcomes. *Pediatr Anesth.* 2014;24(6):608–613.
2. Ramchandren S, Jaiswal M, Feldman, E. Effect of pain in pediatric inherited neuropathies. *Neurology.* 2014;82:793–797.
3. Sahenk Z, Galloway G, Clark K, et al. AAV1.NT-3 Gene Therapy for Charcot–Marie–Tooth Neuropathy. *Mol Ther.* 2014;22(3):511–521.
4. van den Bosch GE, Baartmans MG, Vos P, et al. Pain insensitivity syndrome misinterpreted as inflicted burns. *Pediatrics.* 2014;133(5):e1381–e1387.
5. Burrow TA, Bailey LA, Kinnett D, et al. Acute progression of neuromuscular findings in infantile Pompe disease. *Pediatr Neurol.* 2010;42(6):455–458.
6. Landrieu P, Baet J, De Jonghe P. Hereditary motor-sensory, motor and sensory neuropathies in childhood. In: Dulac O, Lassonde M, Sarnat HB. eds. *Handbook of Clinical Neurology. Pediatric Neurology Part III.* Vol 113 (3rd series). Amsterdam: Elsevier BV;2014.
7. Johnson-Kerner B, Roth L, Greene JP, et al. Giant axonal neuropathy: an updated perspective on its pathology and pathogenesis. *Muscle Nerve.* 2014;50:467–476.
8. Brandow A, Farley R, Panepinto J. Neuropathic pain in patients with sickle cell disease. *Pediatr Blood Cancer.* 2014;61:512–517.
9. Ryan, Monique M. Pediatric Guillain-Barré syndrome. *Curr Opin Pediatr.* 2013;25(6):689–693.
10. Renthal W, Marin-Valencia I, Evans P. Thiamine deficiency secondary to anorexia nervosa: an uncommon cause of peripheral neuropathy and Wernicke encephalopathy in adolescence. *Pediatr Neurol.* 2014;51(1):100–103.
11. Fusco C, Frattini D, Pisani F, et al. Isolated vitamin E deficiency mimicking distal hereditary motor neuropathy in a 13-year-old boy. *J Child Neurol.* 2008;23(11):1328–1330.
12. Jain P, Gulati S, Seth R. Vincristine-induced Neuropathy in Childhood ALL (Acute Lymphoblastic Leukemia) Survivors: Prevalence and Electrophysiological Characteristics. *J Child Neurol.* 2014;29(7):932–937.
13. Mah JK, Pacaud D. Diabetic neuropathy in children. In Zochodne DW, Malik RA, Eds. *Diabetes and the Nervous System. Handbook of Clinical Neurology.* Vol. 126 (3rd series). Amsterdam: Elsevier BV;2014.

EMG in Pediatric Brachial Plexopathy

Jaime R. López, MD

Peripheral nerve injury can occur at any age and as such can involve a variety of structures including the brachial plexus. Brachial plexopathy is a general term used to indicate injury to the brachial plexus. The term does not specify the cause of the injury, and the etiology could be traumatic, vascular, inflammatory, or other. It also does not specify the specific anatomic area of the brachial plexus that is involved. However, of all of the plexopathies, brachial plexopathies are the most common and represent a variety of disorders. Electrodiagnostic testing is an important component in the clinical assessment of brachial plexopathies and can provide accurate localization of the brachial plexus regions affected and shed light on the possible pathophysiologic processes involved. Recognized as an extension of the neurologic examination, electrodiagnostic testing can provide objective evidence of specific muscle involvement that is not always clinically obvious, provide objective confirmation of abnormal muscles identified on physical examination, show active denervation and reinnervation changes in affected muscles, identify patterns consistent with demyelinating and axonal pathology, estimate severity of the pathology, and also provide for the possibility of serial examinations over time to objectively assess clinical progress and help with guiding management and establishing prognosis.

Electrodiagnostic testing of the brachial plexus can be a complicated and difficult task precisely because of its complicated anatomy and anatomic location. It is considered to be the most complex peripheral nervous system structure, and its superficial location, relatively large size, and position between the neck and upper extremity places it at risk for a variety of disorders, especially trauma. In order to be able to perform accurate and comprehensive electrodiagnostic testing, a clear understanding of the regional and brachial plexus anatomy is essential. In addition, a working knowledge of the disorders affecting the brachial plexus is helpful in formulating an electrodiagnostic interpretation of the findings.

ANATOMY

When a patient is referred for electrodiagnostic testing of possible brachial plexopathy, the electromyographer can use the tools available, such as sensory and motor nerve conduction studies (NCSs) in conjunction with needle electromyographic (EMG) examination to distinguish between a radiculopathy, plexopathy, a more distal neuropathy, and mononeuropathy multiplex. In the case of a brachial plexopathy, electrodiagnostic testing can localize the lesion within the brachial plexus. In order to be able to do this, the electromyographer must have an excellent understanding of the brachial plexus anatomy. The following will provide an overview of the anatomy of the brachial plexus. It is intended to be a review relevant to electrodiagnostic assessment and not a comprehensive anatomical review, which is beyond the scope of this chapter. For a detailed review of the brachial plexus anatomy, the reader is referred to Wilbourn (1).

The brachial plexus is a triangular-shaped structure, which lies between two mobile structures, the neck and upper extremity. It extends from the spinal cord to the axilla, its average length is 15.3 cm, and it has a 2 to 1 ratio of connective-to-neural tissue composition (2,3). The brachial plexus is derived from the ventral roots of C5 through T1 and is sequentially divided into five components: roots, trunks, divisions, cords, and terminal nerves (Figure 10.1). There are five roots, C5 to T1; three trunks: upper, middle, and lower; six divisions: three anterior and three posterior; three cords: lateral, posterior, and medial; and several terminal branches (Tables 10.1–10.2).

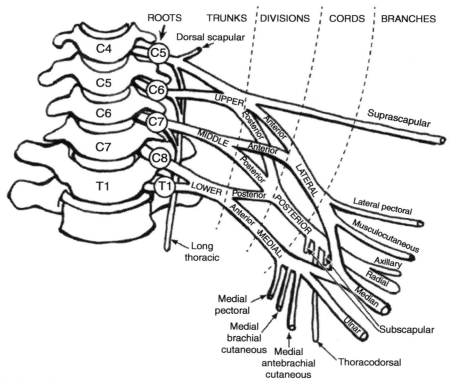

FIGURE 10.1 The components of the brachial plexus: roots, trunks, divisions, cords, and major terminal branches.

Source: From Ref. (4). Simmons Z. Electrodiagnosis of brachial plexopathies and proximal upper extremity neuropathies. *Phys Med Rehabil Clin N Am.* 2013;24:13–32.

TABLE 10.1 Brachial Plexus Composition

NEURAL STRUCTURE	NUMBER	COMPONENT
Roots	5	C5–T1
Trunks	3	Upper, middle, lower
Divisions	6	3 anterior, 3 posterior
Cords	3	Lateral, posterior, medial
Terminal	Several	Nerves

Roots

The neural elements of the brachial plexus have their origin from the C5 through the T1 levels of the spinal cord. The most proximal exit the spinal cord as dorsal and ventral rootlets; they come together, forming the dorsal and ventral roots. Both dorsal and ventral roots then fuse together to form a mixed (sensory and motor fibers) spinal nerve at a point just distal to the dorsal root ganglion (DRG). After exiting the intervertebral foramen, the spinal nerve then branches posteriorly into the posterior primary rami and continues as the anterior primary rami. The anterior primary rami, considered to be the roots of the brachial plexus, are located immediately external to the intervertebral foramina and emerge from between the anterior and middle scalene muscles. In regard to the overall root contribution to the brachial plexus, each of the C6, C7, and C8 roots contributes approximately 25% of its neural elements, and the remainder is provided by the C5 and T1 roots (2). It should also be understood that the percentage of motor and sensory fiber composition of each root varies. Typically, C5 and C6 roots contain the largest percentage of motor fibers, while C7 and T1 have the least. Sensory fibers are found in greatest numbers in the C7 root, followed by C6, C8, T1, and C5, in descending order (3). As is to be expected, anatomic variation exists. "Prefixed plexus" is a term used when there is contribution from C4 and minimal contribution from T1. In these cases, nerve contributions to the brachial plexus are shifted one level superiorly (4). There is also a "postfixed plexus"; this exists when there is minimal contribution of C5 and significant contribution from T2. In this case, nerve contribution to the brachial plexus is shifted one root level inferiorly. Finally, the

TABLE 10.2 Upper Extremity Nerves With Corresponding Cord Origin

LATERAL CORD	MEDIAL CORD	POSTERIOR CORD
Lateral pectoral	Medial pectoral	Upper subscapular
Musculocutaneous	Medial brachial cutaneous	Lower subscapular
Lateral antebrachial cutaneous	Medial antebrachial cutaneous	Thoracodorsal
	Ulnar	Axillary
Median		Radial

brachial plexus is considered expanded when root contribution comes from C4 through T2. It is important to note that there are two nerves that originate directly from the nerve roots:

1. Long thoracic nerve; origin: directly from C5, C6, and sometimes from C7 anterior primary rami; innervation: serratus anterior muscle.

2. Dorsal scapular nerve; origin: C5 root and can sometimes have contribution from C4 or C6; innervation: levator scapulae and major and minor rhomboid muscles.

Important note: Clinical involvement of these muscles, in the form of weakness and/or EMG abnormalities, indicates a very proximal lesion, usually at the root level. From an EMG perspective, it is important to recall that the cervical paraspinal muscles are innervated by the posterior primary rami, indicating that their innervation comes directly from the root level.

Preganglionic sympathetic fibers reach the sympathetic ganglia after exiting via the anterior primary rami and white rami communicantes.

Sympathetic ganglia send postganglionic fibers to C5 through T1 spinal nerves via gray rami communicantes.

Trunks

The three trunks (upper, middle, and lower) are located in the posterior cervical triangle behind the clavicle and sternocleidomastoid. The upper trunk is formed by the union of the C5 and C6 anterior primary rami. The middle trunk is the continuation of the C7 anterior primary ramus, whereas the lower trunk is formed by a merger of the C8 and T1 anterior primary rami. There are two terminal nerves originating from the upper trunk: the suprascapular nerve and the nerve to the subclavius muscle. No significant terminal branches originate from the middle or lower trunks.

Divisions

Progressing distally, each trunk divides into an anterior and posterior division, all located behind the clavicle. There are no terminal nerve branches that arise from the divisions.

Cords

There are three cords, which are formed from the six divisions. Their names are derived from their location in relation to the course of the second segment of the axillary artery. The cords begin at or just distal to the clavicle and lie below the pectoralis major in the proximal axillary region, near the axillary lymph node chain and the major vascular structures to the arm. The cords are formed in the following manner:

Lateral Cord

▨ Upper trunk anterior division

▨ Middle trunk anterior division

▨ Contains C6 to C7 sensory and C5 to C7 motor fibers

▨ Has no C5 sensory fibers

Medial Cord

■ Lower trunk anterior division

■ C8 and T1 sensory fibers present

■ C8 and T1 motor fibers present

Posterior Cord

■ Upper, middle, and lower trunk posterior divisions

■ C5 to C7 sensory fibers present

■ C5 to C8 motor fibers present

■ No C8 sensory fibers present

Several nerves arise from the cords and these are summarized in Table 10.2.

Terminal Nerves

The location of these neural structures is in the distal axilla and includes the median, ulnar, and radial nerves and in some descriptions, also includes the musculocutaneous and axillary nerves (3). There is no clear consensus regarding when the terminal nerves become peripheral nerves. However, this has been defined as 3 cm beyond the cord or at the point where the nerves exit the axilla (5,6).

Brachial Plexopathy Classification

Although brachial plexopathies can arise from many causes and be classified in several ways, perhaps the best method of classification is according to the area of involvement. One method is to divide the plexopathies in the following manner:

1. Supraclavicular

    a. Roots

    b. Trunks

2. Retroclavicular

    a. Divisions

3. Infraclavicular

    a. Cords

    b. Terminal nerves

This classification scheme has practical, clinical utility because the incidence, severity, prognosis, and lesion type vary according to the area involved (3).

■ Supraclavicular are more common and

    ■ Are usually due to closed traction injuries

▦ Tend to be more severe as greater force is required to produce these injuries

▦ Are associated with poor outcome; except for those involving the upper trunk from which patients tend to have better recovery

Supraclavicular plexus lesions are further subdivided into

1. Upper

   a. C5 and C6 roots

   b. Upper trunk

      i. More commonly due to demyelinating conduction block

      ii. Closer to the muscles innervated

      iii. Extraforaminal

2. Middle

   a. C7 root

   b. Middle trunk

3. Lower

   a. C8 and T1 roots

   b. Lower trunk

Infraclavicular plexus lesions are not further divided because there appear to be no regional differences in lesion type, severity, incidence, and prognosis.

PATHOPHYSIOLOGY

Injury to the brachial plexus is caused by a variety of disorders similar to those of the other peripheral nervous system structures. The type of pathologic injury can be classified into two main types: axon loss and demyelination. As a result, these can produce three types of pathophysiologic changes: conduction slowing, conduction block, and conduction failure (7).

Axonal Degeneration and Axon Loss

In general, and regardless of the region affected, axon loss is the most common pathology encountered in brachial plexopathies. Essentially, any type of injury, if sufficiently severe, can destroy nerve fibers, regardless of size and of whether the axons are myelinated or unmyelinated. When considering focal lesions producing axonal loss, it is important to take into account the concept of Wallerian degeneration. Because the entire axonal segment of the axon distal to the lesion is separated from the cell body, it undergoes Wallerian degeneration. Obviously, this will affect all the structures innervated by those axons. Clinically, the symptoms associated with axon loss can be conceptualized as negative and positive. Negative symptoms can be thought of in terms of losing function such as weakness and atrophy if motor axons are lost. Sensory loss of all modalities occurs if sensory axons are lost. Positive symptoms of motor axon loss include fasciculations, myokymia, and cramps. Pain can be observed as a result of small-fiber sensory axon loss and paresthesia from large-fiber sensory axonal injuries.

In the case of a complete axonal lesion, conduction block is present at the site, and electrical stimulation of the neural structure will yield the following:

▨ Proximal stimulation generates no response

▨ Distal stimulation generates responses, which decrease in amplitude with each succeeding day

   ▨ Motor fibers 2 to 3 days

   ▨ Sensory fibers 5 days

This phenomenon is present as long as the distal nerve stump is capable of impulse conduction; 6 days for motor fibers and 8 to 9 days for sensory fibers. At approximately day 11, conduction failure is present, and no motor or sensory responses are elicited due to the advanced degeneration of the distal stump.

Focal Demyelination

Injuries that are of a type insufficient to produce axon loss may still be sufficient to produce injury to myelinated axons, causing focal demyelination. This type of pathology is localized and does not affect other, proximal or distal, areas of the nerve segment. However, conduction slowing and conduction block can arise from this type of pathology, and the resulting conduction abnormality depends on the severity of the demyelination.

Focal demyelinating conduction slowing is less severe and is further characterized by:

▨ All nerve impulses cross the lesion, but the impulse transmission velocity is reduced.

▨ Weakness, atrophy, or sensory deficits are not seen because the nerve impulses are able to reach their destination.

▨ It can produce positive phenomena such as fasciculations, myokymia, cramps, and paresthesias.

▨ If differential slowing is present along the nerve, then nerve impulse synchrony will be affected, and this can manifest as altered vibration, position, and light touch sensation, as well as changes in muscle stretch reflexes. This occurs because these require synchronized volleys.

Focal demyelinating conduction block is a much more severe condition because it blocks nerve impulses from crossing the lesion. This condition is similar to conduction failure encountered with axonal degeneration, and the clinical manifestations are essentially the same. It can involve any area of the plexus. Although in many cases it is clinically indistinguishable from conduction failure, there are three major differences between the two (Table 10.3):

Causes of Brachial Plexopathies

Brachial plexopathies are caused by a variety of conditions and these can affect any part of the brachial plexus. As such, it is useful to divide the disorders into those, which are localized

TABLE 10.3 Conduction Block Versus Conduction Failure

CONDUCTION ABNORMALITY	ATROPHY	SENSORY	DURATION
Conduction block	Rare	Restricted to large myelinated fibers resulting in position, vibration, and touch abnormalities. There is no effect on pain and temperature	Short, with faster full recovery due to lack of Wallerian degeneration
Conduction failure	Yes	Yes, all modalities	Long and slow, with imperfect recovery

to the supraclavicular region and those localized to the infraclavicular regions. Some common brachial plexus disorders, not limited to children, affecting these regions are listed in Table 10.4.

TABLE 10.4 Brachial Plexopathies in Adults

COMMON ETIOLOGIES OF BRACHIAL PLEXOPATHY
Traction
▪ Fall
▪ Trauma
▪ Sports
▪ Motor vehicle accidents
▪ Surgery
Compression
▪ Backpacks
▪ Crutches
▪ Hematoma, aneurysm, arteriovenous malformation
Lacerations from penetrating injuries
▪ Gunshot
▪ Knife
Ischemia
Radiation therapy
Thoracic outlet syndrome
Brachial neuritis
▪ Parsonage-Turner syndrome

In regard to children, Table 10.5 shows the diagnoses reported in the literature with the number and percent, as appropriate, identified at Children's Hospital, Boston, in over a 15-year period (n = 54) (8). Other causes not listed in Table 10.5 have been reported in the literature such as bilateral thoracic outlet syndrome (due to anterior scalene muscle impingement) (9), axillary nerve injury (10), and aortic stent implantation (11). In the pediatric population, similar to the adult population, trauma is recognized to be the most common cause of brachial plexopathies. As opposed to the numerous causes of adult traumatic brachial plexopathy, the etiology in children is most commonly due to one condition, obstetric brachial plexus palsy (OBPP). This is by no means the only cause, but it is the most common, with others occurring primarily in adolescence. OBPPs occur in 0.5 to 5.1 per 1,000 newborns (12). The most common type of OBPP is Erb's palsy, resulting in damage to the upper trunk or lateral cords. Klumpke's palsy, isolated hand paralysis combined with Horner's syndrome, is due to lower trunk or medial cord (C8–T1) injury and occurs much less frequently. Some have questioned its existence as an OBPP disorder. In their review of the literature, which included 3,508 cases of brachial plexus palsy, Al-Qattan and colleagues (13) found only 20 cases (0.6%) labeled as Klumpke's palsy. In addition, they found none in the 235 cases they reviewed from their own center. Their conclusion was that Klumpke's palsy is a rare phenomenon and that recovering global brachial plexus palsy can be misdiagnosed as Klumpke's palsy (14). However, a recent report provides excellent documentation of this condition in a 3.5-year-old child born via vaginal delivery with his right arm in a compound presentation, his arm presented along with his head (12).

TABLE 10.5 Pediatric Brachial Plexus Lesions

DIAGNOSIS/PATHOLOGY	BOSTON EXPERIENCE (%)
Perinatal onset (OBPP)	36/54 (66%)
Osteomyelitis associated (proximal humerus)	1/54 (2%)
Battered child/child abuse	1/54 (2%)
Idiopathic brachial plexopathy (neuralgic amyotrophy)	
Hereditary brachial plexopathy	
Hereditary neuropathy with liability to pressure palsies	
Trauma—cycling	4/54 (7%)
Trauma—falls	2/54 (4%)
Trauma—automobile	1/54 (2%)
Trauma—sports	1/54 (2%)
Trauma—backpacks	
Trauma—gunshot	1/54 (2%)
Crutches	1/54 (2%)
Miscellaneous—heroin	
Indeterminate	6/54 (11%)

Abbreviation: OBPP, obstetric brachial plexus palsy.

Obstetric brachial plexopathies are typically identified at birth. Nerve fiber involvement corresponds to five patterns (15):

1. C5 to C6: Erb's palsy, approximately 50%

2. C5 to C7: Erb's-plus palsy; "waiter's tip" position

    a. Adduction and internal rotation of arm

    b. Forearm extension and pronation

    c. Wrist and finger flexion

    d. Approximately 35%

3. C5 to T1: Some finger flexion sparing

4. C5 to T1: Flail arm and Horner's syndrome

5. C8 to T1: Klumpke's palsy (isolated hand paralysis and Horner's syndrome)

Of note, root avulsion is more common in lesions involving C8 to T1 fibers, while postganglionic lesions are more common with lesions involving C5 to C7 fibers.

In general, weakness on neurologic examination follows the following pattern of altered movement in the newborn:

1. Shoulder abduction: deltoid; C5

2. External rotation: infraspinatus; C5

3. Elbow flexion: biceps: C5 to C6

4. Forearm supination: supinator; C5 to C6

5. Wrist and finger extensions: C6 to C7

The biceps reflex is absent, and it is difficult to ascertain sensory deficits at this age. Diaphragmatic weakness will be present if the C4 root is involved; if so, it is usually right sided.

Even though OBPP has been known for many years, first described in 1764, management of this disorder is controversial (3). The pathophysiologic mechanism of injury ranges from mixed demyelination and axon loss to avulsion, which is complete axon loss. Fortunately, these injuries in children are less severe than traction injuries in adults. Some reviews suggest that spontaneous recovery occurs in over 90% of the cases, but the range reported from full recovery extends from 4% to 95.7% (16). Much of this discrepancy is due to the variations in the definition of full recovery. Regardless, it is safe to say that the natural history of this disorder is unknown (15). Nonetheless, electrodiagnostic studies, specifically EMG, can have a role in guiding therapy.

The two major concerns regarding OBPP are etiology and prognosis. Historically, EMG has not been as helpful as one would expect regarding these two issues. EMG can identify the pathophysiologic mechanisms of injury to the nerve, such as demyelination and axon loss, but it does not provide a direct clinical diagnosis of the cause of the pathophysiologic changes. In many cases, EMG can provide an estimate as to when the injury likely occurred, which can help in searching for the cause of the injury. However, in regard to OBPP, EMG has not provided a clear indication as to the onset of injury. In adults, fibrillations are typically detected at 10 to 14 days, with maximal loss of compound muscle action potential (CMAP) at 4 to 5 days and of the sensory nerve action potential (SNAP) at 10 days. Unfortunately, this does not appear to hold true for the neonate. It is postulated that fibrillations could appear at 1 to 2 days after injury, the CMAPs maximally reduced within 24 hours, and the SNAPs at 48 hours (16) (Table 10.6).

The reasons postulated for the differences noted between neonates and adults are that the time of fibrillation appearance is in inverse correlation to the volume of denervated nerve segment distal to the lesion. Calculations based on known nerve lengths and diameters in babies indicate that the appearance of fibrillations may be shortened by a factor of 7.5 to 10 times compared to adults (15). Animal studies also show that active denervation changes are seen within 24 hours of brachial plexus section in 2-day old piglets and 5 to 8 days in adult pigs (16). There seems to be no controversy regarding needle EMG findings of changes. Thus, if these changes were seen in the first week after birth, they would indicate a likely prenatal cause.

Historically, using EMG to assess prognosis has been difficult and the results unreliable. Being able to establish prognosis is important in the management of patients with OBPP and critical when identifying those who will require surgical intervention. Obviously, surgeons would like to avoid operating on patients whose lesions are likely to heal spontaneously and reserve surgery for those who are unlikely to recover. The currently accepted practice is to clinically follow the patients and assess for improvement. If there is no useful function of the biceps at 3 months after birth, then surgery should be performed. At best, this clinical practice delays surgery for 3 months, which is unfortunate because if surgery could be done earlier, then better outcomes would likely occur. Unfortunately, EMG is not a popular prognostic tool because the findings have been inaccurate. In many cases, the EMG findings at 3 months after birth in children without deltoid and bicep function have been referred to as "overly optimistic" because the EMG often shows a sporadic or mixed pattern without the usual findings of active denervation such as profound fibrillations, positive sharp waves, and absent motor unit action potentials (MUAPs). Therefore, the recruitment pattern can have enough activity so as not to recommend surgery. One reason attributed to this discrepancy is that the recording area of the EMG needle is as large in infants as in adults, such that approximately 11 times more MUAPs will be recorded in an infant, given the same proportion of functional motor units and discharge rates (17). Regardless, this discrepancy has limited the use of EMG in many of these cases. However, a recent study using EMG demonstrated that absence of MUAPs in the deltoid

TABLE 10.6 Onset of EMG and NCS Changes: Adults and Neonates

EMG/NCS CHANGES	ADULTS	NEONATES
Fibrillations	10–14 days	1–2 days
CMAP maximal reduction	4–5 days	24 hours
SNAP maximal reduction	10 days	Approximately 48 hours

Abbreviations: CMAP, compound muscle action potential; SNAP, sensory nerve action potential.

and biceps at 1 month of age correlated strongly with lack of recovery of biceps function at 3 months of age (18). This further suggests that EMG can be an objective and earlier predictor of biceps function at 3 months. This may allow for expansion of the role of EMG and encourage earlier referral for EMG testing and perhaps eventually lead to earlier surgical intervention in these patients with poor prognosis for recovery.

ELECTRODIAGNOSTIC STUDY OF THE BRACHIAL PLEXUS

In regard to electrodiagnostic studies, I will limit the discussion when using this term to the use of EMG and NCS. When evaluating the brachial plexus using electrodiagnostic techniques, extensive testing using NCS (motor and sensory) and needle EMG is required, including comparing results to the contralateral involved limb. This is the typical strategy in adults and with varying success in adolescents. However, extensive testing in an infant is usually not possible unless done under anesthesia. In infants, the choice of which muscles to sample is critical. If the infant has an upper plexus lesion on neurologic exam, then testing the deltoid, biceps, and triceps muscles should be done first. Comparing deltoid and biceps can help differentiate between root and plexus lesions.

▓ In C5 to C6 root lesions, deltoid and biceps will be abnormal.

▓ In plexus lesions, only one of the muscles (deltoid/biceps) may be abnormal.

If the neurologic exam points to a lower brachial plexopathy, then a distal muscle, such as the first dorsal interosseous muscle, should be tested first. Once this has been done, further needle examination of other muscles will be needed as well as motor and sensory NCSs. I will outline a general protocol for the electrodiagnostic study of the brachial plexus.

Performing EMG and NCS in children presents a different set of challenges than those encountered in adults. Infants and toddlers have reduced tolerance to pain, move and withdraw during the procedure, and are unable to relax their muscles to command. Adolescents are able to understand the purpose of the testing and can cooperate with the instructions provided during the procedure. However, some may still have difficulty in fully relaxing their muscles, especially the paraspinal muscles, during needle EMG testing. Topical anesthetic creams, which can help reduce the pain, are used in some laboratories. However, dependent on the age of the child, ability to cooperate, pain tolerance, and overall clinical state of the patient, conscious sedation and, rarely, general anesthesia may be necessary to obtain reliable data. Nonetheless, in the great majority of cases, it is possible to perform an adequate study yielding reliable data.

Electrodiagnostic study of brachial plexopathies requires extensive NCS and needle EMG. In addition, contralateral studies, to compare side-to-side results, are frequently necessary. Unfortunately, because of technical limitations, testing may be much reduced in children. Regardless, an adequate electrodiagnostic examination requires NCS of motor and sensory nerves as well as needle EMG. This is important because each of those different modalities provides different and unique information. For example, root avulsion is felt to exist if the SNAPs are preserved in a patient with clinical sensory loss. However, in some children with traumatic brachial plexopathies, the injury may affect both the nerve roots and plexus. In this situation, the SNAPs may be absent because the plexus is involved even though root avulsion is present (8).

Motor NCSs

Motor NCSs are primarily useful for assessing motor nerve axonal loss or dysfunction. The CMAP is a good indicator of the degree of axonal injury or associated demyelination. It is important to recall that in plexopathies, the motor NCS will only be abnormal if the nerve originates from the affected trunk or cord. In many instances, motor NCSs require testing of nerves not routinely examined. As an example, routine examination of upper limb motor nerves involves testing of the median and ulnar nerves. Both of these nerves provide information only of the lower trunk, medial cord, and C8 to T1 nerve roots. Therefore, motor NCS of other less commonly tested nerves may be necessary. Information on the upper trunk, lateral cord, and C5 to C6 roots can be obtained by testing the musculocutaneous nerve and recording from the biceps. These studies can be technically more challenging, especially in infants and have a wider range of amplitude responses, making interpretation more difficult. In addition, motor NCSs are usually normal in plexopathies but may have reduced CMAP amplitude due to axonal loss or conduction slowing. Thus, comparing CMAP amplitude to the contralateral uninvolved side is useful. A 50% amplitude reduction of the involved side compared to the same nerve on the contralateral side is considered abnormal (19). Table 10.7 shows the motor nerves and corresponding muscle recording sites where NCS can be performed. Unfortunately, some of these less commonly performed motor NCSs cannot be adequately performed in infants due to the

TABLE 10.7 Motor Nerves and Corresponding CMAP Recording Sites

AREA OF THE BRACHIAL PLEXUS	MUSCLE RECORDING SITE
Upper trunk	
▦ Musculocutaneous	Biceps
▦ Axillary	Deltoid
▦ Lateral cord-musculocutaneous	Biceps
Middle trunk/posterior cord	
▦ Axillary	Deltoid
▦ Radial	Anconeus, extensor digitorum communis, extensor indicis proprius
Lower trunk/medial cord	
▦ Median	Abductor pollicis brevis
▦ Ulnar	Abductor digiti minimi, first dorsal interosseous
Lower trunk/posterior cord	
▦ Radial	Extensor indicis proprius

short distances between the stimulation and recording sites. In these situations, assessment of motor involvement relies on needle EMG.

Sensory NCSs

In addition to motor NCS, testing sensory nerves is essential in assessing brachial plexopathies. Typically in injuries to the plexus, SNAP amplitudes are abnormally reduced. This is due to the sensory fibers being injured distal to the DRG. This is in contrast to nerve root injuries where the injury occurs proximal to the DRG, thus preserving the SNAP. However, as previously mentioned, combined root and plexus lesions resulting from trauma can occur, especially in infants and children.

Similar to motor NCS, SNAP amplitude change is the most common parameter affected in plexopathies. Side-to-side comparisons are also important, especially when trying to identify mild abnormalities. A 50% amplitude reduction of the SNAP compared to the same from the uninjured nerve contralateral limb is considered to be abnormal. This holds true even if the absolute amplitude is in the normal range (19). Of course, the determination of which sensory nerve to study should reflect the clinical findings and the dermatome involved. As is the case in most conditions in neurology, a careful neurologic examination, including the distribution of sensory loss, muscle stretch reflex changes, and muscle weakness, will guide the electromyographer regarding which nerve to test.

When choosing which sensory nerve to test, it is important to understand the innervation pattern of each nerve, which can be a complex task. Each of the commonly tested nerves, which include the median, ulnar, superficial radial, and lateral antebrachial cutaneous (LAC), have specific neural pathway innervations patterns, which are useful in localizing the area of the plexus involved. For example, NCS of the LAC assesses the pathway, which extends from the lateral cord to the upper trunk, the C6 anterior primary ramus, the spinal nerve, and finally the DRG. All the other sensory nerves have distinct neural pathways, with the median nerve being the most complicated through the brachial plexus (3). The following, Table 10.8, summarizes the innervation pathway patterns of the different sensory nerves, including the percentage of root contribution.

In comparison to routine median and superficial radial nerve (SRN) SNAPs recorded from digit 2 and snuffbox, respectively, the median and LAC SNAPs recorded from digit 1 are more sensitive for detecting abnormalities. This occurs because the middle trunk contributes fibers to the median nerve innervating digit 2 and the SRN innervating the snuffbox. Superficial radial SNAP can help distinguish upper trunk from lateral cord lesions, especially when used in conjunction with median nerve SNAPs recorded from the thumb. In this case, the routine median nerve SNAP will be abnormal in both upper trunk and lateral cord injuries, but if the SRN SNAP is preserved, then it indicates that the lesion involves the lateral cord, since it does not contribute to the SRN SNAP.

For lower trunk lesions, the ulnar and medial antebrachial cutaneous (MAC) are the most important nerves to test. Both are derived from the lower trunk and medial cord (see Table 10.8), and the ulnar SNAP is as sensitive as the MAC in identifying lower trunk lesions. In cases of separate ulnar neuropathies, MAC SNAPs can be used to assess for lower trunk or medial cord lesions. When assessing the less frequently tested nerves, LAC and MAC, SNAPs should be

TABLE 10.8 Sensory Nerve Innervation Pathway Patterns

TRUNK ELEMENT	DRG	CORD ELEMENT	DRG
Upper trunk		Lateral cord	
■ LAC	C6 (100%)	■ LAC	C6 (100%)
■ Median (thumb)	C6 (100%)	■ Median (thumb)	C6 (100%)
■ Superficial radial	C6 (60%)	■ Median (index finger)	C6 (100%)
■ Median (index finger)	C6 (20%)	■ Median (middle finger)	C6 (80%)
■ Median (middle finger)	C6 (10%)	■ Superficial radial	C6 (60%)
Middle trunk		Posterior cord	
■ Median (index finger)	C7 (80%)	■ Superficial radial	C7 (40%)
■ Median (middle finger)	C7 (70%)		
■ Superficial radial	C7 (40%)		
Lower trunk		Medial cord	
■ Ulnar (little finger)	C8 (100%)	■ Ulnar (little finger)	C8 (100%)
■ MAC	T1 (100%)	■ MAC	T1 (100%)
■ Median (middle finger)	C8 (20%)	■ Median (middle finger)	C8 (20%)

Abbreviations: LAC, lateral antebrachial cutaneous; MAC, medial antebrachial cutaneous.

obtained from the corresponding nerves from the uninvolved contralateral limb to allow for side-to-side comparisons.

Electromyography

Needle EMG is an important, essential, and critical component of the electrodiagnostic assessment of brachial plexopathies. It provides complementary information to that obtained by motor and sensory NCS and together can provide a more thorough evaluation of brachial plexopathy. Whereas NCS limits our ability to completely assess the brachial plexus, there is no such limitation with EMG. There are sufficient and multiple muscles available to allow assessment of each anatomic region of the brachial plexus (Table 10.5). EMG can provide objective evidence regarding the presence and extent of a lesion; estimate severity; detect active, ongoing denervation; identify the presence or absence of reinnervation, in many instances before it can be identified on physical examination; and help in determining prognosis.

In order to more precisely localize the abnormal brachial plexus region, extensive needle EMG testing is often needed. Generally, in older children and adolescents, this is possible at a level similar to adults. However, because of poor cooperation, this is not usually possible in young children and in infants. In addition, needle EMG testing of paraspinal muscles to screen for nerve root involvement is a necessary part of the EMG assessment of brachial plexopathies. Although in infants the information obtained from testing of the paraspinal muscles may be more important due to the possibility of nerve root avulsion due to OBPP, infants and toddlers are the age group where this examination is the most challenging. The difficulty in performing needle EMG in this group lies in attempting to assess insertional activity for the presence of active denervation changes such as fibrillation and positive sharp waves, as well as in analyzing MUAPs during voluntary muscle activation. The goal of EMG in brachial plexopathy is to show the involvement of multiple muscles innervated by a common brachial plexus element but different nerves. Obviously, muscles corresponding to neural innervations outside of the brachial plexus region identified should also be studied so as to exclude other conditions such as multiple mononeuropathies, polyneuropathies, or radiculopathies. To briefly review, in axonal injuries, the earliest finding on needle EMG is decreased MUAP recruitment, followed by denervation changes (fibrillation potentials and positive sharp waves). The temporal onset of these changes was discussed earlier in this chapter (see Table 10.6). Reinnervation changes, characterized by long-duration, high-amplitude, polyphasic MUAPs can be typically detected within 3 to 6 months after an acute injury. In some instances, serial EMG studies are necessary in order to assess for reinnervation or any evidence of recovery. In cases where recovery is not occurring, surgical exploration for possible nerve grafting is an option. Intraoperative testing using a variety of electrophysiologic techniques can be used to assess nerve function and help localize lesions.

SPECIFIC DISORDERS OF THE BRACHIAL PLEXUS

As previously noted, trauma is the most frequent cause of brachial plexopathies in children, with most being diagnosed as OBPP. This condition was discussed earlier and will not be reviewed here. This is also not intended to be a detailed, comprehensive account of all or a majority of the causes of brachial plexopathies. Instead, this will be a brief review of some of the brachial plexopathies, which have been reported in the past.

Trauma

Head and arm position is important in determining susceptibility of the different brachial plexus structures to traumatic closed injury.

■ When the arm is positioned to the side of the body and there is a force that causes excessive shoulder depression, this force will be transmitted to the upper trunk (C5–C6 roots).

■ If the force is applied to the axilla while the arm is overhead, then the force is directed and transmitted to the lower (C8–T1) roots.

In older children, especially teenagers, traumatic brachial plexopathies are due to a variety of different causes, with cycling accidents, falls, motor vehicle accidents, and sports being the most common (8). Football is associated with a specific type of brachial plexopathy, the "burner" or "stinger." These typically occur with tackling or blocking where the shoulder is depressed by the impact. The head often is deviated to the contralateral side. The characteristic symptoms are burning shoulder pain, which radiates to the arm and hand, lasting 3 to 10 seconds, followed by a few minutes of weakness. In a study by Robertson and colleagues (20) of 10 college football players, they found that mild weakness of external rotation and abduction of the arm was detected on physical examination. Nine patients had mild biceps weakness and moderate-to-severe weakness of external rotation, and arm abduction was seen in two patients. In addition, mild-to-minimal weakness lasting up to 9 months was seen in three patients. Median and ulnar motor and sensory NCS were normal as was needle EMG of cervical paraspinal muscles in all patients. However, in all patients, fibrillations and sharp waves were seen in one or more muscles. Overall, the results of the clinical examination and EMG indicated injury to the upper trunk of the brachial plexus. The authors indicated that the mechanism of injury was traction and stretch of the upper trunk of the brachial plexus. Interestingly, they also reported that approximately 50% of the 65 players on their traveling football squad experienced one or more episode of burning paresthesia during a season.

Another cause of traumatic brachial plexopathy in children, which may not be initially considered, is physical abuse. This usually occurs as an acute brachial plexopathy in younger children where no clear predisposing condition, such as febrile illness or independently witnessed accident, is present. Jones (1996) described a case of traumatic brachial plexus injury in a 15-month-old infant with sickle cell trait with a history of a fall. Median and ulnar NCS were normal, but fibrillations and decreased MUAPs were seen in the right biceps and deltoid and normal findings in the triceps and infraspinatus. Neurologic examination 3 months later was normal. However, 5 months after the initial presentation, the mother reported that the child had recurrent right arm weakness, and physical examination identified severe biceps and deltoid weakness with moderate triceps weakness. Although trauma was denied, the social worker confirmed recurrent child abuse, described as the child being picked up by the arm, twirled overhead and then being thrown by the parent. As this case dramatically illustrates, physical abuse should be considered, especially in cases of recurrent, unexplained episodes of brachial plexopathies.

Idiopathic Brachial Plexopathy

Idiopathic brachial plexopathy (IBP) differs from the more common causes of brachial plexopathies due to structural injuries or lesions. Although no etiologies are clearly implicated in this condition, it is considered to be an immune-mediated disorder. IBP has a characteristic clinical pattern and can affect multiple nerves but predominantly affects nerves innervating the shoulder girdle. Approximately a third of the patients can have bilateral involvement. There often are minimal sensory abnormalities and, as opposed to structural lesions, the sensory NCS may be normal.

Hereditary Brachial Plexus Neuropathy

Hereditary brachial plexus neuropathy (HBPN) is an autosomal dominant disorder with onset usually between 6 and 18 years of age but can occur as early as 3 years of age. Children with this disorder can have recurrent episodes of pain in the shoulder and arm, followed by weakness and atrophy, and then gradual recovery. Although the clinical features of this disorder are similar to those of IBP, there are clear differences. Dunn and colleagues (21) described this disorder in 12 members of three families and found the following differences: close-set eyes; recurrent attacks of brachial plexopathies, which are rare in adults with sporadic brachial plexus neuropathy; initial manifestation in childhood, which is unusual in the sporadic condition; and males and females equally affected, in contrast to a predominance of males in the nonfamilial condition. They also reported electrodiagnostic findings of normal motor conduction velocities in affected nerves or mild slowing in the peripheral segments. However, the median and radial nerve SNAPs showed abnormally low amplitude in the acutely affected arms. In addition, denervation was seen in the acutely weak muscles in some patients. In some cases, evidence of denervation associated with normal motor nerve conduction was found, likely due to a proximal lesion.

CONCLUSION

Even though brachial plexopathies are not very common in children they, nonetheless, exist, and electrodiagnostic testing with NCS and EMG is very useful in helping establish a diagnosis, assisting in guiding therapy, and assessing prognosis. It is also important to emphasize that proper interpretation of these studies requires understanding and knowledge of brachial plexus anatomy and how lesions within the brachial plexus affect NCS and EMG findings. Although its utility in OBPP, the most common type of childhood brachial plexopathy, has been questioned, more recent data suggests that EMG may provide an earlier, objective predictor of poor recovery and help identify these children at an earlier stage for consideration of surgical intervention. In older children, EMG and NCS are useful in helping localize the area of abnormality within the brachial plexus, providing functional and pathophysiologic information, and assisting with treatment and management of the underlying disorder. Overall, EMG and NCS are indispensable components in the evaluation of brachial plexopathies in children, and despite perceptions of technical difficulties and limitations in infants and toddlers, these studies are necessary in order to provide a comprehensive assessment.

REFERENCES

1. Wilbourn AJ. Mechanical compression, traction, electrical radiation and neoplastic infiltration of the brachial plexus. In: Dyck PJ, Thomas PK, eds. *Peripheral Neuropathy.* 4th ed. Philadelphia, PA: Saunders;2005:1339–1373.
2. Slingluff CL, Terzis JK, Edgerton MT. The quantitative microanatomy of the brachial plexus in man: reconstructive relevance. In: Terzis JK, ed. *Microreconstruction of Nerve Injuries.* Philadelphia, PA: WB Saunders;1987:285–324.
3. Ferrante MA. Brachial plexopathies: classification, causes and consequences. *Muscle Nerve.* 2004;30:547–568.
4. Simmons Z. Electrodiagnosis of brachial plexopathies and proximal upper extremity neuropathies. *Phys Med Rehabil Clin N Am.* 2013;24:13–32.
5. Narakas AO. Traumatic brachial plexus lesions. In: Dyck PJ, Thomas PK, Lambert EH, Bunge R, eds. *Peripheral Neuropathy.* Philadelphia, PA: WB Saunders;1984:1393–1409.
6. Wilbourn AJ. Brachial plexopathies. In: Katirji B, Kaminski HJ, Preston DC, et al. eds. *Neuromuscular Disorders in Clinical Practice.* Boston, MA: Butterworth-Heinemann;2002:884–904.
7. Wilbourn AJ. Plexopathies. *Neurol Clin.* 2007;25:139–171.
8. Jones HR. Plexus and nerve root lesions. In: Jones HR, Bolton CF, Harper CM, eds. *Pediatric Clinical Electromyography.* Philadelphia, PA: Lippincott-Raven;1996:123–169.
9. Khan A, Rattinalli RR, Hussain N, et al. Bilateral thoracic outlet syndrome: an uncommon presentation of a rare condition in children. *Ann Indian Acad Neurol.* 2012;15:323–325.
10. Dahlin LB, Coster M, Bjorkman A, et al. Axillary nerve injury in young adults - an overlooked diagnosis? Early results of nerve reconstruction and nerve tranfers. *J Plast Surg Hand Surg.* 2012;46:257–261.
11. Sabiniewicz R, Erecinski J, Zipser M. Brachial plexus injury as an unusual complication after aortic stent implantation. *Cardiol Young.* 2011;21:227–228.
12. Buchanan EP, Richardson R, Tse R. Isolated lower brachial plexus (Klumpke) palsy with compound arm presentation: case report. *J Hand Surg.* 2013;38A:1567–1570.

13. Al-Qattan MM, Clarke HM, Curtis CG. Klumpke's birth palsy: does it really exist? *J Hand Surg Br.* 1995;20(1):19–23.

14. Al-Qattan MM. Obstetric brachial plexus palsy associated with breech delivery. *Ann Plast Surg.* 2003;51(3):257–264.

15. Van Dijk JG, Pondaag W, Malessy MJA. Obstetric lesions of the brachial plexus. *Muscle Nerve.* 2001;24:1451–1461.

16. Pitt M, Vredeveld J-W. The role of electromyography in the management of the brachial plexus palsy of the newborn. *Clin Neurophysiol.* 2005;116:1756–1761.

17. Van Dijk JG, Malessy MJ, Stegeman DF. Why is the electromyogram in obstetric brachial plexus lesions overly optimistic? *Muscle Nerve.* 1998;21:260–261.

18. Van Dijk JG, Pondaag W, Buidenhuis SM, et al. Needle electromyography at 1 month predicts paralysis of elbow flexion at 3 months in obstetric brachial plexus lesions. *Dev Med Child Neurol.* 2012;54:753–758.

19. Acosta JA, Raynor EM. Electrophysiology of brachial and lumbosacral plexopathies. In: Blum AS, Rutkove SB, eds. *The Clinical Neurophysiology Primer.* Totowa, NJ: Humana Press;2007:299–311.

20. Robertson WC, Eichmann PL, Clancy WG. Upper trunk brachial plexopathy in football players. *J Am Med Assoc.* 1979;241:1480–1482.

21. Dunn HG, Daube JR, Gomez MR. Heredofamilial brachial plexus neuropathy (hereditary neuralgic amyotrophy with brachial predilection) in childhood. *Dev Med Child Neurol.* 1978;20:28–46.

Intraoperative Considerations in the Pediatric Patient

Gloria M. Galloway, MD, FAAN

CNS MYELINATION

The value of neurophysiological intraoperative monitoring (NIOM) in reducing the risk of injury to neural structures has been well documented in the literature (1,2). However, performing NIOM in young children and infants requires special considerations as compared to those of adults. Central nervous system (CNS) myelination is not complete until approximately age 3 years, and in this age group, there is also significant sensitivity to the effects of volatile anesthetic agents.

MULTIMODALITY MONITORING

The use of multimodality monitoring in a variety of surgeries, including complex spinal deformity surgeries, has become the standard of care at most institutions. Multimodality indicates that several different methods for monitoring pathways are utilized, often monitoring different or complementary pathways as listed in Table 11.1. The goal of multimodal monitoring is increased sensitivity and specificity in detecting changes during the operative procedure from baseline values, thereby helping to prevent neurological impairment (1). In a large retrospective review by Emerson, multimodality monitoring and monitoring of selected modalities in pediatric orthopedic spinal cases demonstrated "accurate detection of permanent neurologic status in 99.6% of 3,436 patients and reduced the total number of permanent neurologic injuries to 6" (2). Intraoperative considerations in the use of these modalities in cases of pediatric NIOM comprise the topic of this chapter.

Multimodality monitoring can be used in the resection of intramedullary spinal cord tumors, accounting for less than 10% of CNS tumors in the pediatric population. They can

TABLE 11.1 List of Monitoring Modalities for use in the OR

MONITORING MODALITIES
SSEP
TcES
BAER
EMG
Cortical stimulation
EEG

Abbreviations: BAER, brainstem auditory evoked response; EEG, electroencephalogram; EMG, electromyogram; OR, operating room; SSEP, somatosensory evoked potential; TcES, transcranial electric motor stimulation.

involve any area of the spinal cord as well as the cervical-medullary junction (3). NIOM using multimodalities is sensitive in determining the potential for neurological compromise. Modalities include dorsal column mapping, somatosensory evoked potentials (SSEPs), and transcranial motor evoked potentials (4). Modalities chosen are similar to those for adult patients, but increased stimulus intensity and, in the case of transcranial electric motor stimulation (TcES), use of longer pulse trains may be needed in the very young due to immaturity of the involved tracts.

Somatosensory Evoked Potentials

SSEPs are elicited by electrical stimulation to a mixed peripheral nerve usually and recorded over the dorsal root entry zone, brainstem, and sensory cortical areas. SSEPs correspond to the posterior column medial lemniscus spinal system. This system has synaptic connections in the ventral posterior lateral (VPL) nuclei of the thalamus. From the VPL, fibers traverse the internal capsule to the primary sensory cortex at the postcentral gyrus. Upper extremity representation is along the lateral cortex and representation of the lower extremities is along the medial and parasagittal area. The effect of anesthesia on NIOM is particularly apparent with SSEPs, in which amplitude is reduced and latency is prolonged as an effect. This is most prominently seen with inhalational agents and the effects are most pronounced for potentials generated from the cortex (cortical potentials), with potentials arising from brainstem generators (brainstem potentials) being more resistant to the effects of anesthesia. These effects are also more pronounced in children and the very young. Therefore, attention in the operating room (OR) to the choice and dosing of anesthetic agents is important in order to have successful NIOM in this age group.

Transcranial Electric Motor Stimulation

TcES of the motor cortex is accompanied by recording from peripheral extremity muscles after stimulation. Due to lack of complete myelination of the corticospinal tracts in very young patients, higher-voltage thresholds and longer pulse trains during TcES are generally needed. Additional limitations include the inability to use needle or screwlike electrodes in a child if the anterior fontanelle is not closed, which occurs typically by 18 months of age. Additionally, TcES generally should not be performed in the presence of a ventriculoperitoneal (VP) shunt or other intracranial hardware or in patients with poorly controlled seizures due to the slightly increased risk of seizures in certain patients with transcranial stimulation. Additionally, it may also be necessary to evaluate further the infant or child suspected of having other CNS or genetic disorders, which may interfere with the ability to perform NIOM or to obtain adequate responses. The usefulness of neurophysiological monitoring has been shown during complex spine procedures in cases of congenital deformities given the significant potential for neurological compromise. In these cases, monitoring with TcES occurs with comparison to baseline amplitude of ongoing motor potentials obtained during the surgery. TcES under general anesthesia during surgery requires the use of several pulses given as a train or multipulse stimulation in order to elicit a response in the peripheral muscle being recorded. Using TcES may result in modification of the surgical case especially when a greater than 50% decrement is seen in motor evoked potential (MEP) amplitude compared to baseline values. Modifying the surgery based on the neurophysiological monitoring can result in reduction in neurological weakness postoperatively (5).

Brainstem Auditory Evoked Responses

Brainstem auditory evoked responses (BAERs) involve an acoustic stimulus and recording of several waveforms (I–V are typically used in clinical practice) recorded from the scalp. Each waveform has several generators, but for clinical purposes, each is predominately attributed to a specific anatomic source allowing for reasonable interpretation of findings. Because myelination is not complete at a younger age, these waveforms do not reach adult values until approximately age 3 years. Intraoperatively, this may not be significant as long as the waveform is recordable; then subsequent recording will be compared to that baseline value. In cases of Arnold Chiari 2, malformation repair with decompression brainstem auditory monitoring may be useful (6), and in some neurophysiology reports, the use of the blink reflex is considered useful for monitoring as well (7).

Cortical Stimulation

In clinical settings in which epilepsy surgery and brain mapping is needed, higher-intensity stimulation protocols than those in adults will likely be needed in pediatric patients in order to identify the eloquent cortex. For the same reasons outlined earlier when using TcES on a young patient, cortical stimulation requires higher stimulation parameters due to lack of complete myelination of cortical tracts in this age group.

EMG Monitoring

Electromyogram (EMG) monitoring can be done with different approaches. One method is monitoring of evoked muscle responses during surgical manipulation in order to identify whether the surgical manipulation is too close in proximity to neural tissue. The other method is one in which a stimulus evoked response is given in order to elicit a muscle response. In order for reliable monitoring of EMG signals during NIOM, it is imperative that no neuromuscular blockade be given. Most anesthetic agents can be used safely; however, propofol has been reported to cause the development of intense muscle spasms during selective dorsal rhizotomy (SDR) procedures.

Selective Dorsal Rhizotomy

More commonly in pediatric patients, a procedure referred to as selective dorsal rhizotomy (SDR) is utilized in cases of spasticity nonresponsive to medical management and often in the case of spastic cerebral palsy. At spinal levels L2 to S2, the surgeon divides each dorsal root into individual rootlets followed by selective stimulation of each rootlet in sequence. Neurophysiologic monitoring is performed so that as each rootlet is stimulated, the response can be graded as to the degree of abnormality seen both clinically and by EMG recording. Depending on the degree of abnormality, the surgeon will selectively sever dorsal rootlets in order to decrease facilitatory afferent input. SDR partially removes sensory input so the degree of motor tone is reduced but the patient is not left hypotonic.

Pedicle Screw Placement

Another situation in which EMG monitoring is utilized in pediatric patients involves scoliosis repair typically involving spinal fusion along with pedicle screw placement. In this situation, EMG is recorded from muscles innervated at the levels in which the pedicle screws are placed. The presence of an EMG response or compound muscle action potential (CMAP) after stimulation of the pedicle screw indicates that a breach within the pedicle wall is present and readjustment of the pedicle screw is needed. An intact pedicle wall should not allow the production of a CMAP after stimulation of the screw.

EMG recording from muscles of the lower limbs and anal sphincter may be useful in cases of tethered cord repair and can be used along with SEP recording of the lower limbs.

Tumor Resection

Additionally, EMG monitoring with free-run EMG recording or after nerve stimulation may be used in cases in which cranial or peripheral nerves are at risk of injury such as with tumor resection. In these cases, avoidance of neuromuscular blockade and anesthetic considerations as in other situations in a pediatric patient are needed. In these situations, recording of EMG activity indicates to the surgical team that their surgical interventions are in close proximity to or risking the integrity of neural tissue and that adjusting surgical exploration or resection away from that area would avoid neural injury.

EEG Monitoring

Pediatric AVM

Endovascular treatment of pediatric arteriovenous malformations (AVM) can incorporate multimodality monitoring using SSEPs, brainstem auditory evoked potentials (BAEPs), MEPs, electroencephalography (EEG), and in some cases EMG in order to monitor and help localize motor cranial nerves and nuclei. Intra-arterial amobarbital sodium injection of a feeding vessel is done prior to embolization of that vessel, and if this injection results in a significant change in the evoked potentials (EPs), EEG, or the patient's physical examination, then a different vessel is instead evaluated for embolization. The assumption is that the change in EPs or EEG occurred after testing because that vessel was likely supplying normal brain and should not be embolized (8).

Pediatric Moyamoya Disease

Pediatric Moyamoya disease is a progressive occlusive disease involving the terminal internal carotid artery (ICA) but can be extensive and involve the proximal middle cerebral artery, anterior cerebral artery, and posterior cerebral artery resulting in cerebral ischemia. There may be enlargement of perforating vessels in the basal ganglia in order to compensate for the occlusive disease.

In order to increase cerebral blood flow, revascularization is done most commonly by anastomosing the superior temporal artery to a branch of the middle cerebral artery. During this revascularization procedure, there is significant risk of cerebral ischemia; so multimodality monitoring with EEG and SSEPs can be utilized to assess cortical function during the anastomosis and allow for surgical modifications if needed (8). In the very young patient, EEG patterns vary in regard to rate and amplitude compared to adult patients. In recanalization procedures, the ongoing EEG is compared to the patient's own baseline intraoperative study for detection of any changes.

Congenital Cardiac Disease

Congenital cardiac disease is a leading cause of mortality in the pediatric population. The incidence of congenital heart defects is 2% to 10% per 1,000 live births. Despite the advancements in technique, congenital heart disease still remains the leading cause of death in all patients with congenital defects and responsible for 10% to 60% rate of neurological compromise during cardiac surgery (9). Cardiopulmonary bypass surgery (CPB) utilizing intraoperative EEG recording along with other measures of functional status have demonstrated usefulness in improving neurological outcomes. EEG is a useful monitoring modality; as it is a sensitive measure of the effects of cerebral blood flow, it can be applied noninvasively and continuously recorded. This appears to be supported by a study by Kimatian and colleagues (10). Their evidence suggested that the addition of NIOM to EEG was associated with a significant change in the intraoperative management of pediatric patients on CPB. Their findings indicated that increases to the use of donor blood were made during the surgery in order to maintain a higher hematocrit level during the bypass period, and this decision was based upon the neurophysiological data. They also noted improvements in postoperative neurologic function with these higher hematocrit levels. Higher hematocrit levels between 25% and 35% have been shown to be associated with improvements in neurological development at 1 year in infants after CPB. The researchers indicated that there were behavioral changes in the surgical team as a result of the NIOM monitoring with a lower tolerance for maintaining a low hematocrit and greater likelihood of using donor blood in these infants during CPB.

Pediatric patients undergoing NIOM require changes to anesthetic technique and in some cases, techniques used for neurophysiologic monitoring as well. Additionally, the clinical scenarios may be particular to their age of onset. In all cases, the goals of NIOM are to reduce the risk of neurological complications and permanent neurological deficit. Selecting the appropriate monitoring modalities, and in many cases multimodality monitoring, is necessary in order to most effectively monitor the neural pathways at risk of injury and prevent neurological compromise.

REFERENCES

1. Francis L, Mohamed M, Patino M, et al. Intraoperative Neuromonitoring in Pediatric Surgery. *Int Anesthesiol Clin.* 2012;50(4):130–143.
2. Mittnacht AJ, Rodriguez-Diaz C. Multimodal neuromonitoring in pediatric cardiac anesthesia. *Ann Card Anaesth.* 2014;17(1):25–32.
3. Emerson R. NIOM for spinal deformity surgery: there's more than one way to skin a cat. *J Clin Neurophysiol.* 2012;29:149–150.
4. Cheng J, Ivan M, Stapleton C, et al. Intraoperative changes in transcranial motor evoked potentials and somatosensory evoked potentials predicting outcome in children with intramedullary spinal cord tumors. *J Neurosurg Pediatr.* 2014;13:591–599.
5. Fulkerson D, Satyan K, Wilder L, et al. Intraoperative monitoring of motor evoked potentials in very young children. *J Neurosurg Pediatr.* 2011;7(4):331–337.
6. Zamel K, Galloway G, Kosnik E, et al. Intraoperative neurophysiologic monitoring in 80 patients with Chiari I malformation: role of duraplasty. *J Clin Neurophysiol.* 2009;26:70–75.
7. Vidmer S, Sergio C, Veronica S, et al. The neurophysiological balance in Chiari type 1 malformation (CM1), tethered cord and related syndromes. *Neurol Sci.* 2011;32(Suppl 3):S311–S316.
8. Lopez J. Neurophysiologic intraoperative monitoring of pediatric cerebrovascular surgery. *J Clin Neurophysiol.* 2009;26:85–94.
9. Jaggers J, Shearer I, Ross M. Cardiopulmonary bypass in infants and children. In: *Cardiopulmonary Bypass Principles and Practice.* Philadelphia, PA; Lippincott Williams & Wilkins; 2000.
10. Kimatian S, Saliba K, Soler X, et al. The influence of neurophysiologic monitoring on the management of pediatric cardiopulmonary bypass. *ASAIO J.* 2008;54:467–469.

Evoked Potentials in Pediatric Brainstem Lesions

Ze Dong Jiang, MD

The human brainstem consists of the midbrain, pons, and medulla, contains 9 of the 12 cranial nerves, and is crossed by the ascending, descending, and cerebellar pathways and their nuclei as well as the reticular formation. Lesions in the brainstem may affect auditory and somatosensory pathways. Evoked potentials (EPs) or evoked responses (ERs) are electrical potentials recorded from the nervous system after the presentation of sensory stimuli. EPs are small electrical events arising from neural tissue and occurring in response to abrupt sensory stimulation. Auditory and somatosensory (and visual) stimuli are the methods of stimulation used commonly for clinical evoked potential studies. They consist of a series of waves that reflect the sequential activation of neural structures along the sensory pathways.

In current clinical application, there are two main types of sensory EPs used to assess the functional status of the brainstem. These are short-latency or brainstem auditory evoked responses (BAERs) and the short-latency somatosensory evoked potentials (SSEPs). BAERs and SSEPs provide sensitive measures of the central conduction functions of the auditory and somatosensory input systems at different levels of the central nervous system (CNS). BAER is the major objective test used in the detection of intrinsic or extrinsic lesions of the brainstem and play a major role in the testing of hearing. SSEPs have the capacity to evaluate both the peripheral nervous system and CNS from the distal peripheral nerves to the sensory cortex. The other important sensory potentials are visual evoked potentials (VEPs) that are often used in ophthalmologic assessment. In clinical application, evaluation with EPs are often less costly than other evaluation techniques such as MRI.

BAERs are also referred to as brainstem auditory evoked potentials (BAEPs) or auditory brainstem responses (ABRs). The responses have been widely used in pediatric, particularly neonatal, neurology to study and assess the hearing or auditory function and neuropathology that may involve the brainstem auditory pathway (1–3). Following brief acoustic stimuli (usually broadband clicks), the brainstem responses are detected by averaging the electroencephalogram (EEG) immediately after each of several thousand stimuli. The submicrovolt deflections in a recorded BAER occur in the first 10 minutes after the stimuli. The first wave component (wave I) in a BAER waveform recorded in normal adults occurs within 2 minutes after acoustic stimuli, with a cochlear microphonic and subsequent compound action potential from the auditory nerve. The following BAER components (waves II to V) occur within the first 7 to 9 minutes in adults and are of brainstem origin. Although the exact generators of the BAERs are not precisely localized, in general, the waveforms in clinical use are attributed to distinct brainstem regions for applicable purposes of interpretation. Wave III is thought to be of lower pontine generation, and wave V is thought in general to have lower midbrain generation (Figure 12.1). Wave I is a near-field response (meaning that the source of generation is close to the site of recording) and is recorded at the ear or mastoid electrode and generated by the peripheral nervous system. All the following waves are far-field responses (generated far from site of recording), generated

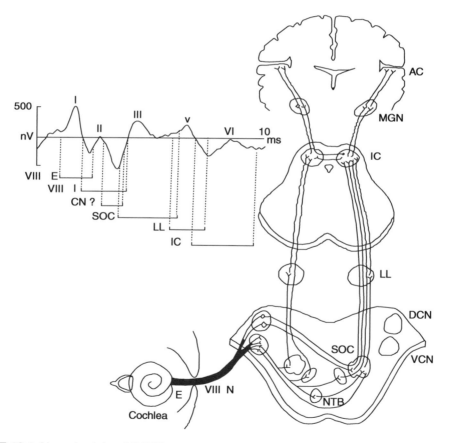

FIGURE 12.1 Neural origin of BAER components.

Abbreviations: VIII N, auditory nerve; AC, auditory cortex; BAER, brainstem auditory evoked response; DCN, dorsal cochlear nucleus; E, extracranial; I, intracranial; IC, inferior colliculus; LL, lateral lemniscus; MGN, medial geniculate nucleus; NTB, trapezoid body; SOC, superior olivary complex; VCN, ventral cochlear nucleus.

in the brainstem but recorded at the scalp. Because of the immaturity of the brainstem auditory pathway, the latencies of BAER wave components in infants are longer than in adults, while the amplitudes are generally smaller than in adults. After birth, over time, BAER wave latencies and interpeak intervals are shortened or decreased while wave amplitudes are increased. This maturational process continues until early childhood.

One important advantage of BAERs is that they are unaffected by sleep state or sedation. This has led to a wide interest in using BAERs in pediatric audiology and neurology to assess the functional status or integrity of both peripheral and central, specifically brainstem, auditory pathways (1–3). In addition to assessing auditory function, the BAERs have been extended to quantitatively evaluate neural integrity and maturation of the immature brainstem and detect brainstem lesions in many pathological conditions that affect the brainstem auditory pathway. More recently, the maximum length sequence (MLS) has been introduced in pediatric neurology to record and analyze BAERs. This relatively new technique, which can exert a more stressful physiological/temporal challenge to brainstem auditory neurons, has been documented to improve the detection of brainstem lesions in pediatric, particularly neonatal, neuropathology (1,2,4).

SSEPs are also used to evaluate brainstem function. They can be elicited by mechanical stimulation, but in clinical application, SSEPs are elicited by electrical stimulation of peripheral nerves, which produces larger and more robust responses than mechanical stimulation. The stimulation sites typically used for clinical diagnostic SSEP studies are the median nerve at the wrist, the common peroneal nerve at the knee, and/or the posterior tibial nerve at the ankle. Recording of the SSEPs to stimulation of the ulnar nerve at the wrist is useful for intraoperative monitoring when the midcervical spinal cord or parts of the brachial plexus are at risk. Recording electrodes are placed over the scalp, spine, and peripheral nerves proximal to the stimulation site. The series of waves generated in a SSEP waveform reflect the sequential activation of neural structures along the somatosensory pathways. SSEPs are used for clinical diagnosis in patients with various neurologic diseases that affect the somatosensory pathways and for intraoperative monitoring during surgeries that place parts of the somatosensory pathways at risk. An abnormal SSEP can result from dysfunction at the level of the peripheral nerve, plexus, spinal root, spinal cord, brainstem, thalamocortical projections, or primary somatosensory cortex. The SSEP components generated in the brainstem and in the cerebral cortex are mediated entirely by the dorsal columns (posterior columns) of the spinal cord, the fasciculus cuneatus for upper limb SSEPs and the fasciculus gracilis for lower limb SSEPs. Lesioning of the dorsal columns of the spinal cord rostral to the root levels where the afferent somatosensory activity enters the spinal cord abolishes the SSEPs generated in the brain. However, the SSEPs can persist, following lesions of the anterolateral spinal cord. Diseases of the dorsal columns in which joint position sense and proprioception are impaired are invariably associated with an abnormal SSEP.

The latencies of SSEP components are, in general, shorter in infants and children than in adults and change progressively with growth and maturation. The latency changes predominantly reflect linear growth with elongation of the peripheral nerves and central somatosensory pathways. These effects are counterbalanced partially by myelination and increase in fiber diameters, which produce faster conduction velocities, and partially by maturation of synaptic transmission. The latter effects operate until age 6 to 8 years, at which time central conduction times (CCTs) have reached adult levels, and further latency changes are due to changes in stature.

SSEP test is an accurate clinical tool to measure somatosensory conduction. The findings can inform us about the presence and extent of a particular disease or injury that affects the somatosensory nerve system. It can be used to monitor the progression of neurological disease and neuropathology, and a patient's status during surgery near the spinal cord or in the intensive care unit in cases of brain injury. SSEPs are also a valuable electrophysiological tool to evaluate brainstem lesions that affect the somatosensory pathway in the brainstem.

The advance of sophisticated neuroradiologic imaging has had a great impact on the clinical use of EPs, with fewer diagnostic EP studies performed than in the pre-MRI and early MRI era. Nevertheless, EPs remain valuable as electrophysiological diagnostic measures in many clinical situations. Among the EPs, BAERs are most affected by brainstem lesions. Over the last three decades, BAERs have been the focus of noninvasive electrophysiological examinations of the functional integrity of the brainstem in pediatric neurology. Compared with SSEPs, VEPs, and the long- and middle-latency auditory evoked potentials (LAEPs and MAEPs), BAERs are simpler to record and are unaffected by sleep state or sedation, which makes the responses particularly suitable for use in very young infants and sick children. Numerous clinical studies have documented that BAERs are an important tool and adjunct to detect neuropathology that involves the brainstem auditory pathway in a wide range of pediatric and neonatal diseases. This chapter is mainly focused on the clinical application of BAERs in the diagnosis and management of brainstem lesions in some common pediatric, particularly neonatal, problems.

TECHNICAL FACTORS IN THE ASSESSMENT OF BAERS

Click Intensity and Repetition Rate

For the purpose of neurologic assessment, it is crucial to clearly and reliably identify wave I in the recorded BAER waveforms, which will allow accurate calculation of I-III interpeak interval and I-V interpeak interval—the so-called brainstem conduction time (BCT) and the most important and commonly used BAER variable to reflect brainstem function. Wave I can be enhanced by changing the stimulus parameters (eg, increasing stimulus intensity, decreasing stimulus repetition rate), using an ear canal or tympanic electrode or transtympanic electrocochleography (ECochG). In patients with peripheral auditory deficits, the simple way to enhance wave I is to increase stimulus intensity. For infants with a BAER threshold within the normal range (≤20 dB nHL), the intensity of click stimuli used to elicit conventional BAERs is usually between 70 and 80 dB nHL. For infants with a BAER threshold greater than 20 dB nHL, the intensity of clicks should be increased as appropriate in order to collect a well-formed BAER waveform.

For MLS BAER testing, the click repetition rates used are much higher than those used in conventional BAER, ie, the BAERs obtained using conventional averaging methods. This results in an increased perception of loudness of the stimulus trains due to temporal integration. Therefore, the click intensity should be relatively lower than that used in conventional BAER. A click intensity level at 45 to 55 dB above the BAER threshold of each subject is usually the best method to obtain a satisfactory MLS BAER waveform, with well-formed waves I, III, and V. Thus, 60 or 65 dB nHL is usually best for infants with a normal BAER threshold (≤20 dB nHL) (1,4). For infants with a BAER threshold greater than 20 dB nHL, the intensity of clicks should be increased to at least greater than 40 dB above the threshold of each individual infant. This will ensure BAER waves I, III, and V to be clearly identified in the recorded waveforms. For infants with a threshold greater than 45 dB nHL, however, it is often difficult to obtain well-formed and reliable waves I, III, and V at any high click intensities. For group comparison, it is important to ensure that there is no significant difference between groups in the click intensity level above the threshold of individual subjects in order to compensate for individual differences in hearing sensation and for the influence of sensation level on wave latencies, amplitudes, and interpeak intervals.

In some clinical situations, infants with neuropathology that affects the brainstem auditory pathway may not show any apparent BAER abnormalities at conventionally used repetition rates of clicks, eg, 11/sec or 21/sec. Increasing the stimulus rate could be a useful "stimulus challenge test" to improve the detection of some neuropathology that may not be shown by the BAERs recorded with relatively slow stimulus rates (1,4). However, a significant increase in click rate, eg, 91/sec, in conventional BAERs can degrade the recorded BAER waveform morphology, and, in turn, can cause difficulty in accurate and reliable identification and measurement of BAER wave components.

MLS Technique

The MLS is a relatively new technique to record and analyze BAERs (1,2,4–10). It can exert a more stressful physiological/temporal challenge to brainstem auditory neurons, thus potentially improving the detection of neuropathology that may not be detected by conventional BAERs (1,4). The MLS technique allows the presentation of stimuli at much higher rates (up to 1,000/sec or even higher) than is possible with conventional averaging methods. Since the higher rates provide a much stronger temporal/physiological challenge to auditory neurons and permit a more exhaustive sampling of physiological recovery or "fatigue" than is possible with conventional stimulation, this technique can potentially enhance the sensitivity of BAERs in the diagnosis of neuropathological conditions. In the past decade, MLS has been documented to be a valuable technique to enhance the diagnostic value of BAERs, particularly for some early or subtle neuropathology, which may not be detected by conventional examination and investigations (1,4,6–16).

The repetition rates of clicks for eliciting MLS BAERs are usually 91/sec, 227/sec, 455/sec, and 910/sec (1,4). Jiang proposed that in terms of detecting neuropathology that involves the brainstem auditory pathway, MLS BAER abnormalities are better detected with high-rate stimulation, typically 455/sec and 910/sec. The highest rate of 910/sec is very "stressful." However, this rate can cause some alteration in the elicited MLS BAER waveform, which may result in difficulty in accurate and reliable identification and measurement of waves I and V. The rate 455/sec usually elicits well-formed MLS BAER waveforms, and appears to be "stressful" enough for the brainstem auditory neuron as to significantly enhance the detection of neuropathology. Therefore, 455/sec is the preferred rate of the four click repetition rates for clinical application (1). Due to temporal integration, the perception of loudness of the stimulus trains increases as the repetition rate is increased. Thus, a click intensity of 80 dB nHL or higher is intolerable for subjects with normal hearing. Even 70 dB nHL tends to be too loud for some subjects, particularly when the test is of a long duration (2,6). In addition, at such high click intensities, the recorded MLS BAER waveforms are often distorted or deteriorated.

Measurement of BAER Variables

The schematic measurement of various BAER components in children and adults is shown in Figure 12.2. Usually, the major point on a wave component that produces the greatest amplitude

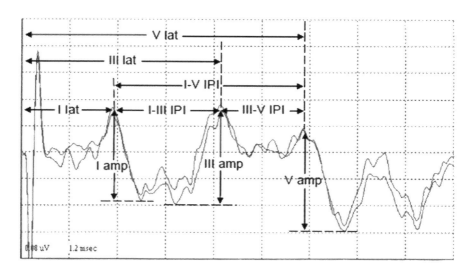

FIGURE 12.2 Measurement of (MLS) BAER wave components in children.

Abbreviations: amp, amplitude; BAER, brainstem auditory evoked response; IPI, interpeak interval; lat, latency; MLS, maximum length sequence.

is selected as the peak of the wave. In some recordings, the top portion of a BAER wave is rounded or consists of a couple of small peaks, and there is no sharp peak of maximum amplitude that can be picked as the wave peak. A general solution is to extend lines from the two slopes of the wave component to a point where the two lines intersect. This point is then taken as the peak of the wave. There are several other methods to pick the peak, but all have certain limitations. The selection of methods is largely dependent on the particular waveform.

The latency of a BAER wave is the time interval between the onset of the stimulus presentation and the appearance of a wave peak in the waveform. There are three major BAER wave latencies (wave I, III, and V latencies). Interpeak interval is the relative measure calculated as the time between the peaks of two different BAER waves. There are three interpeak intervals, including I-V, I-III, and III-V, and an interval ratio of III-V over I-III intervals (ie, III-V/I-III interval ratio) to reflect the relative changes in the two small intervals. The amplitude of a BAER wave is the measurement of the voltage difference between the peak and the preceding or following trough of a wave. The amplitude of wave I is measured from the positive peak of wave I to the negative trough immediately after the peak. Since the trough after wave III is considerably variable, it is not reliable to use the trough to measure the amplitude of wave III. Instead, the amplitude is measured between the peak of wave III and the immediate preceding trough of wave III. The amplitude of wave V is measured from the positive peak of wave V to the major negative trough immediately after the peak. With the amplitudes of BAER waves I, III, and V, relative amplitude ratios (ie, V/I and V/III amplitude ratios) are then calculated to reflect the relative changes in these amplitudes. In newborns and young infants, there is often considerable variation in the amplitude of wave I, which in turn significantly affects the reliability of the diagnostic value of the V/I amplitude ratio (13). To minimize this variation, the amplitude of wave I in young infants is measured from its peak to the lowest trough between waves I and III. The amplitude of wave III in young infants is measured from the peak of wave III to the lowest trough between waves I and III (1,13).

BAER Abnormalities in Brainstem Lesions

In brainstem lesions, the typical BAER abnormality is an abnormal increase in I-V interpeak interval, along with an increase in wave V latency. Intervals I-III and/or III-V may also be increased, depending on the location of the lesion in the brainstem and the nature of the pathology. For instance, wave V latency and I-V interval were found to be significantly increased in both infants with chronic lung disease (CLD) and infants after perinatal asphyxia (14). CLD infants showed a significant increase in the III-V interval but a generally normal I-III interval at all click rates, whereas infants after asphyxia showed a significant increase in both III-V and I-III intervals. Interval I-III was shorter and the III-V/I-III interval ratio was greater in CLD infants than in asphyxiated infants. Thus, CLD infants had a major increase in the more central BAER component (III-V interval), with no appreciable increase in the more peripheral component (I-III interval). In contrast, asphyxiated infants had a significant increase in both central and peripheral components (I-III and III-V intervals). These differences indicate that neonatal CLD affects the central regions of the brainstem more, whereas perinatal asphyxia affects both peripheral and central regions. This difference is likely related to the difference in the nature of pathology between CLD and asphyxia (14,15).

Compared with BAER wave latencies and interpeak intervals, the amplitudes of BAER wave components have a relatively large intersubject variability. Nevertheless, under well-controlled and consistent testing conditions, the amplitudes of BAER waves, particularly wave V, are useful variables to reflect the functional status of brainstem auditory neurons (17–22). The amplitudes can be reduced in some brainstem lesions, but not in others. For instance, the amplitude of BAER wave V was significantly reduced in perinatal asphyxia, but not in neonatal CLD, suggesting that there is major neuronal impairment in the auditory brainstem in asphyxia but not in CLD (13,19). This difference may be, at least partly, related to the difference in the nature of hypoxia associated with the two problems; the hypoxia in CLD is chronic and sublethal, which does not exert a major effect on brainstem neurons, but the hypoxia, which is associated with ischemia, in perinatal asphyxia is often acute and lethal and is detrimental to brainstem neurons.

HYPOXIC-ISCHEMIC ENCEPHALOPATHY

In infants with hypoxic-ischemic encephalopathy after perinatal asphyxia, lesions of the brainstem can be noted on MRI, with several distributive patterns of hypoxic-ischemic injury. There are often subtle but definite uniform symmetric brainstem lesions (23). Asphyxiated infants can manifest selective brainstem injury and exhibit palsy of the lower brainstem cranial nerves. Early histopathologic studies have shown that following perinatal asphyxia, or hypoxia-ischemia, there are discrete brainstem lesions involving auditory centers, including loss of neurons with gliosis or ischemic cell changes in the inferior colliculus and superior olivary complex (24). In fetal primates, asphyxic injury of the inferior colliculus was found to be one of the earliest effects of acute total asphyxia.

Since the late 1970s, BAERs have been used to examine functional impairment in the neonatal brainstem in infants after perinatal asphyxia. More recently, the responses have also been used to assess some therapeutic (eg, brain cooling) effect on the brainstem after hypoxia-ischemia (25). The BAER abnormalities in infants after hypoxia-ischemia include increased wave latencies and interpeak intervals, reduced wave amplitudes, and decreased V/I amplitude ratio, suggesting hypoxic-ischemic brainstem lesions (18,26). In conventional BAERs, a moderate increase in the click rate from 21/sec to 51/sec may not significantly improve the detection of BAER abnormalities, but a significant increase to 91/sec could (Figure 12.3) (26). In MLS BAER, the abnormalities are more pronounced at very high repetition rates (455/sec and 910/sec) than at lower rates (Figure 12.4) (6,7,13,27,28).

In term infants after hypoxia-ischemia, there are characteristically dynamic changes in the BAERs during the first month after birth, typically seen in the I-V interval (Figure 12.5). Jiang et al found that on the first day after birth, wave III and V latencies and I-V and III-V interpeak intervals are increased significantly, particularly at higher click rates (7,26). The abnormalities reach a peak on the third day after birth. Thereafter, the increased wave latencies and intervals recover progressively. These BAER variables approach normal values on day 15. By the end of the first month, the BAER abnormalities almost completely recover, although III–V and I–V intervals remain slightly increased (7,26). The dynamic changes, which are particularly obvious

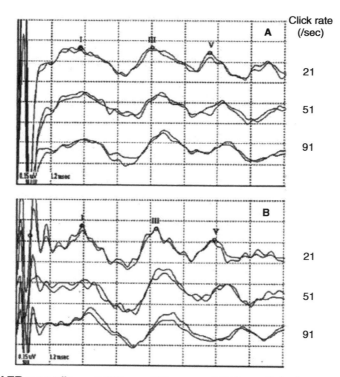

FIGURE 12.3 BAER recordings at 21/sec, 51/sec, and 91/sec clicks in a normal term infant (A) and an asphyxiated term infant (B). Wave latencies and intervals are increased, and wave V amplitude reduced, mainly at 91/sec, in infant B.

Abbreviation: BAER, brainstem auditory evoked response.

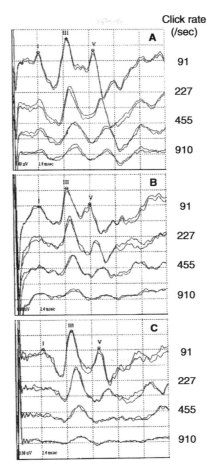

FIGURE 12.4 MLS BAER recordings made from a normal term infant (A) and two term infants after severe asphyxia (B and C) on day 3 after birth. Compared with normal infant A, the amplitudes of waves I, III, and V in infant B are all reduced at all click rates, particularly of wave V at high rates. In infant C, BAER wave latencies, intervals, and wave amplitudes are basically normal at 91/sec clicks. As click rate is increased, the latencies and intervals are increased, and the amplitudes of wave I and, particularly, of wave V are significantly reduced.

Abbreviations: BAER, brainstem auditory evoked response; MLS, maximum length sequence.

in MLS BAER, demonstrate a general trend of functional impairment of the neonatal brainstem after perinatal asphyxia, reflecting a specific time course of pathophysiological changes in the brainstem during the acute phase of hypoxic-ischemic brain damage (7). The impairment progresses shortly after birth, reaches a peak on the third day, and tends to recover progressively thereafter. The first week, particularly the first 3 days, is a critical period of hypoxic-ischemic brainstem damage. Two weeks after birth, the damage recovers significantly and largely returns to normal. By 1 month, the damage almost completely recovers in most cases.

This characteristic time course provides important information for studying and implementing any timing intervention or therapeutic measures to protect the neonatal brain and reduce further hypoxic-ischemic damage (7,26). The progression and deterioration of the abnormalities in BAERs during the first 3 days after birth indicate that early intervention during the critical first few days might prevent further hypoxic-ischemic brainstem damage or reduce the deterioration of damage. The time course could be used as a reference to monitor cerebral function, assess the responses of the brain to neuroprotective and/or therapeutic interventions, and help to judge the value of therapeutic interventions. The time course also provides a valuable time frame for recording BAERs in infants after perinatal hypoxia-ischemia. The first recording can be made on the first day after birth for the early detection of hypoxic-ischemic brain damage and for assessment of the severity of the damage. The second recording can be made at approximately day 3 to examine whether the damage has deteriorated or not. The third recording can be made on days 7 to 10 to assess any significant recovery. The fourth recording can be made at 1 month to examine whether the damage has largely resolved and the MLS BAER has returned to normal.

Figure 12.5 shows dynamic change in the I-V interval of MLS BAER during the first month after birth in a group of term infants after perinatal asphyxia (7). On day 1, the interval increased significantly at all repetition rates of clicks used (91–910/sec), especially the higher

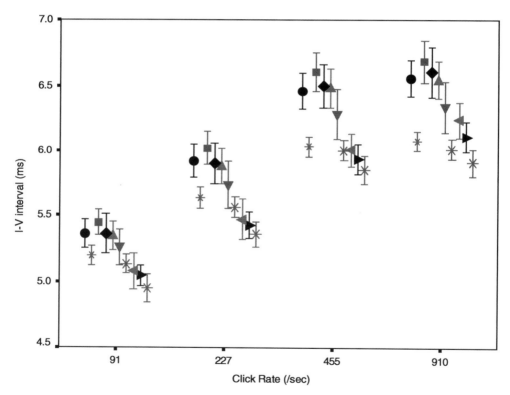

FIGURE 12.5 Means and standard errors of the I-V interval at different repetition rates of clicks (≥40 dB above BAER threshold) during the first month after birth in term infants after hypoxia-ischemia. The symbols in sequence from left to right represent the data of infants after hypoxia-ischemia on day 1, normal control infants on days 1 to 3, infants after hypoxia-ischemia on days 3, 5, 7, and 10, the control infants on days 10 to 15, infants after hypoxia-ischemia on days 15 and 30, and the controls on day 30.

Abbreviation: BAER, brainstem auditory evoked response.

rates. On day 3, all these latencies and intervals increased further and differed more significantly from the normal controls. Thereafter, the latencies and intervals decreased progressively. On day 7, wave V latency and all intervals still differed significantly from the controls. These dynamic changes were more significant at higher rates of clicks than at lower rates. On days 10 and 15, all intervals decreased significantly. On day 30, all wave latencies decreased to the values in the normal controls on the same day. The intervals also approached normal values, although III-V and I-V intervals still increased slightly. These dynamic changes demonstrate a general time course of brainstem pathophysiology after perinatal asphyxia; the hypoxic-ischemic brain damage persists during the first week, with a peak on day 3, and recovers progressively thereafter. By 1 month, the damage has largely resolved. The first week, particularly the first 3 days, is a critical period of hypoxic-ischemic brain damage, and early intervention may prevent or reduce deterioration of the damage.

There are limited reports that used SSEPs to assess perinatally hypoxic-ischemic brainstem lesions. Gibson et al. (1992) studied the median nerve SSEPs in 30 asphyxiated term infants over the course of their encephalopathy and until discharge (29). Three types of responses were noted: normal waveform, abnormal waveform, or absence of cortical response. During the follow up, nine infants died of their asphyxial illness and one of spinal muscular atrophy. Of the 20 survivors, 3 had cerebral palsy (CP), 4 had minor abnormalities, and 13 were neurodevelopmentally normal. The early SSEP results were closely correlated with the outcome. All 13 infants with normal outcome had normal SSEPs by 4 days of age, whereas those with abnormal or absent responses beyond 4 days had abnormal outcomes.

Using multimodality evoked potentials (MMEPs), Scalais et al. (1998) assessed cerebral function in 40 hypoxic-ischemic term or near-term neonates during the first week of life in order to predict the neurological outcome (30). A three-point grading system registered mild, moderate, or severe abnormalities in SSEPs, BAERs, and VEPs. At 24 months of corrected age, the infants were assessed with a blind protocol to determine neurological development. Grade 0 fVEPs and SSEPs were associated with a normal neurological status in 100% of the infants. Abnormal SSEPs or a total grade (VEPs + SSEPs) >1 were not associated with normal outcomes. Normal BAERs did not predict a normal outcome, but severely abnormal BAERs did predict an abnormal outcome. There was a significant correlation between EP (VEPs + SSEPs) grade, Sarnat stage, and clinical outcome. Compared with Sarnat scoring, both fVEPs and SSEPs are more accurate as prognostic indicators. EPs (VEPs + SSEPs) also are more accurate in predicting the ultimate neurological outcome.

The predictive value of early EP testing for neurodevelopmental outcome after perinatal asphyxia seems to be rather limited. Recently, Julkunen et al. (2014) studied SSEPs, BAERs, EEG, and Doppler in 30 asphyxiated term infants during the first 8 days (31). Cerebral blood flow velocities (CBFVs) were measured from the cerebral arteries using pulsed Doppler at 24 hours of age. EEG, EPs, Doppler findings, symptoms of hypoxic-ischemic encephalopathy, and their combination were evaluated in predicting a 1-year outcome. An abnormal EEG background predicted a poor outcome in the asphyxia group with a sensitivity of 67% and 81% specificity and an abnormal SSEP with 75% and 79%. Combining increased systolic CBFV with abnormal EEG or SSEP improved the specificity, but not the sensitivity. The predictive values of abnormal BAER and VEP results were poor. A normal EEG and SSEP predicted a good outcome in the asphyxia group with sensitivities from 79% to 81%. The combination of normal EEG, normal SSEP, and systolic CBFV less than 3 standard deviations (SD) predicted a good outcome with a sensitivity of 74% and 100% specificity. The authors concluded that combining abnormal EEG or EP findings with increased systolic CBFV did not improve prediction of a poor 1-year outcome in asphyxiated infants. A normal SSEP and normal EEG combined with systolic CBFV less than 3 SD at about 24 hours can be valuable in the prediction of normal 1-year outcome for term infants after asphyxia.

BILIRUBIN ENCEPHALOPATHY

Infants with bilirubin encephalopathy are lethargic, hypotonic, or hypertonic. They manifest a high-pitched cry, opisthotonus, seizures, and may even die. Patients surviving kernicterus have severe permanent neurologic symptoms (choreoathetosis, spasticity, hearing loss, ataxia, mental retardation). Less severe injury is associated with mild neurological abnormalities, including hearing loss. BAER has long been used as an important tool to study and evaluate bilirubin neurotoxicity in the brain and the auditory system and assess therapeutic (phototherapy and exchange transfusions) effect on the impaired brainstem and auditory function in neonatal hyperbilirubinemia (32–38). The majority of investigators found an increase in wave latencies and the I-V interval, although a few others reported no significant BAER abnormalities. In our BAER study of 90 term neonates with hyperbilirubinemia, 18% had an abnormal increase in the I-V interval, suggesting brainstem impairment (39). We further noticed that the increase is more significant in MLS BAERs than in conventional BAERs (Figure 12.6) (40). Both I-III and III-V intervals were increased significantly at higher rates of 455/sec and 910/sec. These BAER abnormalities were generally more significant at higher levels of total serum bilirubin

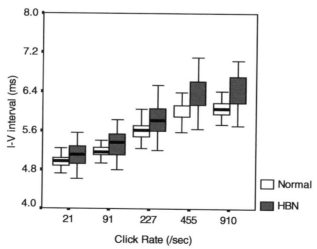

FIGURE 12.6 Boxplot of I-V interpeak intervals (bold line across the box, median; box, 25th and 75th centile; extensions, the largest and smallest values) at various click rates in neonates with HBN and age-matched normal controls. The I-V interval is longer in neonates with HBN than in age-matched normal controls at all click rates, which was particularly obvious at 455/sec and 910/sec.

Abbreviation: HBN, hyperbilirubinemia.

than at lower levels (Figure 12.7), suggesting that the severity of BAER abnormalities and, in turn, auditory brainstem impairment is related to, though not completely in parallel with, the severity of hyperbilirubinemia. In addition, BAER wave amplitudes in neonates with hyperbilirubinemia are often reduced, suggesting that brainstem auditory electrophysiology is depressed (20,41). These BAER abnormalities are valuable markers or indicators of bilirubin ototoxicity or neurotoxicity. The degrees of these abnormalities are correlated with the severity of neonatal hyperbilirubinemia, though they may not precisely indicate the severity. The neurotoxic effect of hyperbilirubinemia on the auditory system could be transient, provided prompt treatment is initiated. Following exchange transfusions, the BAER abnormalities in infants with severe hyperbilirubinemia usually promptly returns to normal or near normal (37,42,43). The prompt recovery of BAERs following the decrease in the level of blood bilirubin further indicates that BAER is a sensitive test to assess the neurotoxic effect of neonatal hyperbilirubinemia and provide a valuable guide for early recognition and close monitoring of bilirubin neurotoxicity.

There is controversy over the use of SSEPs in assessing bilirubin neurotoxicity, as the lemniscal pathways that generate the SSEPs are not involved in kernicterus. Silver et al. (1996) described postnatal development of SSEPs in Gunn rats and the effect of jaundice (44). They found no effect of jaundice on the SSEPs in young jaundiced (jj) rats (16–28 d). However, adult (3–4 months) jj rats had prolonged latencies and decreased amplitudes of the P2 component of the SSEPs compared with adult nonjaundiced (Jj) rats. These changes in the SSEPs of jaundiced rats may reflect a synaptic lesion in these animals, possibly due to cumulative and/or progressive damage induced by bilirubin during the first 3 months of life. After sulfadimethoxine administration, marked latency prolongations (2%–6%) were observed in the early components of SSEPs in young (3-wk-old) jj (but not Jj) rats, as early as 2 hours after injection. These changes, which

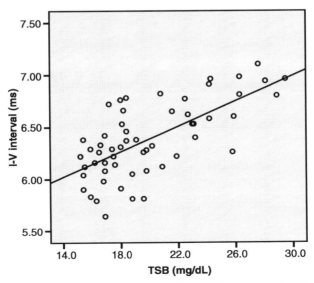

FIGURE 12.7 Scatterplot of the I-V interval at 455/sec, with regression line against TSB. The interval is increased with the increase in TSB level.

Abbreviation: TSB, total serum bilirubin.

became more severe (4%–10%) with time, seem to be mostly peripheral. It appears that the SSEP may be a sensitive marker for the massive entry of bilirubin into the nervous system and could serve as part of an evoked potential battery (in addition to VEPs and BAERs) in assessing bilirubin-induced neurotoxicity in jaundiced newborns and infants (44).

In 16- to 17-day-old jaundiced (jj) Gunn rats, Shapiro (2002) analyzed serial BAERs and SSEPs up to 8 hours after acute bilirubin toxicity (45). SSEPs to median nerve stimulation were recorded from surface electrodes over the brachial plexus (Erb's) and contralateral parietal cortex and subtracted to obtain CCT. No significant change was seen in CCT in the SSEPs, whereas the BAERs were significantly abnormal and even abolished in some rats. When the injection of sulfonamide induced significant peripheral and central BAER abnormalities in jaundiced rats, no SSEP abnormalities occurred. The authors concluded that the SSEPs can assess proprioception but not other somatosensory functions or sensory integration, and BAER findings can sensitively reflect selective acute bilirubin toxicity for the auditory brainstem.

BRONCHOPULMONARY DYSPLASIA

Neonatal CLD, particularly bronchopulmonary dysplasia (BPD)—a severe type of CLD, is a major lung disease and one of the greatest risk factors of neurologic impairment and developmental deficits in very preterm or very low-birth-weight infants (46,47). BAERs were not studied in neonatal CLD or BPD until recent years (14,15,19,48). In conventional BAERs, infants with neonatal CLD show an increase in wave V latency and in I–V and III–V interpeak intervals (Figure 12.8) (48). In MLS BAERs, although there are no major abnormalities in wave

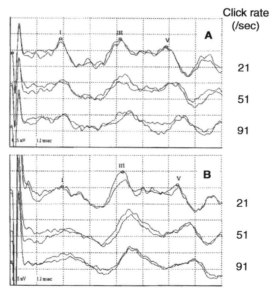

FIGURE 12.8 BAER recordings at term at different rates of clicks in a normal term infant (A, female) and a very preterm infant with neonatal CLD (B, female, 29-wk gestation). Compared to the recordings in the term infant, the very preterm infant with CLD shows an increase in wave V latency, I-V, and, particularly, III-V intervals at all the 21/sec, 51/sec, and 90/sec clicks, with no abnormality in the amplitudes of BAER waves I, III, and V at any click rates.

Abbreviations: BAER, brainstem auditory evoked response; CLD, chronic lung disease.

I and III latencies and I–III intervals, wave V latency, I–V and particularly III–V intervals, and III–V/I–III interval ratios are all increased significantly (Figures 12.9 and 12.10) (14,15). The fundamental abnormality is a significant increase in III-V interval, a BAER variable that reflects the functional status of the more central regions of the brainstem. These abnormal findings in BAER and particularly MLS BAER indicate that CLD or BPD exerts a major damage to myelination and synaptic function of the more central regions of the immature brainstem (14,15). On the other hand, peripheral neural function is relatively intact, suggesting normal neural conduction along the more peripheral or caudal regions of the brainstem. No major abnormality can be seen in the amplitudes of MLS BAER wave components (Figures 12.9 and 12.10). It appears that neonatal CLD or BPD does not cause any major damage to neuronal function. The abnormalities in CLD infants mostly resolve several weeks after term.

Jiang et al. found distinct differences in the BAER and MLS BAER abnormalities between neonatal CLD or BPD and perinatal asphyxia. In infants after asphyxia, there is a significant increase in both peripheral (I-III interval) and central (III-V interval) components of BAERs and MLS BAERs (Figure 12.10) (6,7,14,26). This indicates that perinatal asphyxia affects both the peripheral and central regions of the brainstem, whereas neonatal CLD or BPD affects the more central regions of the brainstem, with no significant effect on the peripheral regions (14,15,48). In addition, infants after perinatal asphyxia show significant reduction in the amplitude of wave V at higher rates of clicks. This suggests that there is also major neuronal impairment in the brainstem after asphyxia, in contrast to no major neuronal impairment in CLD or BPD (13,19).

BRAINSTEM GLIOMAS

Brainstem gliomas are tumors arising from glial cells and mostly seen in children or adolescents. The tumors account for approximately three-fourths of the brainstem tumors in children. They are highly invasive, infiltrating the brainstem, which often makes total surgical removal impossible. BAER test is a valuable neurodiagnostic method, particularly when auditory pathways are primarily involved and when diagnosis via neuroradiology or clinical findings is not conclusive. BAERs and SSEPs, as electrophysiological measures, provide information on the functional status of the CNS, specifically the brainstem, whereas CT and MRI, as conventional neuroradiology, shows the structure.

BAERs are useful in follow up of the effect of the preoperative chemotherapy or the progression of the inoperable tumors. BAERs also proved effective in the assessment of postoperative neurological complications. For example, bilateral symmetrical prolongation of interpeak intervals and wave V reduction occur in postoperative occlusive hydrocephalus, with clinical signs of increased intracranial pressure. Unilateral prolongation of interpeak intervals occurs during irradiation or chemotherapy after medulloblastoma removal as signs of cerebral edema.

From mid-1970s till late 1990s, there were a number of reports on BAERs and SSEPs in pediatric patients with brainstem tumors. When the lesion involved the pons, almost all cases showed abnormal BAERs. For example, Nodar et al. (1980) described BAERs in seven children (aged 2.5 to 13 years) with diagnosed brainstem neoplasms, including one with astroependymoma, one with medulloblastoma, one with intraparenchymal ependymoma, and two with glioma (49). No tumor type was specified for the other two patients. All children showed some of the following BAER abnormalities, including absolute wave latency, wave latency difference

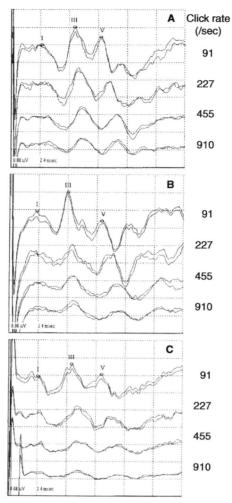

FIGURE 12.9 MLS BAER recordings from a normal control (A), an infant with CLD (B), and an infant after perinatal asphyxia (C). Compared to the control (A), the infant with CLD (B) shows a significant increase in I-V and, particularly, III-V intervals, but no major amplitude reduction for all waves I, III, and V; the infant after asphyxia (C), however, shows a significant increase in all I-V, I-III, and III-V intervals and a major amplitude reduction for all waves, particularly for wave V at very high rates (455/sec and 910/sec).

Abbreviations: BAER, brainstem auditory evoked response; CLD, chronic lung disease; MLS, maximum length sequence.

between ears, wave I-V interval, response stability, amplitude, morphology, and presence of waves. In each case, the BAER test results clearly indicated the site of the lesion as determined by CT and observation during surgery. In 14 children with clinical and radiological evidence of brainstem glioma, Weston et al. (1986) found that all with pontine involvement (13 of the 14) had abnormalities of wave V (delayed latency, reduced or absent amplitude) (50). BAER abnormalities were consistently found in the stimulus ear ipsilateral to the tumor, though they were not invariably related to tumor size. The findings were consistent with intrinsic brainstem

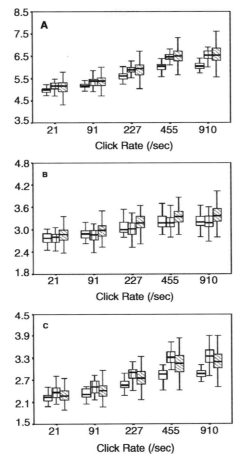

FIGURE 12.10 Boxplot of BAER interpeak intervals (bold line across the box, median; box, 25th and 75th centile; extensions, the largest and smallest values) at various click rates in normal term infants (A), infants with CLD (B), and infants after asphyxia (C). Interval I-V is similar in CLD infants and asphyxiated infants, although the interval in both groups is significantly longer than in normal controls (A). Interval I-III in asphyxiated infants is significantly longer than in CLD infants whose I-III interval is similar to that in normal controls at all click rates 21/sec to 910/sec (B). In contrast, the III-V interval in CLD infants is significantly longer than in asphyxiated infants at all click rates 21/sec to 910/sec, although the interval in both groups is significantly longer than in normal controls (C).

lesions in all except one case with a glioma, which was shown to be located predominantly in the medulla oblongata.

Rotteveel et al. (1985) reported their comprehensive clinical study of the contribution of SSEPs and BAERs in the primary diagnosis and follow-up of 26 children with infratentorial and supratentorial tumors (51). The 14 infratentorial tumors included six medulloblastomas (all but one in the fourth ventricle), four gliomas, two arachnoid sarcomas, two astrocytomas, and a ganglioneuroblastoma. The 12 supratentorial tumors were three craniopharyngiomas, three astrocytomas (grade I, II, and III) in different regions, an optic nerve astrocytoma, a lipoma, an ependymoma, a chromophobe adenoma, a germinoma, and an unspecified tumor in the left thalamus. Occasional BAER abnormalities in the supratentorial group were associated with brainstem dysfunction secondary to intracranial pressure effects (eg, compression of inferior colliculus). The majority of children in the infratentorial group had BAER abnormalities, including delayed interpeak intervals and total absence of waves. Abnormalities were not uncommon for BAERs elicited by stimulation of the ear contralateral to the tumor (pressure of effect). Tumors near the eighth nerve typically produced asymmetric findings, whereas symmetric findings were related to tumors in the midline fourth ventricle region. Serial BAERs had clinical value in documenting the progression of pathophysiologic changes, including development of hydrocephalus. The authors emphasize the clinical importance of BAERs by stating that large tumors are easy to detect, but removal surgically is difficult or impossible. With BAERs, it may be possible to detect small tumors in some cases, which permits effective surgical therapy. The BAERs were sensitive for supratentorial pressure effects and for local and distant posterior fossa tumor effects. The SSEPs, especially the specific complex, showed a latency increase in patients with supratentorial and brainstem mass lesions involving, directly or distantly, the somatosensory tracts. In the follow-up of children, EPs offer a good method of detecting tumor recurrence, whereas neuroradiological procedures may be obscured by surgical or radiation artifacts.

Fischer et al. (1982) summarized BAER findings for a group of 66 patients with various CNS tumors, including eight meningiomas, two fourth ventricle ependymomas, five cerebellar tumors, two third ventricle colloid cysts, a craniopharyngioma, a cyst, a pinealoma, an astrocytoma, a germinoma, and over 40 unspecified tumors involving the brainstem (52). The effect of posterior fossa meningiomas and cerebellar tumors on the BAERs depended on the size of the tumor and its location relative to auditory structures. CT information was generally more useful than BAERs in characterizing location and size. The authors stated that useful, and sometimes unique, diagnostic information was obtained from BAERs for 36 patients, including the evidence of a tumor by BAERs before CT scanning.

In 1997, Fukuda et al. described SSEPs elicited by median nerve stimulation in 17 patients with brainstem tumor (53). Of a total of 35 SSEP records in these patients, 13 had a normal CCT; eight, prolonged CCT; nine, abolished N20 potential; four, abolished N20 and N18 potentials; and one, abolished N20, N18, and P14 potentials. These SSEP groups were correlated with the size and location of the brainstem tumor on MRI. N20 potentials were unchanged in latency in patients with small localized gadolinium (Gd)-enhanced lesions, but were abolished in patients with tumors extending to the dorsal pons and the upper medulla oblongata. The extent of nonenhanced low-intensity lesions did not correlate with the changes in the N20 potentials. The degree of the impairment of the N20 potentials reflected the severity of the clinical symptoms. The N20 potential can evaluate brainstem dysfunction caused by brainstem tumor. In four patients whose extensive tumors (one Gd-enhanced lesion, three low-intensity lesions) involved not only the pons but also the medulla oblongata, the N18 potentials, probably generated from the medulla oblongata, were abolished.

SUPRATENTORIAL MASS LESIONS

Supratentorial mass lesions may produce neurological dysfunction by two mechanisms: cerebral hemispheric damage from the primary lesion itself and secondary brainstem damage from displacement, tissue compression, swelling, and vascular stasis. Early in 1980, MacKay et al.

(1980) conducted an animal experiment to examine BAER changes due to acutely expanding mass lesions (54). In anesthetized cats, after posterior fossa balloon catheters were inflated slowly, there were reliable BAER changes, which occurred before the Cushing response and were reversible by balloon deflation. Since BAER changes precede the agonal changes of the Cushing response, serial BAER recording in patients with known or suspected posterior fossa masses may be useful in the management of these lesions.

In 1993, Inao et al. quantitatively measured brainstem distortion and neural dysfunction in 25 cases of chronic subdural hematoma (55). The horizontal and rotational brainstem displacements were measured on axial and coronal MRI in all patients preoperatively, and BAERs were obtained in 11 cases. BAER wave latencies and I-V interpeak interval were increased, which was correlated with septum shift. The increased wave V latency indicated that brainstem rotation in the coronal plane reflects upper brainstem dysfunction most closely. The correlation between brainstem displacement shown on MRI and the increase in BAER wave latencies and I-V interval demonstrated a good relationship between anatomical and physiological changes in the brainstem that are associated with supratentorial lesions.

Krieger et al. (1993) examined the clinical relevance of BAERs, along with pupillary responses and intracranial pressure monitoring, in 55 comatose patients (9–70 years) with acute supratentorial mass lesions (56). BAERs were rated "bilaterally normal," "unilaterally abnormal," or "bilaterally abnormal." BAER categories correlated significantly with pupillary abnormalities and increased intracranial pressure but did not predict outcome. Increased intracranial pressure was associated with abnormalities in BAERs. The authors concluded that BAERs can be used to support the clinical relevance of abnormal pupillary status and increased intracranial pressure but have no prognostic value. Examination of BAERs, along with pupillary response and intracranial pressure monitoring, provides useful information for managing patients with supratentorial mass lesions.

Later, Krieger et al. (1995) examined the relevance of serial BAERs and SSEPs and clinical parameters (pupillary response and intracranial pressure) in patients with acute supratentorial mass lesions (57). BAER and SSEP results were ranked into three categories: (a) normal on both sides; (b) abnormal or absent on one side; and (c) EPs on both sides abnormal or absent. BAER results were correlated with intracranial pressure values during and at the termination of intracranial pressure therapy and with pupillary findings only at the time of termination of intracranial pressure therapy. No correlation was found between SSEPs and clinical parameters. Pupillary responses indicated a good or poor recovery during and at the termination of intracranial pressure therapy. BAERs and intracranial pressure values distinguished between good and poor outcome only at the termination of intracranial pressure therapy. SSEPs did not predict outcome. Thus, shortly after the manifestation of supratentorial mass lesions, the results of EPs and clinical parameters indicate increased intracranial pressure and incipient transtentorial herniation but do not predict sequelae. After institution of effective therapy, BAER and pupillary abnormalities are valuable prognostic predictors. In contrast, SSEPs reflect neither therapeutic efficacy nor outcome.

CEREBRAL PALSY (CP)

CP, a motor disease in children, is characterized by nonprogressive but varied neurologic deficits, including cerebellar ataxia, athetosis and spasticity, and sometimes associated neurologic disorders (epilepsy and mental retardation). CP is often associated with various adverse prenatal or perinatal risk factors, eg, asphyxia, extreme prematurity, retarded growth, viral infections in utero, and neonatal meningitis. The most common specific risk factor is cerebral anoxia-hypoxia occurring in utero, at delivery, or immediately following birth. It is important to realize, however, that most children with these risk factors do not have subsequent evidence of CP, and, conversely, most of the children with CP have had none of the risk factors.

As CP is a motor disease, normal findings would be expected for sensory EPs. However, abnormal BAER findings have been reported by some investigators (17,58,59). SSEPs (and VEPs) have also been studied by some investigators in children with CP and some abnormalities were found (60,61). Nevertheless, due to the lack of full cooperation by the children with CP during these tests, it is difficult to obtain reliable SSEP data and the results may vary considerably. By comparison, BAER testing does not necessarily require full cooperation of the subject, which makes it particularly suitable for children with CP who cannot fully cooperate with any test. Using BAERs, some investigators have devoted their studies to detect auditory and brainstem abnormalities or deficits in children with CP (17,58,59,62–64). These investigators have explored some BAER abnormalities in these children. Among the abnormalities, a major finding is an amplitude reduction in BAER late wave components (17,58,59). This interesting finding indicates that brainstem auditory electrophysiology is depressed in children with CP. The amplitude reduction is mainly seen in children who survived perinatal or postnatal asphyxia, though it is also seen in those who had other heterogeneous etiologies.

In children with CP, the BAER waveform, particularly the later components, tends to be depressed, which occurs in about 40% of the children (59). The main response abnormality is a significant reduction in the amplitude of wave V. On the other hand, abnormal findings in the interpeak intervals are rare. These findings are in contrast to common findings in the responses in infants and children with progressive neurologic abnormalities following conditions such as perinatal asphyxia and BPD, whereby the major BAER abnormality is a significant increase in I-V and, particularly, III-V intervals (1). Other abnormalities in children with CP include decreased V/I amplitude ratio, missing waves, prolonged I-V interval, and increased interaural difference in the I-V interval. These findings indicate that some children with CP have a depressed auditory electrophysiology, which may be due to decreased or altered neural firing or synchrony in the auditory brainstem. On the other hand, neural transmission along the auditory brainstem in CP is largely intact and rarely compromised, although it could be damaged at the active stages of original neuropathology such as perinatal asphyxia that results in CP. In infants after perinatal asphyxia, the amplitude reduction in wave V was persistent during the first month after birth. Therefore, the reduction appears to be persistent during the postnatal period in children who have CP. The persistent reduction in wave V amplitude in early life might be a valuable early indicator for developing CP later.

Jiang and Tierney (1996) found that in the majority of children who survive asphyxia, whether it occurred perinatally or postnatally, BAERs were normal, without any significant abnormality. However, a small proportion of the children had BAER abnormality, suggesting a residual brainstem lesion (17). The major abnormality was a reduction in wave V amplitude, followed by a decrease in the V/I amplitude ratio and a prolongation of the I-V interval. Missing waves were also seen in a few children. On the other hand, abnormalities in BAER wave latencies and interpeak intervals were rare. Amplitude reduction was less significant for BAER waves I and III, ie, waves prior to wave V. The abnormal BAER results or patterns could be categorized into five patterns, which are shown in Figure 12.11. The most frequently seen patterns were pattern A (combined wave V amplitude reduction and V/I amplitude ratio decrease) and pattern B (combined wave V amplitude reduction and/or V/I amplitude ratio decrease and I-V interval prolongation). Other abnormal patterns (C, D, and E) were relatively rare. Thus, the commonest BAER abnormality was the amplitude reduction in wave V, often accompanied by a decrease in V/I amplitude ratio or a prolongation in the I-V interval. The prevalence of prolonged I-V interval was less than half of the amplitude reduction in wave V. Apparently, perinatal and postnatal asphyxia can exert a long-term effect on the brainstem, resulting in residual neuronal dysfunction of the brainstem, evidenced by the significant reduction in wave V amplitude, but it does not appear to exert any major long-term effect on neuronal

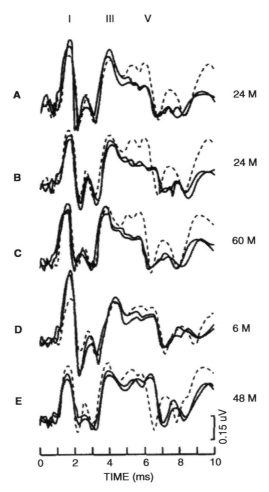

FIGURE 12.11 Abnormal patterns of the central BAER components in children who survive asphyxia. The dashed traces are the age-matched controls. (A) Combined wave V amplitude reduction and V/I amplitude ratio decrease. (B) Combined wave V amplitude reduction and/ or V/I amplitude ratio decrease and I-V interval prolongation. (C) Wave V amplitude reduction only. (D) V/I amplitude ratio decrease only. (E) I-V interval prolongation only.

transmission, evidenced by the normal I-V interval in most cases. These findings are quite different from those seen shortly after the episode of asphyxia where the major abnormality in BAER measures usually is a prolonged I-V interval, followed by reduced wave V amplitude and V/I amplitude ratio. The prolonged I-V interval seen in the acute phase of asphyxia recovers much faster than the reduced amplitude of wave V. It seems that asphyxia is unlikely to exert any major long-term effect on nerve conduction and synaptic transmission or myelination in the brainstem.

Following perinatal asphyxia, there are discrete brainstem lesions involving auditory centers, including loss of neurons with gliosis or ischemic cell changes in the inferior colliculus and superior olivary complex (24). The major underlying mechanism for the persistent reduction of wave V amplitude is most likely to be fewer generating neurons and/or fewer fibers conducting the volley in the generators of the BAER wave V following hypoxic-ischemic insults to the brainstem. Wave V originates in the high pons or low midbrain. Compared to the earlier BAER waves I to IV, wave V has its origin in the most rostral part of the auditory brainstem. The persistent reduction of wave V amplitude in children with CP after asphyxia suggests that compared to the more caudal regions, the lesion in the rostral regions of the brainstem is more profound and/or that the recovery of the damaged neurons in the rostral brainstem is more incomplete or retarded.

OTHER DISORDERS

There are a number of other pediatric disorders that may directly or indirectly involve the brainstem, resulting in abnormalities in EPs, particularly BAERs. These include infections and inflammatory diseases (eg, meningitis, brain abscesses, viral infections, Kawasaki disease, fungal infections), neurodevelopmental disorders (eg, hydrocephalus, myelomeningocele and Arnold-Chiari malformation, autism), metabolic diseases (eg, storage diseases, phenylketonuria, diabetes mellitus, maple syrup urine disease, mitochondrial encephalomyopathies), degenerative diseases (eg, sclerosing panencephalitis, hereditary motor sensory neuropathy [Dejerine-Sottas disease]). In the following text are two samples of storage diseases: Leigh's syndrome and Gaucher's disease.

Leigh's Syndrome

Mitochondrial disorders are a varied collection of progressive diseases that have in common morphological, biochemical, and/or genetic abnormalities of the mitochondria. Features include the accumulation of mitochondria and metabolic disorders. Among the others, Leigh's syndrome (a subacute necrotizing encephalopathy that can affect the brainstem tegmentum) has been widely studied with BAERs (65–69). The responses are often markedly abnormal, including prolonged wave latencies and interpeak intervals. Sakai et al. (2004) reported two sisters (age 4 and 11 years) with Leigh's syndrome with a T8993G point mutation of mitochondrial DNA (67). Clinical medical findings included low-density areas in the basal ganglia and posterior limb of the internal capsule by CT, high levels of lactate and pyruvate in the spinal fluid, muscle weakness, ataxia, retinitis pigmentosa, epileptic seizures, and mental retardation. The children were referred to the authors because they responded poorly to sounds. The older sister yielded essentially normal BAER findings. Hearing sensitivity, however, progressively worsened in the younger sister, associated with delayed BAER latencies. BAER threshold fluctuated remarkably during a 3-year follow-up, suggesting that her hearing problems may well have been caused by both cochlear nerves and retrocochlear or brainstem lesions.

In 1993, Yoshinaga et al. described a case of a 7-month-old girl with Leigh's syndrome diagnosed with neurophysiologic, radiologic, enzymatic, biochemical, and molecular studies (68). Over time, the patient developed additional clinical symptoms of brainstem dysfunction (irregular respiration and dysphagia), hypotonia, and then seizures and tonic spasms. Blood analysis showed elevated levels of lactate and pyruvate and a mitochondrial DNA point mutation at 8993 in the patient and the mother. BAER abnormalities were among the first clinical signs found in this patient. Later in 2003, to assess the utility of BAERs in diagnosing brainstem changes in patients with Leigh's syndrome, Yoshinaga et al. performed a longitudinal study of five patients with Leigh's syndrome using both BAER and neuroimaging techniques (CT and MRI; 69). The brainstem components of the initial BAERs were abnormal in all five patients. In four patients, these abnormal findings preceded any clinical signs of brainstem impairment. Improvements in clinical findings were reflected in improvements in BAER findings in three patients. In one of these three patients, improvements in clinical findings were also reflected in improvements in MRI findings. In the other two patients, MRI findings showed no improvements, despite the improvements in clinical findings. In two of the patients, BAERs clearly revealed functional improvements in the brainstem, which were not revealed by MRI. Therefore, BAERs are an essential diagnostic technique for patients with Leigh's syndrome.

With SSEPs and BAERs, Araki et al. (1997) evaluated brainstem dysfunction in a girl with Leigh's syndrome (65). Serial analysis of BAERs and SSEPs showed progressive disturbances of the brainstem wave components. The authors also performed neuroradiological and other neurophysiological tests, including brain MRI, single-photon emission computed tomography, electrically elicited blink reflexes, and all-night polysomnography and detected many abnormalities. They concluded that the multimodality tests in combination with neuroradiologic examinations are useful for assessing brainstem dysfunction in patients with Leigh's syndrome.

Gaucher's Disease

This is a rare lipid storage disease due to an enzyme deficiency and the accumulation of ganglioside (cerebroside) in the nervous system as well as the viscera (liver, spleen, lungs). There is diffuse neuronal damage and progressive and marked CNS dysfunction (eg, muscle paralysis), which usually commences at 6 months of life. The infants often die at 1 year. The patients show gross BAER abnormalities (70–74). Kaga et al. (1982) recorded serial BAERs from an infant with Gaucher's disease (72). The disease started at 3 months. The infant first showed stridor, strabismus, failure to thrive, and inguinal hernia, and then muscular rigidity, ocular palsies, and respiratory failure. The initial BAER recordings at 6 months revealed a prolongation or increase in the latencies of waves I, II and III, and disappearance of waves after wave IV. Subsequent BAER recordings at 8 months showed that these wave latencies became further prolonged and wave components after wave III disappeared as neurologic status deteriorated. He died of respiratory failure due to central origin developed. In autopsy, there was no obvious structural damage in the auditory brainstem, suggesting that metabolic and electrophysiologic changes precede histopathologic changes. In a later study, Kaga et al. (1998) correlated abnormal BAER findings (only wave I and wave II were recorded) with neuropathology (73). An autopsy revealed there were Gaucher's cells in the cerebrum and thalamus, dorsal brainstem gliosis, and pathologic cells in the superior olivary complex with marked gliosis in the cochlear nucleus.

In eight children with type III Gaucher's disease, Campbell et al. (2003) found a diverse collection of BAER abnormalities, including absence of all waves except wave I (a common pattern) and delays in later waves (III and V; 70). The abnormalities progressively deteriorated, reflecting underlying subclinical brainstem deterioration. To detect early subclinical nervous dysfunction in Gaucher's disease type 1, Perretti et al. (2005) examined multimodality EPs in 17 patients with the disease. Five patients (31.2%) showed clear BAER abnormalities, the most frequent abnormality being a bilateral increased I-III interpeak latency (75). SSEP abnormalities were seen in three patients (18.7%), including an increased N13-N20 interval in two patients and an irreproducible N13 wave in one patient. In addition, the authors found a delayed latency of the P100 wave in VEPs in four patients (25%), and the central motor evoked potential was abnormal in nine patients (69.2%). The multimodal evoked potential approach provides information about nervous subclinical damage in Gaucher's disease type 1 and helps early detection of subclinical neurologic dysfunction.

CONCLUSION

Lesions in the human brainstem may affect the auditory and somatosensory pathways. BAERs and SSEPs are the two main types of ERs to evaluate the functional status of the auditory and somatosensory input systems at different levels of the CNS. In clinical application, evaluation with the two methods are often less costly than other evaluation techniques such as MRI. BAERs are the most commonly used electrophysiological test to detect intrinsic or extrinsic lesions of the brainstem and has been widely used in pediatric, particularly neonatal, clinics. The BAERs are unaffected by sleep state or sedation. This significant advantage has led to the wide use of BAERs in pediatric neurology to assess the functional integrity of the brainstem and detect brainstem lesions in many pathological conditions that affect the brainstem auditory pathway. SSEPs are useful for clinical diagnosis of brainstem lesions in patients with various neurologic diseases that affect the somatosensory pathways in the brainstem. The SSEP components generated in the brainstem are mediated entirely by the dorsal columns (posterior columns) of the spinal cord, the fasciculus cuneatus for upper limb SSEPs and the fasciculus gracilis for lower limb SSEPs. Diseases of the dorsal columns in which joint position sense and proprioception are impaired are invariably associated with an abnormal SSEP.

Among the EPs, BAERs are most affected by brainstem lesions. Over the last three decades, BAERs have been the focus of noninvasive electrophysiological examinations of the functional integrity of the brainstem in pediatric neurology. Compared with SSEPs (and other evoked potentials, eg, VEPs), BAERs are simpler to record and are unaffected by sleep state or sedation. These advantages make BAERs particularly suitable for use in very young infants and sick children. Numerous clinical studies have documented that BAERs are an important tool and adjunct to assess and detect neuropathology that involves the brainstem auditory pathway in a wide range of pediatric diseases. As a relatively new technique, the MLS BAER has recently been introduced in pediatric, particularly neonatal, neurology. There is increasing evidence suggesting that the MLS is a promising technique to enhance the diagnostic value of BAERs for brainstem lesions in pediatric neuropathology and to provide valuable information for the clinical management of brainstem lesions. In terms of simplicity of clinical application, conventional BAERs remain a very useful test for pediatric brainstem lesions, whereas MLS BAER is recommended to enhance the detection of some early or subtle neuropathology that may not be detected with conventional BAERs (1,4). More clinical studies of MLS BAER are warranted in a wide range of pediatric diseases that may result in brainstem lesions.

REFERENCES

1. Jiang ZD. Brainstem auditory evoked response in neonatal brain damage. *Curr Trends Neurol.* 2013;7:1–14.
2. Wilkinson AR, Jiang ZD. Brainstem auditory evoked response in neonatal neurology. *Semin Fet Neonatol Med.* 2006;11:444–451.
3. Hall III JW. ABR: Pediatric clinical application and populations. In: Hall III JW, ed. *New Handbook of Auditory Evoked Responses.* Boston, MA: Pearson Education; 2007:313–365.
4. Jiang ZD. Maximum length sequence technique improves detection of brainstem abnormalities in infants. In: Lawson PN, McCarthy EA, eds. *Pediatric Neurology.* New York, NY: Nova Science Publishers; 2012:1–38.
5. Jirsa RE. Maximum length sequences-auditory brainstem responses from children with auditory processing disorders. *J Am Acad Audiol.* 2001;12:155–164.
6. Jiang ZD, Brosi DM, Shao XM, Wilkinson AR. Maximum length sequence brainstem auditory evoked response in term infants after perinatal hypoxia-ischaemia. *Pediatr Res.* 2000;48:639–645.
7. Jiang ZD, Brosi DM, Wang J, et al. Time course of brainstem pathophysiology during first month in term infants after perinatal asphyxia, revealed by MLS BAER latencies and intervals. *Pediatr Res.* 2003;54:680–687.
8. Jiang ZD. Neural conduction impairment in the auditory brainstem and the prevalence in term babies in intensive care unit. *Clin Neurophysiol.* 2015;126:1446–1452.
9. Lasky RE, Perlman J, Hecox K. Maximum length sequence auditory evoked brainstem responses in human newborns and adults. *J Am Acad Audiol.* 1992;3:383–389.
10. Picton TW, Champagne SC, Kellett AJC. Human auditory potentials recorded using maximum length sequences. *Electroencephalogr Clin Neurophysiol.* 1992;84:90–100.
11. Jiang ZD, Brosi DM, Li ZH, et al. Brainstem auditory function at term in preterm babies with and without perinatal complications. *Pediatr Res.* 2005;58:1164–1169.
12. Jiang ZD, Xu X, Brosi DM, et al. Sub-optimal function of the auditory brainstem in term neonates with transient low Apgar scores. *Clin Neurophysiol.* 2007;118:1088–1096.
13. Jiang ZD, Brosi DM, Shao XM, Wilkinson AR. Sustained depression of brainstem auditory electrophysiology during the first month in term infants after perinatal asphyxia. *Clin Neurophysiol.* 2008;119:1496–1505.
14. Jiang ZD, Brosi DM, Wilkinson AR. Differences in impaired brainstem conduction between neonatal chronic lung disease and perinatal asphyxia. *Clin Neurophysiol.* 2010;121:725–733.
15. Wilkinson AR, Brosi DM, Jiang ZD. Functional impairment of the brainstem in infants with bronchopulmonary dysplasia. *Pediatrics.* 2007;120:362–371.
16. Jiang ZD, Wang C, Chen C. Neonatal necrotizing enterocolitis adversely affects neural conduction of the rostral brainstem in preterm babies. *Clin Neurophysiol.* 2014;125:2277–2285.
17. Jiang ZD, Tierney TS. Long-term effect of perinatal and postnatal asphyxia on developing human auditory brainstem responses: brainstem impairment. *Int J Pediatr Otorhinolaryngol.* 1996;34:111–127.
18. Jiang ZD, Brosi DM, Wilkinson AR. Comparison of brainstem auditory evoked responses recorded at different presentation rates of clicks in term neonates after asphyxia. *Acta Paediatr.* 2001;90:1416–1420.
19. Jiang ZD, Brosi DM, Chen C, Wilkinson AR. Brainstem auditory response amplitudes in neonatal chronic lung disease and differences from perinatal asphyxia. *Clin Neurophysiol.* 2009;120:967–973.
20. Jiang ZD, Brosi DM, Wilkinson AR. Changes in BAER wave amplitudes in relation to total serum bilirubin level in term neonates. *Eur J Pediatr.* 2009;168:1243–1250.
21. Jiang ZD, Wu YY, Liu XY, Wilkinson AR. Depressed brainstem auditory function in children with cerebral palsy. *J Child Neurol.* 2011;26:272–278.

22. Jiang ZD, Zhou Y, Yin R, Wilkinson AR. Amplitude reduction in brainstem auditory response in term infants under neonatal intensive care. *Clin Neurophysiol.* 2013;124:1470–1476.

23. Sugama S, Eto Y. Brainstem lesions in children with perinatal brain injury. *Pediatr Neurol.* 2003;28:212–215.

24. Leech RW, Alvord EC Jr. Anoxic-ischemic encephalopathy in the human neonatal period: the significance of brain stem involvement. *Arch Neurol.* 1977;34:109–113.

25. Mietzsch U, Parikh NA, Williams AL, et al. Effects of hypoxic-ischemic encephalopathy and whole-body hypothermia on neonatal auditory function: a pilot study. *Am J Perinatol.* 2008;25:435–441.

26. Jiang ZD, Yin R, Shao XM, Wilkinson AR. Brainstem auditory impairment during the neonatal period in infants after asphyxia: dynamic changes in brainstem auditory evoked responses to clicks of different rates. *Clin Neurophysiol.* 2004;115:1605–1615.

27. Jiang ZD, Brosi DM, Wilkinson AR. Impairment of perinatal hypoxia-ischaemia to the preterm brainstem. *J Neurolog Sci.* 2009;287:172–177.

28. Jiang ZD, Brosi DM, Wilkinson AR. Depressed brainstem auditory electrophysiology in preterm infants after perinatal hypoxia-ischemia. *J Neurolog Sci.* 2009;281:28–33.

29. Gibson NA, Graham M, Levene MI. Somatosensory evoked potentials and outcome in perinatal asphyxia. *Arch Dis Child.* 1992;67:393–398.

30. Scalais E, François-Adant A, Nuttin C, et al. Multimodality evoked potentials as a prognostic tool in term asphyxiated newborns. *Electroencephalogr Clin Neurophysiol.* 1998;108:199–207.

31. Julkunen MK, Himanen SL, Eriksson K, et al. EEG, evoked potentials and pulsed Doppler in asphyxiated term infants. *Clin Neurophysiol.* 2014;125:1757–1763.

32. Ahlfors CE, Parker AE. Unbound bilirubin concentration is associated with abnormal automated auditory brainstem response for jaundiced newborns. *Pediatrics.* 2008;121:976–978.

33. Ahlfors CE, Amin SB, Parker AE. Unbound bilirubin predicts abnormal automated auditory brainstem response in a diverse newborn population. *J Perinatol.* 2009;29:305–309.

34. Amin SB, Ahlfors C, Orlando MS, et al. Bilirubin and serial auditory brainstem responses in premature infants. *Pediatrics.* 2001;107:664–670.

35. Funato M, Tamai H, Shimada S, Nakamura H. Vigintiphobia, unbound bilirubin, and auditory brainstem responses. *Pediatrics.* 1994;93:50–53.

36. Funato M, Teraoka S, Tamai H, Shimida S. Follow-up study of auditory brainstem responses in hyperbilirubinemic newborns treated with exchange transfusion. *Acta Paediatr Jpn.* 1996;38:17–21.

37. Hung K L. Auditory brainstem responses in patients with neonatal hyperbilirubinaemia and bilirubin encephalopathy. *Brain Dev.* 1989;11;297–301.

38. Wennberg RP, Ahlfors CE, Bickers R, et al. Abnormal auditory brainstem response in a newborn infant with hyperbilirubinemia: Improvement with exchange transfusion. *J Pediatr.* 1982;100:624–626.

39. Jiang ZD, Liu TT, Chen C, Wilkinson AR. Changes in BAER wave latencies in term neonates with hyperbilirubinaemia. *Pediatr Neurol.* 2007;37:35–41.

40. Jiang ZD, Wilkinson AR. Brainstem auditory impairment in term neonates with hyperbilirubinemia. *Brain Dev.* 2014;36:212–218.

41. Jiang ZD, Liu TT, Chen C. Brainstem auditory electrophysiology is supressed in term neonates with hyperbilirubinemia. *Eur J Paediatr Neurolog.* 2014; 18:193–200.

42. Yilmaz Y, Degirmenci S, Akdas F, et al. Prognostic value of auditory brainstem response for neurologic outcome in patients with neonatal indirect hyperbilirubinemia. *J Child Neurol.* 2001;16:772–775.

43. Wong V, Chen WX, Wong KY. Short- and long-term outcome of severe neonatal nonhemolytic hyperbilirubinemia. *J Child Neurol.* 2006;21:309–315.

44. Silver S, Sohmer H, Kapitulnik J. Postnatal development of somatosensory evoked potential in jaundiced Gunn rats and effects of sulfadimethoxine administration. *Pediatr Res.* 1996;40:209–214.

45. Shapiro SM. Somatosensory and brainstem auditory evoked potentials in the Gunn rat model of acute bilirubinneurotoxicity. *Pediatr Res.* 2002;52:844–849.

46. Baraldi E, Filippone M. Chronic lung disease after premature birth. *N Engl J Med.* 2007;357:1946–1955.

47. Cristea AI, Carroll AE, Davis SD, et al. Outcomes of children with severe bronchopulmonary dysplasia who were ventilator dependent at home. et al. 2013;132:e727–e734.

48. Jiang ZD, Brosi DM, Wilkinson AR. Brainstem auditory function in very preterm infants with chronic lung disease: delayed neural conduction. *Clin Neurophysiol.* 2006;117:1551–1559.

49. Nodar RH, Hahn J, Levine HL. Brain stem auditory evoked potentials in determining site of lesion of brain stem gliomas in children. *Laryngoscope.* 1980;90:258–266.

50. Weston PF, Manson JI, Abbott KJ. Auditory brainstem-evoked response in childhood brainstem glioma. *Childs Nerv Syst.* 1986;2:301–305.
51. Rotteveel JJ, Colon EJ, Hombergen G, Stoelinga GB, Lippens R. The application of evoked potentials in the diagnosis and follow-up of children with intracranial tumors. *Childs Nerv Syst.* 1985;1:172–178.
52. Fischer C, Mauguière F, Echallier JF, Courjon J. Contribution of brainstem auditory evoked potentials to diagnosis of tumors and vascular diseases. *Adv Neurol.* 1982;32:177–185.
53. Fukuda M, Kameyama S, Honda Y, et al. Short-latency somatosensory evoked potentials in patients with brain stem tumor: study of N20 and N18 potentials. *Neurol Med Chir (Tokyo).* 1997;37:525–531.
54. MacKay AR, Hosobuchi Y, Williston JS, Jewett D. Brain stem auditory evoked response and brain stem compression. *Neurosurgery.* 1980;6:632–638.
55. Inao S, Kuchiwaki H, Kanaiwa H, et al. Magnetic resonance imaging assessment of brainstem distortion associated with a supratentorial mass. *J Neurol Neurosurg Psychiatry.* 1993;56:280–285.
56. Krieger D, Adams HP, Schwarz S, et al. Prognostic and clinical relevance of pupillary responses, intracranial pressure monitoring, and brainstem auditory evoked potentials in comatose patients with acute supratentorial mass lesions. *Crit Care Med.* 1993;21:1944–1950.
57. Krieger D, Jauss M, Schwarz S, Hacke W. Serial somatosensory and brainstem auditory evoked potentials in monitoring of acute supratentorial mass lesions. *Crit Care Med.* 1995;23:1123–1131.
58. Jiang ZD, Liu XY, Shi BP, et al. Brainstem auditory outcome and correlation with neurodevelopment after perinatal asphyxia. *Pediatr Neurol.* 2008;39:189–195.
59. Jiang ZD, Wu YY, Liu XY, Wilkinson AR. Depressed brainstem auditory function in children with cerebral palsy. *J Child Neurol.* 2011;26:272–278.
60. Ghasia F, Brunstom J, Tychsen L. Visual acuity and visually evoked responses in children with cerebral palsy: Gross Motor Function Classification Scale. *Br J Ophthalmol.* 2009;93:1068–1072.
61. Suppiej A, Cappellari A, Franzoi M, et al. Bilateral loss of cortical somatosensory evoked potential at birth predicts cerebral palsy in term and near-term newborns. *Early Hum Dev.* 2010;86:93–98.
62. Kaga K, Ichimura K, Kitazumi E, et al. Auditory brainstem responses in infants and children with anoxic brain damage due to near-suffocation or near-drowning. *Int J Pediatr Otorhinolaryngol.* 1996;36:231–239.
63. Zafeiriou DI, Andreou A, Karasavidou K. Utility of brainstem auditory evoked potentials in children with spastic cerebral palsy. *Acta Paediatr.* 2000;89:194–197.
64. Zhang L, Jiang ZD. Development of the brainstem auditory pathway in low birthweight and perinatally asphyxiated children with neurological sequelae. *Early Hum Dev.* 1992;30:61–73.
65. Araki S, Hayashi M, Yasaka A, Maruki K. Electrophysiological brainstem dysfunction in a child with Leigh disease. *Pediatr Neurol.* 1997;16:329–333.
66. Kaga M, Naitoh H, Nihei K. Auditory brainstem response in Leigh's syndrome. *Acta Paediatr Jpn.* 1987;29:254–260.
67. Sakai Y, Kaga K, Kodama K, et al. Hearing evaluation in two sisters with a T8993G point mutation of mitochondrial DNA. *Int J Pediatr Otorhinolaryngol.* 2004;68:1115–1119.
68. Yoshinaga H, Ogino T, Ohtahara S, et al. A T-to-G mutation at nucleotide pair 8993 in mitochondrial DNA in a patient with Leigh's syndrome. *J Child Neurol.* 1993;8:129–133.
69. Yoshinaga H, Ogino T, Endo F, et al. Longitudinal study of auditory brainstem response in leigh syndrome. *Neuropediatrics.* 2003;34:81–86.
70. Campbell PE, Harris CM, Harris CM, et al. A model of neuronopathic Gaucher disease. *J Inherit Metab Dis.* 2003;26:629–639.
71. Campbell PE, Harris CM, Vellodi A. Deterioration of the auditory brainstem response in children with type 3 Gaucher disease. *Neurology.* 2004;63:385–387.
72. Kaga M, Azuma C, Imamura T, et al. Auditory brainstem response (ABR) in infantile Gaucher's disease. *Neuropediatrics.* 1982;13:207–210.
73. Kaga K, Ono M, Yakumaru K, et al. Brainstem pathology of infantile Gaucher's disease with only wave I and II of auditory brainstem response. *J Laryngol Otol.* 1998;112:1069–1073.
74. Lacey DJ, Terplan K. Correlating auditory evoked and brainstem histologic abnormalities in infantile Gaucher's disease. *Neurology.* 1984;34:539–541.
75. Perretti A, Parenti G, Balbi P, et al. Study of multimodal evoked potentials in patients with type 1 Gaucher's disease. *J Child Neurol.* 2005;20:124–128.

Evoked Potentials in Adolescent Idiopathic Scoliosis: Intraoperative Neurophysiological Monitoring

Ronald G. Emerson, MD

Surgical correction of scoliosis entails the risk of neurological injury. The risk varies with etiology, nature of the curve, and the type of procedure. For adolescent idiopathic scoliosis (AIS), the overall risk of neurological injury is under 0.5%; it is higher when accompanied by hyperkyphosis, a Cobb's angle over 90°, or involves a combined anterior/posterior surgical procedure or revision surgery (1–3). Scoliosis of other etiologies, for example, congenital scoliosis and neuromuscular scoliosis also carry greater risks (4).

Intraoperative neurophysiological monitoring (IONM) has been effective in reducing the risk of neurological injury during spinal deformity surgery by quickly detecting incipient injury and allowing the surgeon and anesthesiologist to take appropriate measures. The Therapeutics and Technology Assessment Subcommittee of the American Academy of Neurology and the American Clinical Neurophysiology Society have affirmed the ability of IONM, with somatosensory evoked potentials (SSEPs) and motor evoked potentials (MEPs), to effectively predict adverse neurological outcomes (5). Early on, Nuwer (6) demonstrated that monitoring of SSEPs during scoliosis surgery was accompanied by a nearly three-fold reduction in the rate of persistent severe postoperative neurological deficits.

SSEP was initially proposed as a monitor of spinal cord function during spinal surgery in 1977 (7). By 1991, SSEPs were recognized as superior to the wake-up test for detection of spinal cord injury during scoliosis surgery (8); a series of 1,168 cases at Royal Orthopedic Hospital, Forbes (8), encountered no false-negatives and suggested that SSEP monitoring was more sensitive than, and should replace, the wake-up test. Nuwer's 1995 multicenter study of over 51,000 monitored cases of scoliosis surgery confirmed the very low (0.063%) false-negative rate of SSEP monitoring.

Occasional false-negatives have occurred, and will occur, during spinal cord monitoring based on SSEPs alone. This happens for two reasons: (a) SSEPs are mediated by the dorsal columns of the spinal cord; SSEP monitoring directly reflects their integrity. SSEPs monitor the function of other pathways, including motor pathways, only indirectly. Ischemia, compression, and blunt trauma generally affect spinal cord function widely, allowing the SSEP to function as an effective surrogate for "global" cord function (9–13). This relationship, however, can fail, causing SSEPs to inadequately detect injury to spinal motor pathways (14). (b) SSEPs can, at times, be difficult to monitor reliably for a variety of reasons, including electrical interference, electromyogram (EMG) artifact, anesthetic effects, and as a consequence of baseline pathology. First described in 1980 by Merton and Morton (15), MEPs are now employed routinely, along with SSEPs, for monitoring spinal cord integrity during scoliosis surgery. The concurrent use of both techniques allows detection of injury confined to either motor or sensory pathways. In addition, they provide an important level of safety through redundancy, should one or the other monitoring modality fail. They also provide complementary information, as they may be differentially affected by, for example, anesthetic agents and blood loss, and can respond with different sensitivity and speed to intraoperative spinal cord injury.

SOMATOSENSORY EVOKED POTENTIALS

Physiological Basis

SSEPs are recorded by stimulating a peripheral nerve, usually the posterior tibial or peroneal nerve for lower extremity (LE) SSEPs and the median or ulnar nerve for upper extremity (UE) SSEPs, and recording over the scalp using electrode derivations designed to selectively record signals generated in the brainstem and in the primary sensory cortex. Cortical SSEPs are acquired using bipolar scalp-to-scalp derivations, whereas brainstem SSEPs are recorded using scalp-to-noncephalic derivations. It is helpful to record both brainstem and cortical SSEP signals because while each can serve as a monitor of dorsal column function, anesthetic agents and electrical interference in the operating room (OR) affect the two classes of signals differently. Cortical SSEPs are relatively resistant to muscle noise and electrical artifacts but can be suppressed by anesthetic agents. Brainstem SSEPs are much more susceptible to electrical noise and EMG artifact, but they are largely unaffected by anesthetic drugs.

Brainstem Signals

Brainstem SSEPs to UE and LE stimulation are quite similar (Figure 13.1), differing largely by latency, which reflects the length of the afferent pathway. SSEPs consist of a positivity, reflecting activity in the caudal medial lemniscus, followed by a longer-duration negativity (P14 and N18 for UE SSEPs, P31 and N34 for LE SSEPs) (16–18). Brainstem SSEP signals are conducted electrically through the brain and cerebrospinal fluid (CSF) to the scalp; they project over the entire scalp, and thus are easily recorded by any scalp electrode referred to any noncephalic electrode.

In the OR, a cervical reference electrode is commonly used for recording brainstem SSEPs. The recorded signal is often called a "cervical" response, reflecting the common misconception that the cervical electrode is the principal "active" electrode in the scalp-cervical pair.

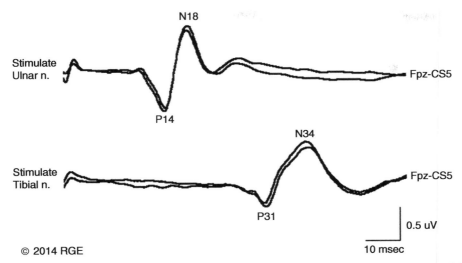

© 2014 RGE

FIGURE 13.1 Upper and lower extremity brainstem somatosensory evoked potentials, recorded from Fpz to a noncephalic reference. The responses are similar in appearance and consist of a positivity (P14 and P31) generated in the caudal medial lemniscus, followed by a negativity (N18 and N34), reflecting synaptic activity in the rostral brainstem.

While for UE SSEPs, an electrode over the lower cervical spine can add a postsynaptic cervical contribution (19), for LE SSEPs, the cervical electrode serves only as an "inactive' noncephalic reference.

Cortical Signals

The scalp topography and polarity of the cortical components of UE and LE SSEPs differ, in part, because of the different locations of the hand and foot regions of the homunculus on the lateral hemispheric convexity and within the interhemispheric fissure, respectively. Cortical activation following median or ulnar nerve stimulation produces a negativity (N20) over the contralateral centroparietal scalp, overlying the hand area. UE SSEPs are recorded from an electrode on the contralateral centroparietal scalp (CPc) referred to a similarly positioned ipsilateral electrode (CPi). This arrangement allows for electronic removal of the underlying brainstem signals, detected by both electrodes, and recording of the cortical signal in isolation (16) (Figure 13.2). CPc-CPz may offer superior performance in the OR (20); the CPz reference provides for similar subtraction of underlying brainstem signals but with lower noise due to the shorter interelectrode distance. CPz-Fz is another commonly employed alternative. In this derivation, N20 signal amplitude may be enhanced by an approximately synchronous positivity often registered by the Fz electrode; in some patients, however, Fz may also introduce "noise" in the form of frontally maximal anesthetic-induced EEG activity (20).

The situation for LE SSEPs is more complicated because the cortical location of the foot area varies considerably between people, from deep within the hemispheric fissure in some to near to the top of the fissure in others. In the former case, the LE cortical SSEP consists of a negativity (N38) over the contralateral hemisphere and a (approximately) simultaneous positivity (P38) over the ipsilateral hemisphere. In the latter situation, only a positivity (P38)

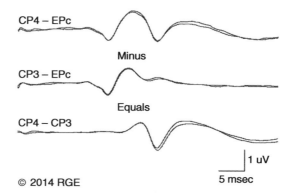

FIGURE 13.2 Left ulnar nerve somatosensory evoked potential (SSEP), recorded referential and bipolar derivations. The bipolar derivation (CP4-CP3) records the cortical SSEP in isolation, by electronically subtracting the brainstem potential (CP3-EPc) from the composite cortical *plus* brainstem potential (CP4-EPc).

is recorded at the vertex (21). LE SSEP scalp topographies of most individuals fall between these two extremes. For this reason, two or more channels are usually devoted to recording LE cortical SSEPs. For standard laboratory recordings, Cz-Fpz and Ci-Fpz are commonly used, selected to ensure detection of the P38 in each of its two extreme positions (Figure 13.3). In the OR, MacDonald observed that optimal recordings are often obtained using Cz-CPc or

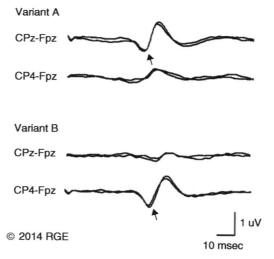

FIGURE 13.3 Two normal topographic variants of the P38 cortical somatosensory evoked potential (SSEP) following right tibial nerve stimulation. In variant A, a prominent positivity is recorded at the vertex, and very little is recorded over the lateral scalp; in variant B, a prominent positivity is recorded over the scalp *ipsilateral* to the stimulated limb and very little is recorded at the vertex. In the latter case, an approximately synchronous negativity (N38) is often recorded over the contralateral *centroparietal* scalp (not shown).

CPZ-CPc derivations. These derivations tend to produce high signal-to-noise ratio recordings because they employ short interelectrode distances, do not use a frontal reference, and often combine contributions from both the P38 and N38 signals (22).

Distal Monitors

The adequacy of peripheral nerve stimulation is confirmed by recordings of the afferent volley, from Erb's point for UE SSEPs and in the popliteal fossa for tibial nerve LE SSEPs. While SSEPs can be recorded from the lumbar spine, reflecting postsynaptic activity in the lumbar enlargement of the spinal cord (N22) (23), and are important for outpatient diagnostic testing, they are not generally used for intraoperative monitoring.

Monitoring Setup

Both UE and LE SSEPs are usually monitored during scoliosis surgery. Since the region of spinal cord at risk is usually below the cervical cord, UE SSEPs function as "systemic" controls, that is, reflecting the effects of anesthesia, hypotension, or hypovolemia, rather than surgically related injury. On occasion, the cervical cord may be within the region at risk, for example, in patients with coexistent cervical cord abnormalities (24) or when orthopedic instrumentation extends to the cervical spine. Additionally, UE SSEPs are effective for detection of brachial plexus injury related to surgical positioning (25,26).

Stimulation

Either surface disk electrodes or subdermal needle electrodes may be used for stimulation. For longer cases, needle electrodes tend to be more reliable; for patients with large circumference extremities, needle electrodes may be necessary for effective stimulation. For UE SSEPs, either median or ulnar nerve SSEPs may be recorded. Median SSEPs generally provide higher-amplitude, more robust signals for monitoring. Ulnar SSEPs can be sensitive to cervical cord injury below C6 that would go undetected by median SSEPs as well as to positioning-related brachial plexus stretch injuries. They are also useful for detecting intraoperative injury of the ulnar nerve at the elbow.

For LE SSEPs, the tibial nerve is stimulated at the ankle. Alternatively, the common peroneal nerve (common fibular nerve) may be stimulated near the fibular head or in the popliteal fossa. The common peroneal nerve stimulation is technically more difficult and causes more patient movement than tibial nerve stimulation. Nonetheless, it can be a suitable alternative if the tibial nerve is difficult to stimulate. Also, it can be useful to record common peroneal SSEPs of patients in whom the popliteal fossa potential to tibial nerve stimulation is difficult to monitor; loss of scalp-recorded tibial SSEPs but preservation of peroneal SSEPs would imply a peripheral problem (eg, stimulation failure) rather than a spinal cord problem related to the surgery.

Constant current simulators are preferred to constant voltage stimulators because of their ability to better compensate for variations in contact resistance. Stimulation rates of approximately 5 Hz are usually optimal (27), avoiding rates that are harmonically related to the power line frequency (60 Hz in North America). Higher rates may be used but they may produce lower-amplitude cortical responses. Lower rates usually offer no advantage and slow signal averaging; occasionally, however, particularly in patients with neurological abnormalities, rates between 1.5 and 3 Hz may improve responses. Stimulation intensity should be supramaximal. In healthy patients, stimulus intensities of 20 mA are often adequate; higher intensities, however, may be used as needed. Interleaved left/right stimulation may be employed, but *simultaneous* right and left stimulation should be avoided.

Recording

Subdural needle electrodes are generally used for recording. They maintain good contact over lengthy operations, and, if dislodged, are easily replaced. Standard EEG disk electrodes may also be used and should be applied with collodion.

Multichannel montages that include both cortical and brainstem channels should be used. It is important to include multiple cortical channels to account for known variations in signal scalp topography and to provide redundancy in case of electrode loss. Similarly, multiple brainstem channels can be helpful as they provide some redundancy for these typically "noisier" electrode derivations. It can be helpful to obtain recordings from a larger number of channels at baseline and then select a montage optimized to the patient's scalp signal topography and to the noise environment (20,22).

For UE SSEPs, a suggested montage is:

CPc-CPi
CPc-Fpz
CPc-CPz
Fpz-CS5
CPi-CS5
EPi-EPc

For LE SSEPs, a suggested montage is:

CPz-Fpz
CPi-CPc
CPz-CPc
Fpz-CS5
CPi-CS5
PF1-PF2

Electrical interference, particularly at the frequency of power line alternating current (60 Hz in the North America), often presents a challenge to obtaining technically satisfactory recording in the OR. Equipment such as blood warmers, motorized patient tables, and operating microscopes are important sources of electrical noise. Care should be taken to run lead wires to avoid proximity to interference sources, when possible. It is often very helpful to twist or braid scalp-recording leads to maximize common mode rejection of power line interference.

Band-pass filters of 30–1,000 Hz (-6 dB) are most commonly employed. However, most of the energy for SSEPs lies between 30 and 500 Hz, and high-frequency filters of 500 or even 300 Hz may be used effectively for monitoring, decreasing noise with only minimal effect of waveform morphology. Lower low-pass settings below 30 Hz offer no advantage and increase noise.

Typically, several hundred trials are averaged per recorded response. The number of trials that must be averaged is determined largely by the amount of noise present. Sometimes, as few as 100 trials will suffice, while at other times, many more will be necessary. If an average becomes contaminated by a particularly high-noise trial, it may be necessary to "clear" the average and begin again.

Anesthesia

Cortical SSEP signals are susceptible to attenuation by general anesthetic agents. Halogenated inhalations agents (eg, isoflurane, desflurane, sevoflurane) attenuate and also increase the latency of the N20 upper and P37 lower extremity SSEPs; nitrous oxide has similar effects (28–31) (Figure 13.4). The combined effect of nitrous oxide and halogenated agents appears to be greater than similarly potent doses of either drug alone (32). Infants and young children tend to be especially susceptible to these effects (33). Most intravenous agents (eg propofol, opioids, dexmedetomidine, benzodiazepines) have similar, but notably less prominent, effects (28,31,34). The degree of attenuation varies with not only the agent and the dose but also varies remarkably among patients (Figure 13.5). In some patients, ketamine and etomidate can be effective for enhancing SSEP cortical signals (35–37).

Brainstem SSEPs signals (P14 and N18 for upper extremities, P31 and N34 for lower extremities), by contrast, are essentially unaffected by anesthetic agents in clinically relevant

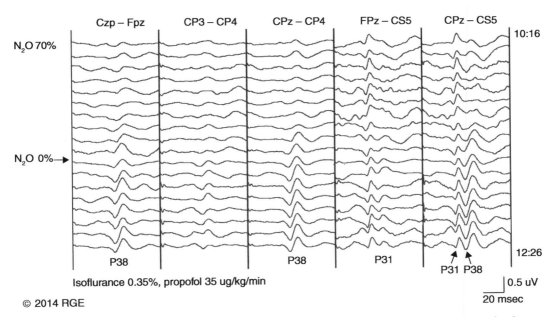

© 2014 RGE

FIGURE 13.4 Effect of nitrous oxide on cortical lower extremity somatosensory evoked potentials (LE SSEPs). In a patient receiving balanced anesthesia with 70% nitrous oxide, 0.35% isoflurane, and propofol 35 ug/kg/min, the P38 cortical signal is barely detectable. When nitrous oxide is decreased to 0%, P38 quickly becomes dramatically larger. Holding nitrous oxide constant and decreasing isoflurane would have had a similar but slower effect, the speed reflecting isoflurane's greater solubility in blood.

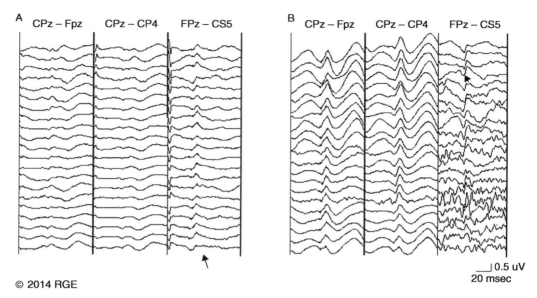

© 2014 RGE

FIGURE 13.5 Interpatient variability of the effect of anesthetic agents on cortical somatosensory evoked potentials (SSEPs). Patients A and B both received balanced anesthesia with 50% nitrous oxide, 0.5% isoflurane, and propofol 35 ug/kg/min. Cortical SSEPs are markedly suppressed in patient A but are sufficiently preserved in patient B to permit effective monitoring. Brainstem signals (arrows) are unaffected in both patients. Patient A received intermittent boluses of vecuronium to eliminate EMG artifact and permit monitoring of the brainstem SSEP.

concentrations (34) (Figures 13.4 and 13.5). Brainstem SSEPs can be technically difficult to monitor, however, being more susceptible to contamination by both electrical noise and muscle artifact. The latter is a consequence of the long interelectrode distances required by scalp-to-noncephalic derivations as well as the location (often on the back of the neck) of the reference electrode. Neuromuscular blocking (NMB) agents can be used to eliminate EMG artifact and are sometimes necessary for monitoring brainstem SSEPs (Figure 13.6). Apart from technical issues, brainstem SSEPs may be difficult to record at baseline in patients with preexistent myelopathies.

Either cortical or brainstem SSEPs can be sufficient for monitoring spinal cord function, as each serves as an indicator of dorsal column function. Their complementary strengths and weaknesses combine to enhance the reliability and flexibility of SSEP monitoring. Although some authors have recommended omitting brainstem SSEPs from routine SSEP monitoring protocols because they often have low signal-to-noise ratios and can be difficult to record (20), routine incorporation of brainstem channels in SSEP monitoring protocols adds flexibility and places fewer constraints on anesthetic choice. If cortical signals are robust, brainstem signals may be disregarded in favor of more rapid surgical feedback based on the cortical signals. If, however, for an individual patient and anesthetic protocol, brainstem responses are the most robust signals, then they should be used preferentially because they will, in fact, provide for the best and most rapid feedback to the surgeon.

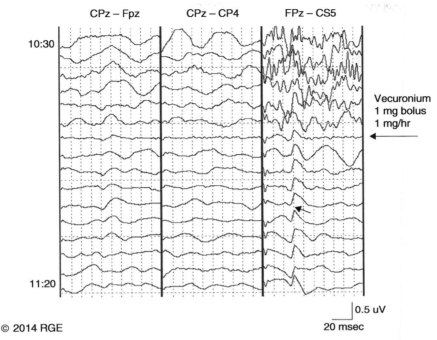

FIGURE 13.6 Use of neuromuscular blocking agents to facilitate monitoring based on brainstem somatosensory evoked potentials (SSEPs) in a 12-year-old with neuromuscular scoliosis and cerebral palsy, undergoing scoliosis surgery. Patient was receiving 0.25% isoflurane along with propofol 100 ug/kg/min. Cortical SSEPs are barely present and not monitorable. Following the administration of vecuronium, muscle artifact in the Fpz-CS5 channel is eliminated and the brainstem SSEP becomes monitorable (arrow).

MOTOR EVOKED POTENTIALS

Physiological Basis

MEP monitoring during spinal surgery is performed by transcranial electrical stimulation of the motor cortex and recording the compound motor potential (CMAP) from muscle (M-wave) in the arms and legs. In direct spinal cord recordings, a single transcranial electrical stimulus can be seen to generate a series of efferent volleys: an initial single D (or direct)-wave followed over several milliseconds by a series of I (or indirect)-waves. D-waves result from direct activation of pyramidal cell *axons*. I-waves, in contrast, reflect firing of pyramidal cells in response to inputs from interneurons, themselves activated by transcranial electrical stimulation (38). Since no synapses are involved in D-wave generation, they are relatively resistant to anesthetic effects; I-waves, in contrast, are suppressed by most general anesthetics.

Under general anesthesia, a single transcranial electrical stimulus is generally insufficient to fire spinal cord alpha motor neurons and elicit an M-wave. Instead, a rapid train of several transcranial electrical stimuli, typically 1 to several milliseconds apart, is required. The stimulus train elicits a corresponding train of D-waves plus some I-waves. The resultant synaptic

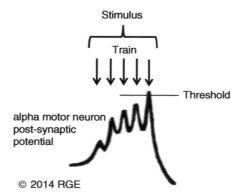

© 2014 RGE

FIGURE 13.7 Temporal summation by a spinal motor neuron. Each volley (corresponding to a D-wave or I-wave) causes further depolarization of the alpha motor neuron until it finally reaches threshold and fires, causing the innervated muscle fibers to fire.

inputs temporally summate, causing alpha motor neurons to reach threshold, fire, and produce the M-wave MEP (39) (Figure 13.7).

Recently, it has been shown that two sequential trains, separated by an appropriate inter-train interval (ITI), can often substantially enhance M-wave MEPs (Figure 13.8). The mechanism for this enhancement likely involves polysnaptic facilitatory circuits, both at the spinal and cortical levels. Proper timing of the trains is important because an incorrectly selected ITI can result in inhibition, rather than facilitation (40).

Monitoring Setup

Both UE and LE MEPs are usually monitored. As is the case with SSEPs, when the region of the spinal cord at risk is below the cervical cord, UE MEPs serve as "systemic" controls, reflecting the effects of anesthesia, neuromuscular blockade, hypotension, and hypovolemia.

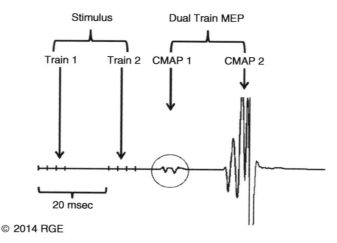

© 2014 RGE

FIGURE 13.8 MEP facilitation by dual-train stimulation. Two stimulus trains are delivered, the second 20 milliseconds after the beginning of the first. Each train elicits an M-wave, the second much larger than the first.

Stimulation

MEP stimulation may be performed using subdermal needle or corkscrew electrodes, or electroencephalogram (EEG)-type disk electrodes secured with collodion. Electrodes are most often placed at C1/C2 or C3/C4 scalp locations (41). C3/C4 locations can be more effective but also tend to elicit more face and jaw movement. Although MEPs are usually generated bilaterally, D-waves and hence M-waves are most reliably elicited by anodal stimulation (42). For monitoring, therefore, stimulator polarity is set so that the anode is contralateral to the recorded muscles; stimulator polarity is then switched when recording from the opposite side. Alternatively, the anode may be placed at Cz, with the cathode at Fz; with this arrangement, both legs may be effectively stimulated simultaneously, but UE muscle activation may be more difficult. In practice, it is useful to test several stimulating electrode placements and select the best one for the individual patient.

M-waves are relatively large signals, often several hundred microvolts, so signal averaging is not needed. On the other hand, M-wave amplitude and morphology can vary from stimulation to stimulation, reflecting spontaneous fluctuation of the motor pool excitability. In some patients, this trial-to-trial variability of M-wave MEPs can be pronounced and can require several repeated stimuli to properly characterize (Figure 13.9).

Either constant-voltage or constant stimulators can be employed; constant-voltage MEP stimulators are more common, largely for historic and regulatory reasons. Pulse train parameters

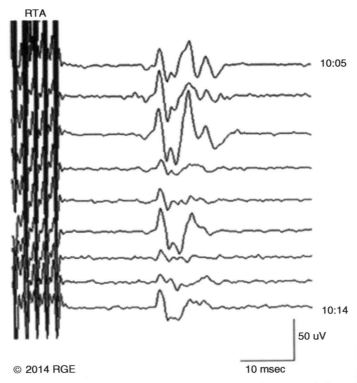

© 2014 RGE

FIGURE 13.9 Variability of motor evoked potentials obtained sequentially under identical anesthetic and hemodynamic conditions. Anesthesia was achieved using propofol 125 ug/kg/min; mean arterial pressure was 60 mmHg.

Abbreviation: RTA, right tibialis anterior.

should be optimized for the patient. In some patients, as few as three pulses may suffice; in others, six to eight may be needed. ITIs of 2 to 4 milliseconds are usually optimal (43–45). For dual-train stimulation, facilitation is greatest with ITIs of 10 to 20 milliseconds and again between 100 and 1,000 milliseconds (40).

Recording

Subdermal or intramuscular needle electrodes, 2 to 3 cm apart, are used to record MEPs from the muscle belly. Belly tendon derivations can be used, but the longer interelectrode distance can be a source of added noise. For spinal cord monitoring, the most robust MEP signals are generally recorded from distal muscles controlled principally by the corticospinal tract. Abductor pollicis brevis and first dorsal interosseus for the upper extremity and adductor hallucis and tibialis anterior for the lower are commonly employed. Reliable MEPs can often be obtained from other muscles as well, and it can be helpful to include these in the selection of muscles for monitoring. For spinal cord monitoring, each muscle MEP serves as a surrogate for motor pathway integrity, probably because of the small size of the corticospinal tract and the likelihood that injury will affect many of its axons.

Specific muscles, including proximal muscles and anal sphincter, can also be monitored for the purpose of detecting nerve root injury. While this can be effective, MEP nerve root monitoring is also more difficult and less reliable than MEP monitoring of spinal cord function. MEP monitoring of nerve root function is heavily dependent upon adequacy and stability of the particular muscle's baseline response; its reliability is further constrained by the confounding effects of multisegmental innervation (46).

Spinal cord D-waves are not monitored during scoliosis surgery because of the possibility of spurious amplitude changes resulting from movement of the epidural recording electrode with respect to the spinal cord during spinal deformity correction (47).

Safety

Transcranial MEP monitoring is a safe procedure. Tongue bite and patient movement are the major risks. Twenty-five instances of tongue laceration were reported in a series of 18,862 MEP cases. Twenty-one were self-limited, requiring no intervention; only four required suturing (48). A soft bite block (eg, rolled gauze pads) should be used to prevent the tongue from coming in contact with the teeth. Patient movement is common with MEP stimulation, although it can often be minimized by appropriate adjustment of stimulation parameters (stimulation intensity, number of pulses). It is important to coordinate stimulation with the surgeon so that movement does not occur, for example, when surgical instruments are close to neural structures. No movement-related injuries were reported in a series of more than 18,000 cases involving MEP monitoring over 15 years (48).

Epilepsy, shunts, cerebral lesions, skull defects close to stimulating electrodes, and implanted devices have been cited in the past as relative contraindications to transcranial electrical MEP (49). None, however, has been proven to result in complications related to MEP monitoring, and in many centers these do not presently preclude MEP monitoring (48,50). For individual patients, of course, the benefits of MEP monitoring need to be assessed, relative to potential risks.

Seizures can theoretically be produced by MEP stimulation. Although after discharges have been reported to occur following transcranial electrical stimulation (51), clinical seizures, if they occur, are very rare. Five seizures were reported, some possibly coincidental, in a review of 15,000 published and unpublished MEP cases (49). No seizures were reported in another series of 18,862 cases, including 35 patients with a history of prior seizures (48). A history of seizure should not ordinarily be considered to be a contraindication to MEP monitoring. The anesthesiologist should, however, be prepared to treat a seizure, should one occur. If a seizure does occur, the risks and benefits of continuing MEP monitoring should be evaluated. At some centers, concurrent EEG monitoring is performed, but its role has not been established.

Anesthesia

While D-waves are largely unaffected by commonly used anesthetics, these agents attenuate cortical I-waves (52) and also suppress spinal motor neurons (53). M-wave MEPs are particularly sensitive to both the halogenated inhalational agents and nitrous oxide (53,54). They are generally less severely affected by propofol and dexmedetomidine, and total intravenous anesthesia (TIVA), based on these agents combined with an opioid (eg, fentanyl, remifentanil) is commonly recommended for MEP monitoring (34,55). Nonetheless, modest doses of halogenated inhalational agents (generally < ½ minimum alveolar concentration [MAC]) or nitrous oxide can often be compatible with MEP monitoring (56–59). In our experience, dual-train MEP stimulation further facilitates flexibility in anesthetic selection (Figure 13.10). Low-dose ketamine can also be helpful, particularly in young children. While ketamine does not directly affect MEPs, it also does not inhibit I-waves. It can facilitate MEP monitoring by allowing lower doses of other anesthetics to be used (59,60). As with SSEPs, sensitivity to the suppressive effects of anesthetic agents varies considerably between patients.

MEPs can be particularly sensitive to changes in anesthetic doses; boluses of anesthetic agents can transiently attenuate or even abolish responses. Even boluses of opioids, which in general only mildly affect MEPs (59), can also occasionally produce transient prominent attenuation. Stable anesthesia is ideal; when anesthetic adjustments are necessary, it is important that these be tracked and correlated with monitoring changes. Anesthetic changes that are likely to attenuate MEPs, and particularly their administration as boluses, are best avoided at times when close monitoring of MEPs is critical.

NMB agents can be useful for improving SSEP signal quality, reducing patient movement, and perhaps reducing the incidence and severity of tongue bite injuries. If neuromuscular blockade is used, it must be partial, and the degree of blockade must be carefully monitored and titrated (48,59,61). The NMB agent should be given by a continuous infusion, because even small boluses tend to obliterate or substantially attenuate MEP signals (Figure 13.11). Most centers avoid the use of NMB agents in conjunction with MEP monitoring (59). In our experience, we have found that very low doses of vecuronium, titrated to three to four twitches on a "train of four" testing, can often notably improve SSEPs, particularly the brainstem signals, while not detracting from the quality of MEP recording (Figure 13.12).

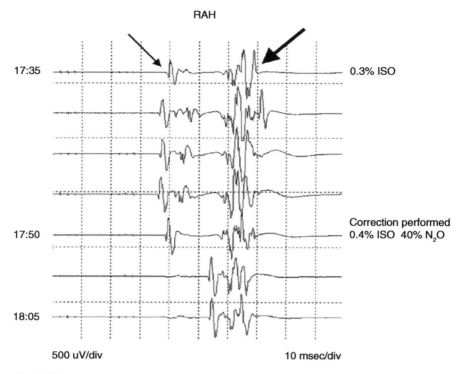

500 uV/div   10 msec/div

© 2014 RGE

FIGURE 13.10 Dual-train stimulation can provide resilience to anesthetic effects on motor evoked potentials (MEPs). In a 12-year-old undergoing scoliosis surgery, anesthesia was provided using propofol 70 ug/kg/min and 0.3% isoflurane. Shortly after correction was achieved, 50% nitrous oxide was added, causing loss of the MEP response to the first train (thin arrow). Confusion, and a possible "false-positive" alert, were avoided by preservation of the response to the second stimulus train (thick arrow).

Abbreviation: RAH, right abductor hallucis.

INTERPRETATION

Preoperative Evaluation

SSEPs are routinely performed extraoperatively as part of the routine clinical evaluation of various neurological disorders. Extraoperative interpretation is based largely on interpeak latencies, reflecting conduction times between the various generators of the SSEPs signals. For UE SSEPs, these include EP-P14, P14-N20, and EP-N20, reflecting conduction times between Erb's point and the lower brainstem, between the lower brainstem and cortex, as well as the overall conduction time between Erb's point and cortex, respectively. For LE SSEPs, these include N22-P31, P31-P38, and N22-P38, reflecting, respectively, conduction times between lumbar spinal cord and lower brainstem, lower brainstem and cortex, and the overall conduction time between the lumbar cord and cortex. Interpretation is based on comparison of a patient's latency values to normative data as well as differences between interpeak latencies measured following right- and left-sided stimulation. While the absence of expected signals also constitutes an abnormality, waveform amplitudes vary considerably among normal individuals and, as such, are generally not used in routine outpatient testing.

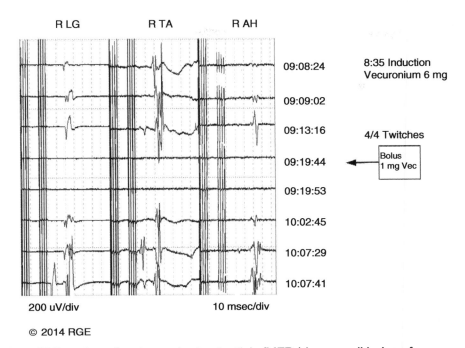

FIGURE 13.11 Obliteration of motor evoked potentials (MEPs) by a small bolus of vecuronium. Forty minutes after receiving 6 mg of vecuronium for intubation, the patient had four of four twitches, and well-formed MEPs were obtained. The MEPs were then transiently abolished by a 1-mg bolus of vecuronium.

Abbreviations: RAH, right abductor hallucis; RLG, right lateral gastrocnemius; RTA, right tibialis anterior.

In the early days of intraoperative monitoring, it was common to obtain extraoperative SSEP recordings as a guide to what to expect in the OR. Although this practice continues to be advocated by some (62), it has been abandoned by many, in favor of simply relying on baselines obtained intraoperatively. This author generally favors the latter practice. In the absence of outpatient sedation, intraoperative recordings are usually of better technical quality; indeed, the brainstem P31 signal is frequently not recordable in unsedated outpatient recordings. Often, the most important information derived from baseline recording relates to the effect of anesthetics agents and can be assessed only in the OR. Preoperative assessment of MEPs, using transcranial magnetic stimulation, has been suggested (63). While this is feasible and could be useful in some cases, Food and Drug Administration (FDA)-approved devices are not currently available.

In patients with AIS, SSEPs and MEPs are generally easy to obtain in the OR. While preoperative SSEPs could detect spinal cord abnormalities, such as Chiari malformations and syrinxes, that are occasionally present in patients with AIS (62), structural assessments are best made by using structural imaging techniques.

That said, baseline latency-based SSEP abnormalities may be common in AIS, their reported prevalence varying from about 15% to nearly 100%. The abnormities appear to be subtle, however, and are best revealed using height-adjusted normative data and specifically evaluating interpeak intervals (62,64,65). Machida reported SSEP abnormalities in 97 of 100

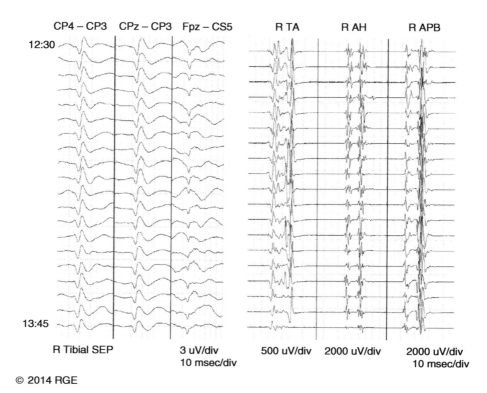

© 2014 RGE

FIGURE 13.12 Motor evoked potentials (MEPs) and somatosensory evoked potentials (SSEPs) recorded during surgery for adolescent idiopathic scoliosis (AIS) in a 12-year-old child receiving a vecuronium infusion at 1 mg/kg/hr, along with propofol and isoflurane. Train-of-four testing demonstrated three to four twitches. Robust MEPs were maintained, and with easily monitored brainstem SSEPs.

Abbreviations: RAH, right abductor hallucis; RAPB, right abductor pollicis brevis; RTA, right tibialis anterior.

AIS patients, finding the P31-P38 interpeak latency to be prolonged following stimulation of the tibial nerve ipsilateral to the concavity of the curve (65). This observation, which suggests a sensory system abnormality rostral to the lower brainstem, may provide an important clue to the pathogenesis of AIS. Indeed, disturbed somatosensory function and balance abnormalities have been described in AIS patients with abnormal SSEPs (64,66).

Intraoperative Interpretation

For intraoperative monitoring, each patient's responses are evaluated with respect to baseline signals, that is, the patient serves as his own control. This contrasts with standard laboratory testing, where patients' responses are evaluated relative to normative population-based data. Baselines are obtained at the beginning of the case; it is often necessary to reestablish the baseline during the case, to account, for example, for changes in anesthesia. Even at constant anesthetic doses, both SSEPs and MEPs can change over time, a phenomenon known as "anesthetic fade." Over hours, SSEP latencies are often seen to gradually increase and amplitudes to gradually decrease (67). Similarly, MEP threshold stimulation voltage commonly increases slowly over hours. The effect can be more striking in myelopathic patients (68). The mechanism for anesthetic fade is uncertain. It is seen both with lipid-soluble (eg, propofol), as well as lipid-insoluble (eg, N_2O) agents, and may be explained by slower time courses for some anesthetic effects, such as prolongation of refectory periods, than others (68).

For SSEPs, the generally accepted "alarm criteria" are a 50% decrease in amplitude or a 10% increase in latency from baseline (69). Loss of SEP amplitude and degradation of signal morphology are the most common consequences of intraoperative spinal cord injury, which causes conduction block or desynchronization; latency changes are distinctly less prominent. In contrast to extraoperative testing, SSEP amplitude is therefore the most important parameter to monitor. It is a serious error to conclude that everything if okay simply because latencies have remained stable.

The 50% amplitude 10% latency alarm criteria are empirically based and are best used as a guide, rather than a strict threshold above which it can be assumed that no adverse events have occurred. For one, noise can make it difficult to reliably distinguish a 60% from a 40% change from baseline. Further, it can be helpful to alert the surgeon to new, albeit smaller, SSEP changes that exceed their observed prior variability during the case. This approach can facilitate more accurate identification of the cause of SSEP changes and better affords the surgeon the option of acting immediately or taking a "wait and see" approach (70).

There is no firm consensus on the alarm criteria for MEP monitoring. Suggested criteria include the presence or absence of a response, various percent loss of response amplitudes, decrease of M-wave complexity or duration, and increase in stimulus intensity required to elicit M-waves (71). Latency criteria are not useful (72). The complexity of MEP interpretation reflects, in part, the integrative role of the motor neurons in generating M-waves, requiring the temporal summation of descending volleys, as well as the trial-to-trial variability of MEPs. Complete loss of M-wave does not necessarily indicate complete loss of spinal cord motor function; indeed, M-waves can be lost when D-wave amplitude decreases by 30% to 50%, often resulting in a transient postoperative motor deficit (72).

Although complete disappearance of the MEP has been a widely employed alarm criterion, once M-waves are lost, it is impossible to judge the degree of D-wave loss without direct spinal cord recording. It would seem, therefore, that a somewhat less strict alarm threshold is desirable to best ensure that the surgeon is notified before a possible "point of no return." Given the commonly encountered degree of MEP variability, a 50% amplitude decrease criterion would likely cause too many false-positive notifications. The American Clinical Neurophysiology Society has suggested amplitude reduction of 75% to 90% as a reasonable threshold for alarm (41).

The combined use of SSEPs and MEPs affords robust monitoring of spinal cord function during spinal deformity surgery. The two modalities rely on different signals, are mediated by different pathways, are monitored using different leads and cables, and may be differentially affected by anesthetic agents. Yet, both are usually affected by traumatic, compressive, and ischemic injury to the spinal cord. This redundancy can be critical to continued monitoring during real-life situations commonly encountered in the OR, which cause one or the other modality to fail or to become unreliable. If, for example, a bolus of propofol obliterates MEPs, monitoring could continue based on subcortical SSEP and perhaps cortical SSEP signals. If muscle or electrical artifact obscures the SSEPs, the much larger CMAP signals would likely permit continued MEP monitoring.

SSEP monitoring does not disturb the surgical field and can be performed continuously; MEP monitoring can produce movement and must be coordinated with the surgeon. On the other hand, feedback to the surgeon based on SSEPs is necessarily delayed by the time required to average a sufficient number of trials to produce an interpretable response; depending on accompanying noise, this can be several minutes. MEP monitoring does not require averaging and results are instantaneous. As such, provided that MEPs are recorded sufficiently frequently, they can provide for quicker and more accurate identification of causes of surgical injury and allow for faster intervention. Additionally, MEPs are often inherently more sensitive, detecting injury before SSEPs are affected (Figure 13A–H); simultaneous loss of SSEPs and MEP may signal a more severe injury. In this manner, the routine combined use of the two modalities contributes importantly to the safety of spinal deformity surgery.

Although, in the past, monitoring has focused on a "critical period" following correction, it is now clear that MEP and SEP changes reflecting incipient spinal cord injury can, and do, occur at any time during spinal deformity surgery. For this reason, monitoring should continue throughout the entire procedure, including during closure (73).

Example Case

Figure 13.13 illustrates a typical case of loss of SSEPs and MEPs during scoliosis surgery, with return of signals following modification of the correction. The patient is a 12-year-old girl undergoing posterior instrumentation for correction of AIS under total intravenous anesthesia, using propofol and fentanyl, plus partial neuromuscular blockade. Well-formed cortical (asterisk) and brainstem (arrow) SSEPs as well as MEPs are present at baseline (9:56, Figure 13A).

By 16:05 (Figure 13B), correction has been achieved with placement of the first rod. As the second rod is placed, MEPs are lost on the left as well as in a single right LE muscle (VL) (arrows). SSEPs are unchanged. The surgeon is informed who begins removing the rods. For spinal cord monitoring, the response from each muscle serves as surrogate for right or left spinal cord motor function. Monitoring of responses from multiple muscles is useful, not only because of redundancy, in case one recording fails but also because responses from the muscles that are more difficult to stimulate (higher stimulation threshold voltage) can be lost first, and provide an "early warning" of possible further deterioration.

Within several minutes (Figure 13C), MEPs are completely lost on both sides, while SSEPs remain unchanged. Only by 16:13 (Figure 13D), 8 minutes after the initial MEP loss, do SSEPs become attenuated bilaterally. MEPs often detect compromise of spinal cord function faster than SSEPs, in part because of the time required for SSEP signal averaging but also because they commonly prove to be more sensitive to spinal cord injury.

By 16:21 (Figure 13E), with rods removed, MEPs have returned, and SSEPs are returning. Note that the first of the three superimposed SSEPs to be acquired (arrows) is of somewhat lower amplitude than the subsequent two recordings. At 16:43 (Figure 13F), the surgeon begins reinserting the rods, now shaped to achieve less aggressive correction of the scoliosis deformity. Six minutes later (Figure 13G), MEPs are again lost bilaterally; SSEPs remain unchanged. The surgeon is informed, the rods are released, and MEPs return (Figure 13H). Note that the first of

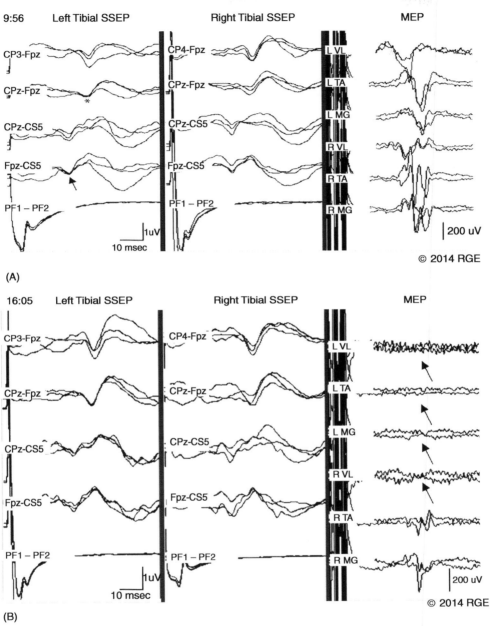

FIGURE 13.13 A series of "screen shots" from a posterior instrumentation and fusion procedure for correction of scoliosis (see text for details). In each figure, three sets of superimposed tibial somatosensory evoked potentials (SSEPs) and two lower extremity motor evoked potentials (MEPs) are shown, with MEPs having been acquired following each of the first two sets of SSEPs. The labeled times correspond to the time of the first MEP. Right and left SSEPs were obtained simultaneously. VL, TA, and MG correspond to vastus lateralis, tibialis anterior, and medial gastrocnemius muscles, respectively. Ulnar SSEPs and abductor pollicis brevis MEPs as "systemic controls" are not shown, and they remained stable throughout the entire case. (*continued*)

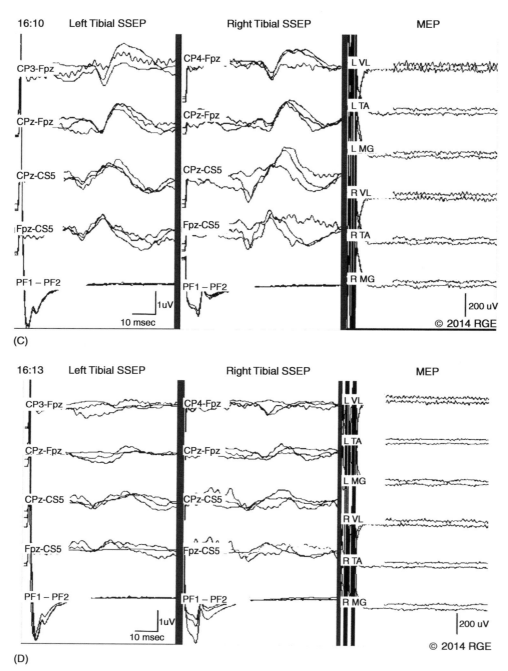

FIGURE 13.13 (*continued*) A series of "screen shots" from a posterior instrumentation and fusion procedure for correction of scoliosis (see text for details). In each figure, three sets of superimposed tibial somatosensory evoked potentials (SSEPs) and two lower extremity motor evoked potentials (MEPs) are shown, with MEPs having been acquired following each of the first two sets of SSEPs. The labeled times correspond to the time of the first MEP. Right and left SSEPs were obtained simultaneously. VL, TA, and MG correspond to vastus lateralis, tibialis anterior, and medial gastrocnemius muscles, respectively. Ulnar SSEPs and abductor pollicis brevis MEPs as "systemic controls" are not shown, and they remained stable throughout the entire case. (*continued*)

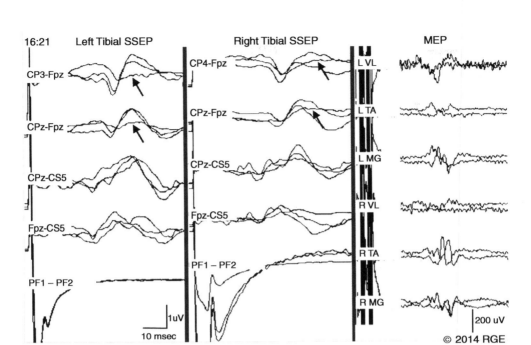

(E)

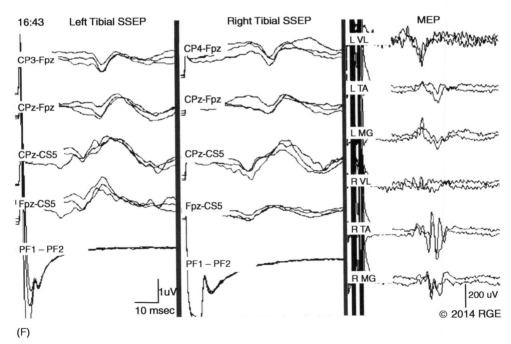

(F)

FIGURE 13.13 (*continued*)

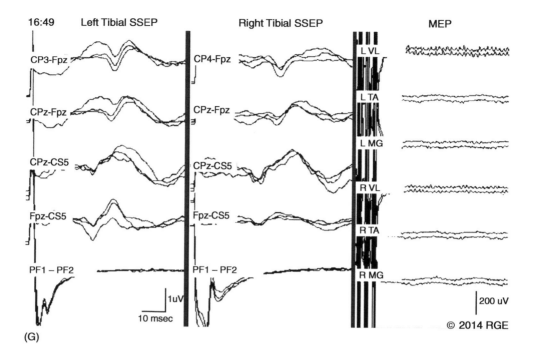

(G)

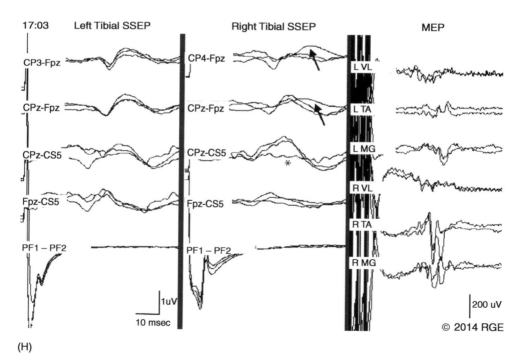

(H)

FIGURE 13.13 (*continued*)

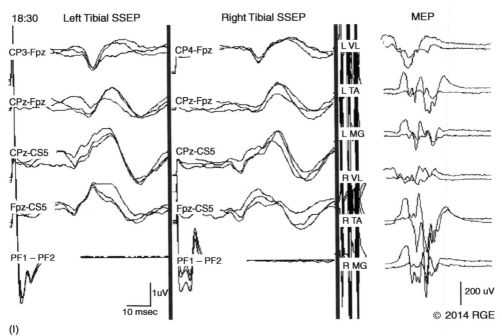

(I)

FIGURE 13.13 (*continued*) A series of "screen shots" from a posterior instrumentation and fusion procedure for correction of scoliosis (see text for details). In each figure, three sets of superimposed tibial somatosensory evoked potentials (SSEPs) and two lower extremity motor evoked potentials (MEPs) are shown, with MEPs having been acquired following each of the first two sets of SSEPs. The labeled times correspond to the time of the first MEP. Right and left SSEPs were obtained simultaneously. VL, TA, and MG correspond to vastus lateralis, tibialis anterior, and medial gastrocnemius muscles, respectively. Ulnar SSEPs and abductor pollicis brevis MEPs as "systemic controls" are not shown, and they remained stable throughout the entire case.

the three superimposed SSEP recordings to be obtained does, in fact, show attenuation of the right brainstem (asterisk) and cortical (arrows) responses.

Rods are then reinserted, configured to achieve still less correction. This time, MEPs and SSEPs remain stable. Signals remain stable through closing (Figure 13I), and the patient awakens from anesthesia with intact spinal cord function.

REFERENCES

1. Coe JD, Arlet V, Donaldson W, et al. Complications in spinal fusion for adolescent idiopathic scoliosis in the new millennium. A report of the Scoliosis Research Society Morbidity and Mortality Committee. *Spine.* 2006;31(3):345–349.
2. Diab M, Smith AR, Kuklo TR, et al. Neural complications in the surgical treatment of adolescent idiopathic scoliosis. *Spine.* 2007;32(24):2759–2763.
3. Qiu Y, Wang S, Wang B, et al. Incidence and risk factors of neurological deficits of surgical correction for scoliosis: analysis of 1373 cases at one Chinese institution. *Spine.* 2008;33(5):519–526.
4. Reames DL, Smith JS, Fu K-MG, et al. Complications in the surgical treatment of 19,360 cases of pediatric scoliosis. *Spine.* 2011;36(18):1484–1491.

5. Nuwer MR, Emerson RG, Galloway G, et al. Evidence-based guideline update: intraoperative spinal monitoring with somatosensory and transcranial electrical motor evoked potentials*. *J Clin Neurophysiol.* 2012;29(1):101–108.

6. Nuwer MR, Dawson EG, Carlson LG, et al. Somatosensory evoked potential spinal cord monitoring reduces neurologic deficits after scoliosis surgery: results of a large multicenter survey. *Electroencephalogr Clin Neurophysiol.* 1995;96(1):6–11.

7. Nash CL, Lorig RA, Schatzinger LA, et al. Spinal cord monitoring during operative treatment of the spine. *Clin Orthop Relat Res.* 1977;(126):100–105.

8. Forbes HJ, Allen PW, Waller CS, et al. Spinal cord monitoring in scoliosis surgery. *J Bone Joint Surg Am.* 1991;73-B:219–220.

9. Deecke L, Tator CH. Neurophysiol assessment of afferent and efferent conduction in the injured spinal cord of monkeys. *J. Neurosurg.* 1973;39:65–74.

10. Baskin DS, Simpson RK Jr. Corticomotor and somatosensory evoked potential evaluation of acute spinal cord injury in the rat. *Neurosurgery.* 1987;20(6):871–877.

11. Shiau JS, Zappulla RA, Nieves J. The effect of graded spinal cord injury on the extrapyramidal and pyramidal motor evoked potentials of the rat. *Neurosurgery.* 1992;30(1):76–84.

12. Machida M, Weinstein SL, Imamura Y, et al. Compound muscle action potentials and spinal evoked potentials in experimental spine maneuver. *Spine.* 1989;14(7):687–691.

13. Fehlings MG, Tator CH, Linden RD. The relationships among the severity of spinal cord injury, motor and somatosensory evoked potentials and spinal cord blood flow. *Electroencephalography and Clincal Neurophysiology.* 1989;74:241–259.

14. Ben-David B, Haller G, Taylor P. Anterior spinal fusion complicated by paraplegia. A case report of a false-negative somatosensory-evoked potential. *Spine.* 1987;12:536–539.

15. Merton PA, Morton HB. Stimulation of the cerebral cortex in the intact human subject. *Nature.* 1980;285(5762):227.

16. Mauguiere F, Desmedt JE. Bilateral somatosensory evoked potentials in four patients with long-standing surgical hemispherectomy. *Ann Neurol.* 1989;26(6):724–731.

17. Mauguiere F, Desmedt JE, Courjon J. Neural generators of N18 and P14 far-field somatosensory evoked potentials studied in patients with lesion of thalamus or thalamo-cortical radiations. *Electroencephalogr Clin Neurophysiol.* 1983;56(4):283–292.

18. Urasaki E, Tokimura T, Yasukouchi H, et al. P30 and N33 of posterior tibial nerve SSEPs are analogous to P14 and N18 of median nerve SSEPs. *Electroencephalogr Clin Neurophysiol.* 1993;88(6):525–529.

19. Emerson RG, Seyal M, Pedley TA. Somatosensory evoked potentials following median nerve stimulation. I. The cervical components. *Brain.* 1984;107(Pt 1):169–182.

20. MacDonald DB, Al-Zayed Z, Stigsby B, et al. Median somatosensory evoked potential intraoperative monitoring: recommendations based on signal-to-noise ratio analysis. *Clin Neurophysiol,* 2009;120(2):315–328.

21. Seyal M, Emerson RG, Pedley TA. Spinal and early scalp-recorded components of the somatosensory evoked potential following stimulation of the posterior tibial nerve. *Electroencephalogr Clin Neurophysiol,* 1983;55(3):320–330.

22. MacDonald DB, Al-Zayed Z, Stigsby B. Tibial somatosensory evoked potential intraoperative monitoring: recommendations based on signal to noise ratio analysis of popliteal fossa, optimized P37, standard P37, and P31 potentials. *Clin Neurophysiol,* 2005;116(8):1858–1869.

23. Emerson RG. Anatomic and physiologic bases of posterior tibial nerve somatosensory evoked potentials. *Neurol Clin.* 1988;6(4):735–749.

24. Maiocco B, Deeney VF, Coulon R, et al. Adolescent idiopathic scoliosis and the presence of spinal cord abnormalities. Preoperative magnetic resonance imaging analysis. *Spine.* 1997;22(21):2537–2541.

25. O'Brien MF, Lenke LG, Bridwell KH, et al. Evoked potential monitoring of the upper extremities during thoracic and lumbar spinal deformity surgery: a prospective study. *J Spinal Disord.* 1994;7(4):277–284.

26. Jones SC, Fernau R, Woeltjen BL. Use of somatosensory evoked potentials to detect peripheral ischemia and potential injury resulting from positioning of the surgical patient: case reports and discussion. *Spine J.* 2004;4(3):360–362.

27. Nuwer MR, Dawson E. Intraoperative evoked potential monitoring of the spinal cord: enhanced stability of cortical recordings. *Electroencephalogr Clin Neurophysiol.* 1984;59(4):318–327.

28. Perlik SJ, VanEgeren R, Fisher MA. Somatosensory evoked potential surgical monitoring. Observation during combined isoflurane-nitrous oxide anesthesia. *Spine.* 1992;17(3):273–276.

29. Browning JL, Heizer ML, Baskin DS. Variations in corticomotor and somatosensory evoked potentials: effects of temperature, halothane anesthesia, and arterial partial pressure of CO2. *Anesth Analg.* 1992;74(5):643–648.

30. Sebel PS, Bowles SM, Saini V, et al. EEG bispectrum predicts movement during thiopental/isoflurane anesthesia. *J Clin Monit.* 1995;11(2):83–91.

31. Clapcich AJ, Emerson RG, Roye DP Jr, et al. The Effects of Propofol, Small-Dose Isoflurane, and Nitrous Oxide on Cortical Somatosensory Evoked Potential and Bispectral Index Monitoring in Adolescents Undergoing Spinal Fusion. *Anesth Analg.* 2004;99:1334–1340.

32. Sloan T, Sloan H, Rogers J. Nitrous oxide and isoflurane are synergistic with respect to amplitude and latency effects on sensory evoked potentials. *J Clin Monit Comput.* 2010;24(2):113–123.

33. Harper CM, Nelson KR. Intraoperative electrophysiological monitoring in children. *J Clin Neurophysiol.* 1992;9(3):342–356.

34. Sloan T, Heyer EJ. Anesthesia for intraoperative neurophysiologic monitoring of the spinal cord. *J Clin Neurophysiol.* 2002;19:430–443.

35. Agarwal R, Roitman KJ, Stokes M. Improvement of intraoperative somatosensory evoked potentials by ketamine. *Paediatr Anaesth.* 1998;8(3):263–266.

36. Schubert A, Licina MG, Lineberry PJ. The effect of ketamine on human somatosensory evoked potentials and its modification by nitrous oxide. *Anesth.* 1990;72(1):33–39.

37. Sloan TB, Ronai AK, Toleikis JR, et al. Improvement of intraoperative somatosensory evoked potentials by etomidate. *Anesth Analg.* 1988;67(6):582–585.

38. Amassian VE, Stewart M, Quirk GJ, et al. Physiological basis of motor effects of a transient stimulus to cerebral cortex. *Neurosurgery.* 1987;20(1):74–93.

39. Jones SJ, Harrison R, Koh KF, et al. Motor evoked potential monitoring during spinal surgery: response of distal limb muscles to transcranial cortical stimulation with pulse trains. *Electroencephalogr and Clin Neurophysiol.* 1996;100:375–383.

40. Journée HL, Polak HE, De Kleuver M. Conditioning stimulation techniques for enhancement of transcranially elicited evoked motor responses. *Neurophysiol Clin.* 2007;37(6):423–430.

41. American Clinical Neurophysiology Society. Guidleine on Transcranial Electrical Stimulation Motor Evoked Potentials (TES-MEP) Monitoring. *ACNS.* 0AD. http://www.acns.org/practice/guidelines. Accessed August 25, 2014.

42. Hern JE, Landgren S, Phillips CG, et al. Selective excitation of corticofugal neurones by surface-anodal stimulation of the baboon's motor cortex. *J Physiol.* 1962;161:73–90.

43. MacDonald DB. Intraoperative Motor Evoked Potential Monitoring: Overview and Update. *J Clin Monit Comput.* 2006;20(5):347–377.

44. Deletis V, Isgum V, Amassian VE. Neurophysiological mechanisms underlying motor evoked potentials in anesthetized humans. Part 1. Recovery time of corticospinal tract direct waves elicited by pairs of transcranial electrical stimuli. *Clin Neurophysiol.* 2001;112(3):438–444.

45. Quinones-Hinojosa A, Lyon R, Zada G, et al. Changes in transcranial motor evoked potentials during intramedullary spinal cord tumour resection correlate with postoperative motor function. *Neurosurgery.* 2005;56:982–893.

46. Lyon R, Gibson A, Burch S, et al. Increases in voltage may produce false-negatives when using transcranial motor evoked potentials to detect an isolated nerve root injury. *J Clin Monit Comput.* 2010;24(6):441–448.

47. Ulkatan S, Neuwirth M, Bitan F, et al. Monitoring of scoliosis surgery with epidurally recorded motor evoked potentials (D wave) revealed false results. *Clin Neurophysiol.* 2006;117:2093–2101.

48. Schwartz DM, Sestokas AK, Dormans JP, et al. Transcranial electric motor evoked potential monitoring during spine surgery: is it safe? *Spine.* 2011;36(13):1046–1049.

49. MacDonald DB. Safety of intraoperative transcranial electrical stimulation motor evoked potential monitoring. *J Clin Neurophysiol.* 2002;19(5):416–429.

50. MacDonald DB, Deletis V. Safety issues during surgical monitoring. In: Nuwer MR, ed. *Monitoring Neurol Function During Surgery, Handbook of Clinical Neurophysiology*. Amsterdam: Elsevier;2008:929–945.

51. Kobylarz EJ, Bilsky MH, Sandhu SK, et al. Monitoring of electroencephalography during transcranial electrical motor evoked potentials. *Epilepsia*. 2005;46(Suppl 8):309–310.

52. Burke D, Hicks R, Stephen J, et al. Assessment of corticospinal and somatosensory conduction simultaneously during scoliosis surgery. *Electroencephalogr Clin Neurophysiol*. 1992;85:388–396.

53. Zentner J, Albrecht T, Heuser D. Influence of halothane, enflurane, and isoflurane on motor evoked potentials. *Neurosurgery*. 1992;31(2):298–305.

54. Zentner J, Ebner A. Nitrous oxide suppresses the electromyographic response evoked by electrical stimulation of the motor cortex. *Neurosurgery*. 1989;24:60–62.

55. Bala E, Sessler DI, Nair DR, et al. Motor and somatosensory evoked potentials are well maintained in patients given dexmedetomidine during spine surgery. *Anesthesiology*. 2008;109(3):417–425.

56. Pelosi L, Stevenson M, Hobbs GJ, et al. Intraoperative motor evoked potentials to transcranial electrical stimulation during two anaesthetic regimens. *Clin Neurophysiol*. 2001;112(6):1076–1087.

57. Kempton LB, Nantau WE, Zaltz I. Successful monitoring of transcranial electrical motor evoked potentials with isoflurane and nitrous oxide in scoliosis surgeries. *Spine*. 2010;35(26):E1627–E1629.

58. Ubags LH, Kalkman CJ, Been HD. Influence of isoflurane on myogenic motor evoked potentials to single and multiple transcranial stimuli during nitrous oxide/opioid anesthesia. *Neurosurgery*. 1998;43(1):90–94.

59. Sloan T. Anesthesia and intraoperative neurophysiological monitoring in children. *Childs Nerv Syst*. 2010;26(2):227–235.

60. Frei FJ, Ryhult SE, Duitmann E, et al. Intraoperative monitoring of motor-evoked potentials in children undergoing spinal surgery. *Spine*. 2007;32(8):911–917.

61. Adams DC, Emerson RG, Heyer EJ, et al. Monitoring of intraoperative motor evoked potentials under conditions of controlled neuromuscular blockade. *Anesth Analg*. 1993;77(5):913–918.

62. Hausmann ON, Boni T, Pfirrmann CWA, et al. Preoperative radiological and electrophysiological evaluation in 100 adolescent idiopathic scoliosis patients. *Eur Spine J*. 2003;12(5):501–506.

63. Galloway GM, Brennan D, Brown JL. Transcranial magnetic stimulation—may be useful as a preoperative screen of motor tract function. *J Clin Neurophysiol*. 2013;30(4):386–338.

64. Guo X, Chau WW, Hui-Chan CWY, et al. Balance control in adolescents with idiopathic scoliosis and disturbed somatosensory function. *Spine*. 2006;31(14):E437–E440.

65. Machida M, Dubousset J, Imamura Y, et al. Pathogenesis of idiopathic scoliosis: SEPs in chicken with experimentally induced scoliosis and in patients with idiopathic scoliosis. *J Pediatr Orthop*. 1994;14(3):329–335.

66. Loa MLM, Chow DHK, Guo X, et al. Impaired dynamic balance control in adolescents with idiopathic scoliosis and abnormal somatosensory evoked potentials. *J Pediatr Orthop*. 2008;28(8):846–849.

67. Kalkman CJ, Brink ten SA, Been HD, et al. Variability of somatosensory cortical evoked potentials during spinal surgery. Effects of anesthetic technique and high-pass digital filtering. *Spine*. 1991;16(8):924–929.

68. Lyon R, Feiner J, Lieberman JA. Progressive suppression of motor evoked potentials during general anesthesia: the phenomenon of "anesthetic fade". *J Neurosurg Anesthesiol*. 2005;17(1):13–19.

69. American Clinical Neurophysiology Society. Guideline 11B: Recommended standards for intraoperative monitoring of somatosensory evoked potentials. *ACNS*. http://www.acns.org/pdf/guidelines/Guideline-11B.pdf. Accessed August 6, 2014.

70. Moller AR, Jho HD, Janetta PJ. Preservation of hearing in operations on acoustic tumors: an alternative to recording brainstem auditory potentials. *Neurosurgery*. 1994;34:688–692.

71. Langeloo DD, Journée HL, De Kleuver M, Grotenhuis JA. Criteria for transcranial electrical motor evoked potential monitoring during spinal deformity surgery. A review and discussion of the literature. *Neurophysiol Clin*. 2007;37:431–439.

72. Deletis V, Sala F. Intraoperative neurophysiological monitoring of the spinal cord during spinal cord and spine surgery: a review focus on the corticospinal tracts. *Clin Neurophysiol*. 2008;119(2):248–264.

73. Kamerlink RJ, Errico T, Xavier S, et al. Major intraoperative neurologic monitoring deficits in consecutive pediatric and adult spinal deformity patients at one institution. *Spine*. 2010;35:240–245.

Autonomic Disorders in Children

Nancy L. Kuntz, MD
Theresa Oswald, BS, MS
Pallavi P. Patwari, MD

In the human body, the autonomic nervous system (ANS) regulates fundamental, involuntary functions. The ANS is involved in temperature regulation, digestion, maintaining upright posture, control of breathing, and circulation. Practitioners of most medical specialties can benefit from understanding autonomic function and from the potential diagnostic insight provided by quantitative autonomic testing. Traditionally, care for children with ANS dysregulation (ANSD) has been distributed among a variety of subspecialists based on the primary affected organ system. As understanding of ANSD in children expands, so does the need for pediatric-focused autonomic specialists and centers.

Over the past several decades, objective and noninvasive techniques have been developed and standardized in adults to evaluate the functioning of cardiovagal, adrenergic, and sudomotor aspects of the ANS (1). With this review, we aim to provide an overview of existing experience with noninvasive testing of autonomic function in children and to outline areas of promising future development.

SPECIAL CONSIDERATIONS FOR AUTONOMIC TESTING IN CHILDREN

At different ages, children and adolescents are frequently unable or unwilling to provide a cogent description of their clinical symptoms. In the youngest children, the barrier is frequently limited by expressive language. In school-aged children, their primal need to not embarrass themselves and to avoid being "different" creates a barrier to their self-reporting. Adolescents tend to be extraordinarily self-absorbed, reporting all of the innate sensations occurring in their bodies making it difficult, given their different personalities, to know whether the reported symptoms are normal or alarming. It is in this context that laboratory testing of autonomic function in children and adolescents becomes important. Objective findings that can demonstrate normal or altered function in one of the autonomic pathways can be helpful diagnostically. This data can also serve to monitor changes in function over time. An understanding of the child's age and developmental stage are key to anticipating a child's ability to tolerate and cooperate with autonomic testing. For example, certain aspects of testing include lying completely still during the application of low currents to the skin (sudomotor testing) or maintaining sustained increase in intrathoracic pressure (Valsalva maneuver)—tasks that can sometimes be challenging for cooperative adults. Further, during analysis and interpretation of results, consideration should be given to the developmental and maturational changes in the nervous system from infancy through adolescence. The development of age- and gender-matched normative data has been and remains a central goal. The organ systems and types of autonomic testing pertinent to children and adolescents are listed in Table 14.1.

To be maximally useful in children, autonomic testing should be brief, have instructions that are easy to understand and carry out, and be nonintrusive/nonpainful. This is particularly important as there is much work to be accomplished establishing normal control values in healthy children under 10 years of age.

TABLE 14.1 ANS Regulation by System and Available Autonomic Testing

ORGAN SYSTEM	ANS COMPONENT	AUTONOMIC TEST
Cardiovascular	Cardiovagal	- HR_{DB}, HR_{ST}, HR_{SQ}
		- VR
		- HRV
	Adrenergic	- Valsalva maneuver
		- HUT
		- SSR
		- Biochemical (catecholamine levels)
	Vasomotor	- Digit wrinkle
Respiratory	Control of breathing including chemoreception	- Exogenous ventilatory challenges
		- Awake and asleep physiologic testing
Skin	Sudomotor	- QSART
		- TST
Ophthalmologic	Pupillary	- Pupillography
Gastrointestinal	Enteric	- Gastric scintigraphy
		- Colonic transit
Urologic	Sympathetic	- Urodynamics
	Parasympathetic	- Bladder US

Abbreviations: ANS, autonomic nervous system; HR_{DB}, heart rate response to deep breathing; HR_{SQ}, heart rate response to squatting; HR_{ST}, heart rate response to standing (30:15 ratio); HRV, heart rate variability; HUT, head up tilt; QSART, quantitative sudomotor axon reflex test; SSR, sympathetic skin response; TST, thermoregulatory sweat test; US, ultrasound; VR, Valsalva ratio.

RATIONALE FOR AUTONOMIC TESTING IN PEDIATRICS

Quantitative ANS testing allows for the development of a deeper understanding of the inter-relationship of multisystem features of ANSD and the associated clinical significance of dysfunction in these physiologically intertwined systems. Laboratory autonomic testing is most effective when it is paired with a clinical evaluation that includes ANS-focused questions. Based on the preliminary evaluation, the pediatric clinician may find that there are children in whom the diagnostic question is related to autonomic control over a specific organ system or that broad screening of autonomic function is appropriate in order to determine whether a symptom is due to isolated, widespread, and/or evolving autonomic dysfunction. Autonomic testing is indicated in congenital autonomic disorders as well as for the growing number of recognized diseases for which autonomic dysfunction is an acquired phenomenon (Table 14.2).

TABLE 14.2 Classification of Pediatric Autonomic Nervous System Dysregulation

CLASSIFICATION	EXAMPLES OF DISORDERS/DIAGNOSES
Developmental/genetic	Alacrima, anhidrosis, adrenal insufficiency (AAAS)
	Congenital central hypoventilation syndrome (CCHS)
	Dopamine beta-hydroxylase (DBH) deficiency
	Fabry's disease
	Hereditary sensory and autonomic neuropathies, including familial dysautonomia
	Hirschsprung's disease
	Menkes syndrome
	Norepinephrine transporter (NET) deficiency syndrome
	Rett syndrome
	Shapiro's syndrome
Acquired	
Autoimmune	Guillain-Barré syndrome
	Autoimmune neuropathy/ganglionopathy
	Postural orthostatic tachycardia syndrome
Paroxysmal disorders	Autonomic storm (post central nervous system insult)
	Mast cell disorders
	Recurrent syncope
	Pheochromocytoma
	Postural orthostatic tachycardia syndrome
	Abdominal migraine, cyclic vomiting

(continued)

TABLE 14.2 Classification of Pediatric Autonomic Nervous System Dysregulation (*continued*)

CLASSIFICATION	EXAMPLES OF DISORDERS/DIAGNOSES
Disorders with associated autonomic dysregulation	
	Autism
	Chronic fatigue syndrome
	Cyclic vomiting syndrome
	Diabetes mellitus
	Migraine
	Mitochondrial cytopathies
	Rapid-onset obesity with hypothalamic dysfunction and autonomic dysregulation

The development of noninvasive, child-friendly autonomic testing methods and obtaining normative data for children of both genders is ongoing. As this is accomplished, we need to acknowledge that the process of performing autonomic testing can change autonomic tone in children and adolescents and use care when selecting the test to be performed and the normal values to be used (2).

TEST DESCRIPTIONS

Cardiovagal

Cardiovagal function refers to the dynamic, coordinated impact of the parasympathetic component of the autonomic system in regulating heart rate (HR) and blood pressure (BP) in response to challenges. These physiologic challenges effect changes in cardiac output and venous return, while being affected by intravascular volume and posture. Standardized testing methods include measurement of HR and BP responses to deep breathing, Valsalva maneuver, and position change (sit to stand, stand to squat, and squat to stand).

Heart Rate Response to Deep Breathing

The HR response to deep breathing (HR_{DB}) essentially provides a systematic and objective measure of the normal physiologic change in HR in response to breathing ("sinus arrhythmia"). With a combination of verbal coaching and visual pacing, subjects are asked to breathe slowly and deeply at 5 to 6 times per minute. HR during eight cycles (inspiration and expiration each taking 5 seconds) is recorded and the largest five consecutive responses are marked (Figure 14.1). HR_{DB} is calculated as the mean of the consecutive differences between maximal and minimal HR. Normative values exist for ages greater than 9 years, with reported inverse relationship of HR_{DB} with age (1,3). Specifically, normative values from 10 to 29 years of age in the Mayo Autonomic Lab are 14 to 41 (5th and 95th percentile, respectively) (1). HR_{DB} has been used to identify children with presymptomatic trypanosomiasis infections in Peru (4).

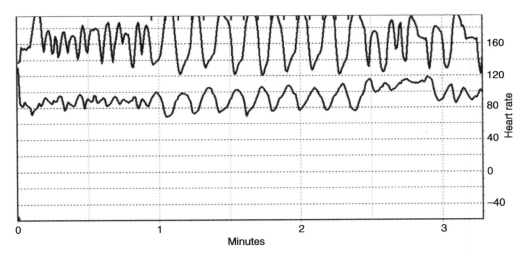

FIGURE 14.1 shows an HR$_{DB}$ recording in a normal 7-year-old girl with respiration monitored on the top trace and heart rate on the lower trace.

Valsalva Ratio

A stereotyped Valsalva maneuver must be performed to calculate the Valsalva ratio (VR), which measures the vagal component of the baroreflex. For this test, the subject is resting and supine, with continuous HR and finger BP monitoring and is then asked to maintain a fixed expiratory pressure (40–50 mmHg) for 15 seconds by blowing into a mouthpiece with a partial air leak. The VR is the ratio between the maximum HR occurring during the maneuver and the lowest HR occurring within 30 seconds of the maximal HR. VR appears to be a less sensitive measure of cardiovagal dysfunction than HR$_{DB}$ in adults. Normal values are 1.5 to 2.9 (5th and 95th percentile, respectively) and do not vary with age or gender in adults (1). In children, normative data for healthy children appear to be similar to reported values in adults with Longin et al. finding the 5th and 95th percentile values to be 1.4 and 2.7, respectively, for 6- to 11-year-old children and 1.3 and 2.8, respectively, for 12- to 15-year-olds (5). Other pediatric investigators report slightly lower VR values with a mean of 1.65 in 6- to 15-year-olds (4) and a mean value of 1.5 in 10- to 17-year-olds (3). In pediatric practice, it is important to consider that small finger size may limit ability to obtain BP values and that children may have difficulty with maintaining the sustained intrathoracic pressure required to successfully complete this test.

HR Response to Standing

For this test, the subject has his/her HR continuously monitored in a supine position for a baseline interval, then gets to an upright position without assistance, followed by continued cardiac monitoring for 2 minutes. The HR response to standing (HR$_{ST}$ or 30:15 ratio) is the ratio between the R-R interval at the 30th beat while standing and the 15th beat while standing. This has not been used as widely as the HR$_{DB}$. Though children tend to stand up quickly and more uniformly (as compared to adults who have notable variability in time to stand), they also tend to be more fidgety, causing variability in response due to altered venous return from muscle contraction and to excessive movement causing recording artifact. Normative data (with some variation in protocols) has been published for children as young as 4 years of age (3–5).

HR Response to Squatting

The baroreflex involves a negative feedback response to changes in BP and can be tested noninvasively with continuous HR and finger BP monitoring while asking the patient to change position. With the heart rate response to squatting (HR_{SQ}), the patient is asked to stand for 3 minutes and then squat for 1 minute, which causes an abrupt increase in BP. An attenuated baroreflex response with HR_{SQ} has been shown in adult diabetic patients with autonomic neuropathy (6,7). Another maneuver, which involves starting in a squatting position, then standing for 1 minute can be used to evaluate the baroreflex response for initial orthostatic hypotension (8). There are no published normal values for children.

HR Variability

Measures of HR variability (HRV) are acquired noninvasively through monitoring of electrocardiogram (ECG) for various intervals (from 5 minutes to 24 hours) and analyzing R-R intervals. HRV can be reported as time domain or frequency parameters. HRV reflects the neural influences upon HR at the level of the cardiac pacemaker (sinoatrial node), which are due to naturally opposing sympathetic and parasympathetic signals. These measures are influenced by physiologic state; so, interpretation of HRV values should be made with consideration of behavioral state: active versus quiet sleep and awake versus asleep state. It has been shown that HRV varies with age (8,9), reinforcing the importance of broadly applicable age-matched normal reference values (2,5). HRV can also be evaluated through visualization of Poincaré plots (scatter plots of successive R-R intervals). Decreased HRV, a sign of autonomic dysfunction, would demonstrate a narrow scatter pattern as opposed to a normal "ice cream cone" pattern indicating increased variability at slower HRs with longer R-R intervals (Figure 14.2).

Adrenergic

Head-Up Tilt

Tilt table testing has been widely used by cardiologists and physiologists for the evaluation of orthostatic tolerance. All protocols require that the lower extremities be passively restrained with feet planted on a footboard so that no muscle tension is required to maintain the upright posture as this would affect the physiologic status. Generally with head-up tilt (HUT), the patient is initially at rest, supine for 10 to 30 minutes, then passively elevated (motorized tilt table) to 70° HUT. HR, BP, and clinical status are then monitored for another 10 to 30 minutes. HUT performed in autonomic laboratories tends to be of shorter duration and performed without intravenous (IV) pharmacologic challenges typically used in cardiology testing. Adolescents without history of orthostatic intolerance experience a higher incidence of near fainting during cardiac HUT than adults, particularly when IV lines are placed and IV infusions are used (10,65). Recent studies have demonstrated that the 95th percentile for HR increment was 43 bpm in 106 healthy children from 8 to 19 years of age. While the HR increment was mildly higher in children referred for orthostatic intolerance, there was considerable overlap between controls and patients (11). Galland and coworkers have published data on young infants who

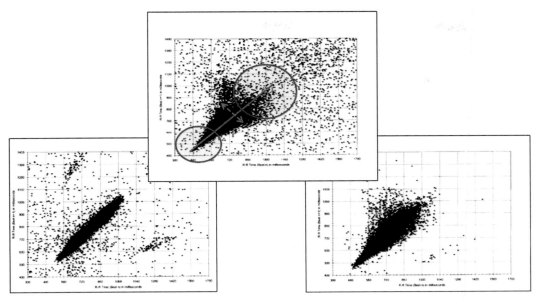

FIGURE 14.2 Poincaré plots. CCHS (left graph): narrow "cigar"-shaped plot (first reported by Marilyn Woo); normal child (middle graph): "ice cream cone"-shaped plot with labels indicating higher heart rates in circle to left, lower heart rates in circle to right, "line of identity" in red; ROHHAD (right graph): narrow plot, note decreased heart rate variability at lower heart rates.

Abbreviations: CCHS, congenital central hypoventilation syndrome; ROHHAD, rapid-onset obesity with hypothalamic dysfunction, hypoventilation, and autonomic dysregulation.

had simulated HUT testing while propped in HUT within their prams (12). They observed the effect of a 60° HUT on 60 full-term infants who were studied at 1 and 3 months of age. They noted that the HRV increased between 1 and 3 months of age, was reduced in prone as compared to supine sleeping position, and higher in active sleep compared to quiet sleep. There was no influence of a maternal history of cigarette smoking.

This data emphasizes the need for the development of normative data and unique diagnostic criteria in children and adolescents (11). Clearly, using adult norms (with 20-bpm increase in HR with upright posture) would create a significant pool of "false-positive" HUT in adolescent subjects.

Our autonomic laboratory monitors oxygen saturation, end-tidal CO_2, respiratory rate, and regional cerebral perfusion (rSO$_2$) via near-infrared spectroscopy (NIRS) as well as beat-to-beat HR and BP during our HUT. These data are very useful as changes in physiology and tendency to progress to syncope have been reported with hyperventilation. Martinon-Torres and colleagues (13) monitored end-tidal CO_2 during HUT in 34 children (mean age 10 yrs) referred for evaluation of syncope and noted that the time from onset of tilt and from onset of clinical symptoms to syncope were both significantly longer in children who were noted to hyperventilate. It was felt that this might identify a subgroup of children who would respond differently to preventive measures. Rao (14) demonstrated failure of cerebral autoregulation in syncope by monitoring NIRS during HUT. In our laboratory, we have demonstrated poor cerebral perfusion during postural orthostatic tachycardia syndrome (POTS)-associated "foggy" mental status with preserved peripheral BP. Figure 14.3 demonstrates the HR, BP, and cerebral perfusion responses to HUT in several adolescents with orthostatic intolerance. Note the wide swings in monitored vital HR and BP in the first and second set of tracings, which are frequently noted in POTS. The third set of tracings demonstrates failure of cerebral autoregulation in an adolescent with POTS.

Valsalva Maneuver (BP Response During Phases II and IV)

A stereotyped Valsalva maneuver (see description under "Valsalva Ratio") can also provide information regarding adrenergic function. In normal individuals, four phases of change in BP are observed: Late phase II and phase IV provide the most information about adrenergic function. Early phase II consists of a decline in BP followed by late phase II, which is an alpha-adrenergic–mediated arterial vasoconstriction leading to recovery of BP toward/above baseline levels. Phase IV consists of a BP overshoot of baseline (beta-adrenergic mediated) followed by gradual return of BP to baseline. With the Valsalva maneuver, BP is affected by a combination of mechanical factors such as intrathoracic and intra-abdominal pressure changes, changes in peripheral vascular resistance, as well as cardiovagal and adrenergic tone. Insight regarding cardiac adrenergic tone can be obtained from qualitative assessment of the arrest of the fall and subsequent increase in BP in late phase II and assessment of the increase in BP (with overshoot past baseline) seen in phase IV. There is limited experience in evaluating this phenomenon in children, as the youngest (and most ill) children have more difficulty in maintaining the required expiratory pressure for 15 continuous seconds. The two lower lines on Figure 14.4 outline systolic and diastolic BP during a Valsalva maneuver in a 7-year-old girl, with arrows noting late phase II and phase IV changes in BP demonstrating intact adrenergic function in this young girl.

Sympathetic Skin Response

The sympathetic skin response (SSR) reflects the degree of activity in the sympathetic nervous system and is based on skin conductance that can be recorded over the palm of the hand and the sole of the foot in response to sensory or electrical stimuli (see Figure 14.5). SSR has been used to establish hearing thresholds after cochlear implants (15) as well as to monitor response to enzyme replacement therapy in individuals with Fabry's disease (16). Assessing SSR with different stimuli (electrical, thermal, inspiratory gasp, or auditory) has been used to objectively identify the preserved sensory fibers in familial dysautonomia (FD or HMSN III) (17) Many factors can affect the SSR such as skin temperature and stimulus strength as well as the patient's emotional state and ability to be surprised (18). A limitation of this test is that the response habituates and tends to be "all or none" rather than a graded response.

Sudomotor

Quantitative Sudomotor Axon Reflex Test

Quantitative sudomotor axon reflex test (QSART) was developed in the Autonomic Laboratory at Mayo Clinic, Rochester, and provides information about sweat glands and postganglionic sympathetic nerve fibers. The QSWEAT is a commercially available, Food and Drug Administration (FDA)-approved device (based on QSART technique), which measures evoked sweat volumes. QSWEAT requires surface placement of quarter-sized disks through which a

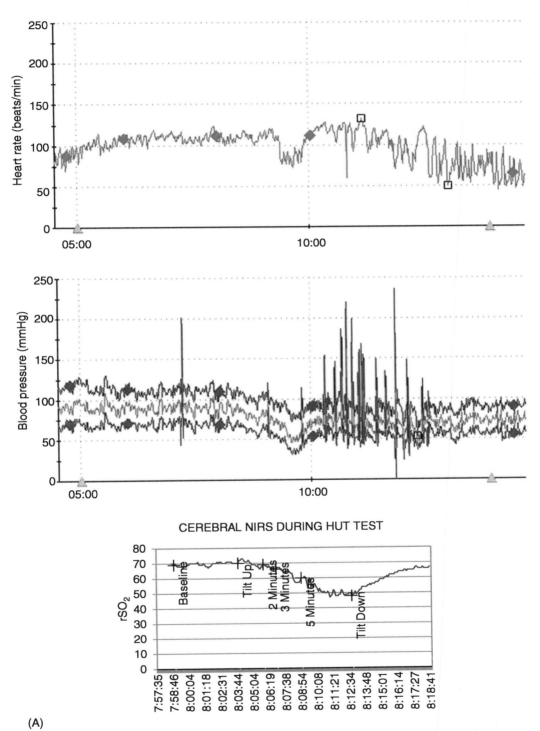

(A)

FIGURE 14.3 (A) Vasovagal response. Ten-year-old male with progressive decline in HR, BP, and cerebral regional saturation values in association with abdominal pain, nausea, and poor color/perfusion of face and neck. (*continued*)

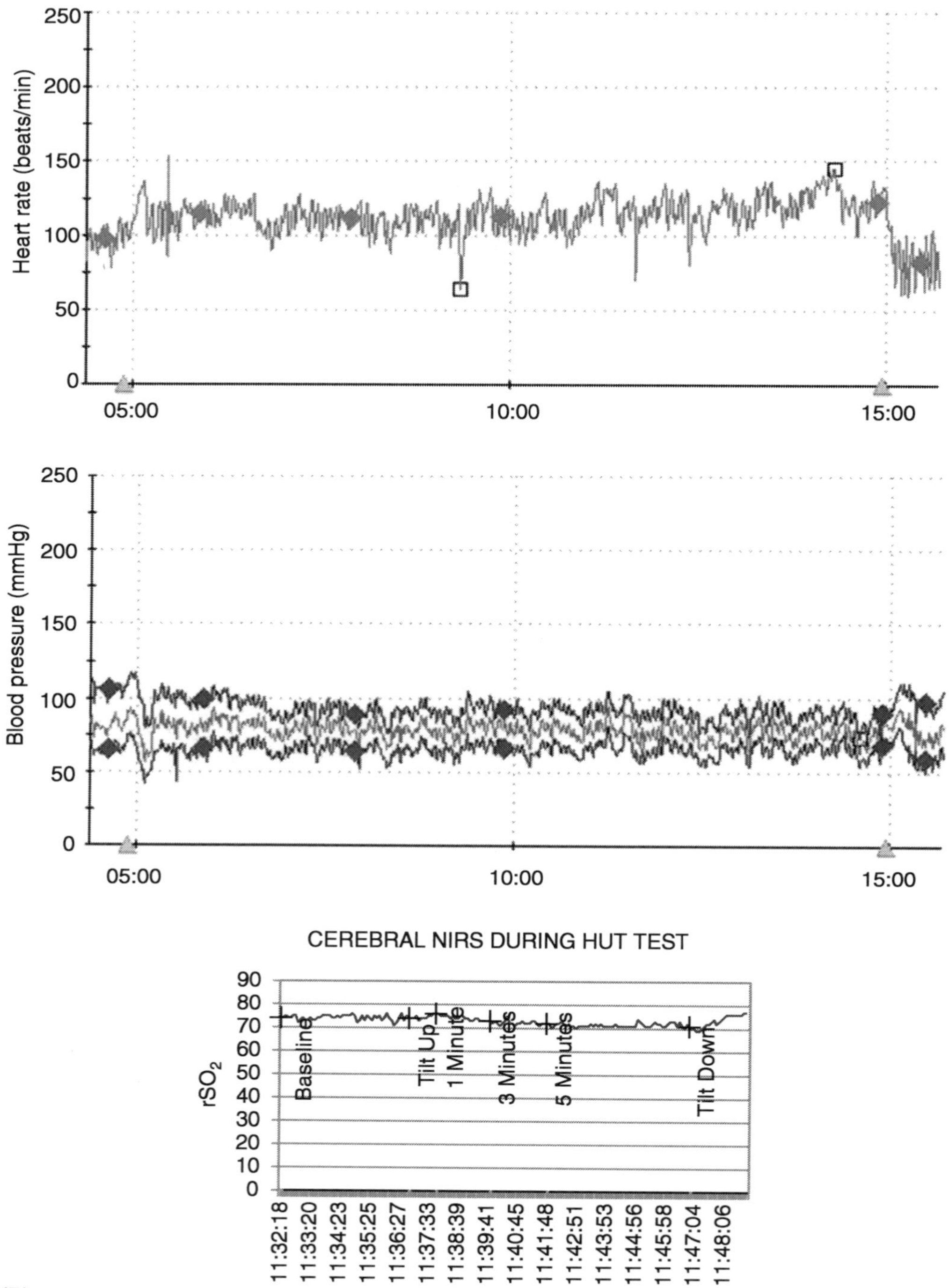

(B)

FIGURE 14.3 (*continued*) (B) Postural orthostatic tachycardia syndrome (POTS). Ten-year-old female demonstrates a 45-bpm increase in HR from baseline with stable BP during HUT. (*continued*)

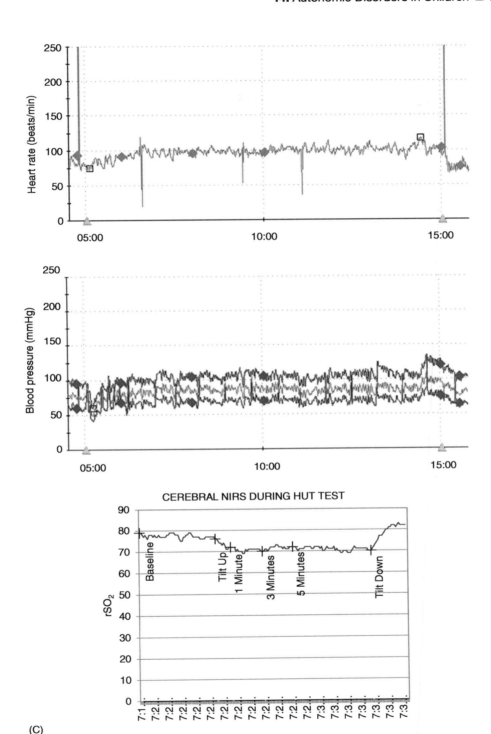

(C)

FIGURE 14.3 (*continued*) (C) POTS with drop in cerebral perfusion. Fourteen-year-old female demonstrating a regional cerebral perfusion (rSO₂) decrease in the first minute of HUT and then rebounding above baseline after return to the horizontal position.

Abbreviations: BP, blood pressure; HR, heart rate; HUT, head-up tilt; NIRS, near-infrared spectroscopy.

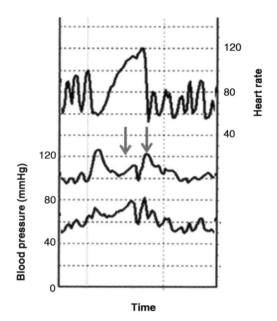

FIGURE 14.4 Upper tracing records heart rate and two lower tracings record beat-to-beat changes in blood pressure during voluntary Valsalva maneuver in a 7-year-old girl.

low-intensity constant current stimulus is passed for iontophoresis of acetylcholine through the skin and stimulation of sudomotor sympathetic axons. The impulse travels antidromically to an axon branch point and then orthodromically back down to synapse on the muscarinic receptor on an eccrine sweat gland. The same capsule is used to provide acetylcholine for iontophoresis, guide the constant current stimulus, and collect data regarding the volume of local sweat production. Capsules are typically placed at four sites (foot, distal leg, proximal leg, and forearm) and simultaneous stimulation provides information regarding sudomotor function along the extremities at various postganglionic axonal lengths (1). However, it is possible to have focal or regional sudomotor dysfunction that will not be identified with this technique. Sweat volumes are affected by age, gender, hydration status, and anticholinergic medication. These techniques have been used diagnostically in children down to 2 years of age (personal observation). However, normative data has not been systematically developed for individuals less than 20 years of age. Staiano et al. reported forearm QSART responses of 2.8 ± 1.3 mV amplitude in 11 healthy children between 4 and 10 years of age and 2.9 ± 1.2 mV amplitude in eight healthy children from 10 to 17 years of age (3).

Thermoregulatory Sweat Test

The thermoregulatory sweat test (TST) is a sensitive, established autonomic test of central and peripheral sympathetic sudomotor function. By applying moisture-sensitive powder to the entire anterior aspect of a body, sweat production over the forehead, lower face, torso, and extremities can be evaluated (see Figure 14.6) (19). It has proven value in the diagnosis of small-fiber neuropathy, autonomic failure, focal and multifocal neuropathies, and

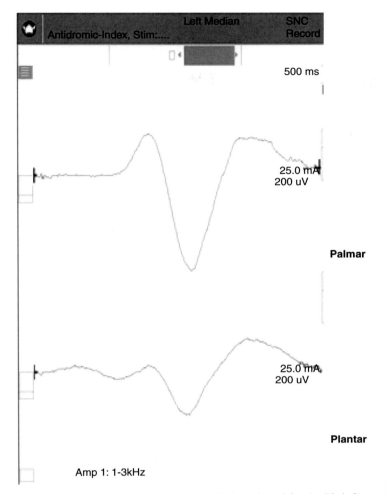

FIGURE 14.5 Sympathetic skin response from right hand and foot with left median nerve stimulation.

ganglionopathies. The utility of this test in the evaluation of pediatric disorders has not been well studied. However, in 2011, Kuntz et al. reviewed the experience at Mayo Clinic, Rochester, relating to TST in over 200 children 2 to 16 years of age—demonstrating that TST was well tolerated in children and adolescents with valid, clinically relevant results obtained in 93.5% of the patients studied (20). TST, in children, was particularly useful in the evaluation of small-fiber peripheral neuropathies, myelopathies, multifocal or patchy peripheral nerve involvement, and disorders of sweating including anhidrosis and hyperhidrosis. In children and adolescents, TST was valuable for the assessment of small-nerve fiber function as it required less cooperation than quantitative sensory testing and was less invasive than multiple epidermal nerve fiber layer biopsies. Figure 14.7 demonstrates how TST can define abnormalities of sweating in children.

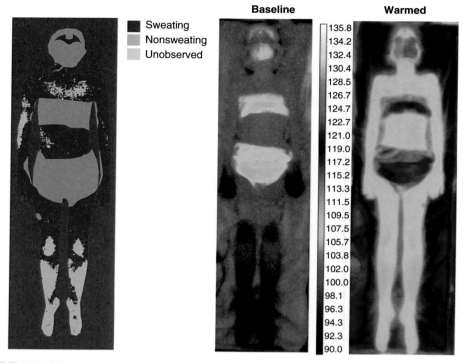

FIGURE 14.6 Fifteen-year-old female with distal anhidrosis suggestive of distal sudomotor or small-fiber nerve dysfunction.

Pupillography

Actions of the smooth muscles of the iris cause changes in pupil size. Pupillometry provides noninvasive, detailed measures of pupil size and response to light, with pupil dilation and constriction, respectively, indicating relative sympathetic and parasympathetic responsiveness

Hyperhidrosis and Anhidrosis

 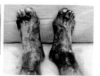 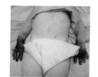

Fourteen-year-old with 5+ years of execessive sweating from hands, feet, and axillae. Images above *taken before-heat*, show the resting sweat distribution in purple. After heating, the remainder of body sweat profusely.
Dx: Primary Focal Hyperhidrosis

Six-year-old female also with excessive hand sweating. Above image taken *after* heat exposure revealed widespread anhidrosis with compensatory hand hyperhidrosis.
Dx: Chronic Idiopathic Anhidrosis

FIGURE 14.7 Examples of thermoregulatory sweat test in children with excessively sweaty hands and feet.

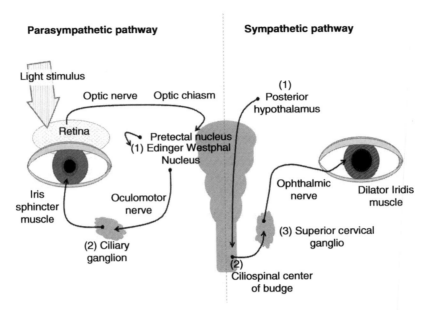

Parasympathetic pathway   **Sympathetic pathway**

FIGURE 14.8 Parasympathetic and sympathetic pathways involved in pupillary control.

Source: Adapted from Patwari PP, Stewart TM, Rand CM, et al. Pupillometry in Congenital Central Hypoventilation Syndrome (CCHS): Quantitative evidence of autonomic nervous system dysregulation. *Pediatr Res.* 2012;71(3):280–285, copyright 2012 by International Pediatric Research Foundation, Inc. (IPRF).

(Figure 14.8). Daluwatte and colleagues (63,64) have published normative values for pupillary responses in children. Accordingly, quantitative pupil measurements have recently been used to evaluate ANSD in various conditions including autonomic neuropathies (21,22), enuresis (23), heart failure (24), diabetes (25,26), and pediatric autonomic disorders such as FD (27) and congenital central hypoventilation syndrome (CCHS) (28).

Studies investigating the use of pupillometry have often used a 30- to 40-millisecond duration light flash (29,30); however, there is the need for a longer flash in some groups of patients. Patients with autoimmune autonomic ganglionopathy (AAG) have been found to have premature pupil redilation (31). These patients require a 2-second flash.

Use of pupillometry to measure autonomic regulation requires attention to ambient room light and ocular pathology or anterior visual pathway disease, which alter the afferent pathways. The patient must be cooperative (able to maintain stable eye position during the recording). Environmental triggers (loud noises or any type of stimulation that can cause anxiety or fear) can affect the sympathetic/parasympathetic balance.

Enteric

The process of eating (from perception of food through digestion to defecation) requires intact autonomic (sympathetic, parasympathetic, and enteric) function. Salivary secretion is under both sympathetic and parasympathetic control with inhibition and stimulation of salivary gland output, respectively. As the parasympathetic system is activated, gastric and pancreatic secretion increases. With elegant coordination, enteric motility is also enhanced. Most often, altered enteric autonomic function becomes apparent through altered gastrointestinal (GI) motility:

delayed or enhanced stomach or intestinal transit time with symptoms of vomiting, early satiety, abdominal distention, abdominal pain, diarrhea, or constipation.

The options for the evaluation of GI transit are increasing as technology advances. For the purposes of this review, we will focus on GI emptying studies and colonic transit studies that can be performed in the pediatric patient. An excellent review of the adult clinical experience with autonomic testing of GI function has been recently published (32).

In children, differential diagnosis needs to include potential congenital anomalies. In children with constipation, GI dysmotility, or unexplained abdominal pain, Hirschsprung's disease (HSCR) (absence of ganglion cells due to failure of migration) needs to be considered. Evaluation for HSCR starts with barium enema to determine the presence and location of a transition zone. If barium enema is suggestive of HSCR, then rectal biopsy is indicated to identify the absence of ganglion cells. A subset of children with HSCR have been found to have signs of ANSD relating to pupillary, cardiovascular, and sudomotor function (3). Further, HSCR can be found in pediatric autonomic disorders, such as in CCHS (33).

Gastric Scintigraphy

For scintigraphy, the patient is required to ingest a standardized amount of radiolabeled solid or liquid material (mixed with palatable items) with sequential imaging to determine the rate of emptying. Gastric scintigraphy would be indicated for the evaluation of unexplained vomiting, early satiety, or food intolerance suggestive of gastroparesis. Small-bowel and colonic scintigraphy can be performed but require longer duration of evaluation and lack standardization with limited normative data even in adults.

Colonic Transit With Radiopaque Markers

Ingestion of radiopaque markers is in use for the evaluation of colonic transit time by following the number of retained markers via abdominal radiograph over several days. Normative values are available for children (34–36).

Urologic

Urodynamic studies including the measurement of postvoid residual volume can be performed in children and adolescents to evaluate sympathetic and parasympathetic function. Recent articles outline the use of videourodynamic studies and uroflow/electromyography (EMG) for differentiating between common voiding disorders in children (37,38). Most interestingly for those interested in autonomic dysfunction in children and adolescents, the commonly observed voiding disorders, which occur without identifiable anatomic lesions of the spinal cord or spinal roots, are termed "nonneurogenic voiding disorders." These disorders appear to involve poor coordination or balance between activation of the bladder smooth muscle, bladder neck, urinary sphincters, and pelvic floor. These would logically be disorders involving some combination of dysfunction in the central and peripheral autonomic pathways controlling voiding. Since "nonneurogenic" is a misleading term, these disorders could be considered autonomic disorders affecting voiding rather than nonneurogenic voiding disorders (personal observation).

Vascular

Skin Wrinkling

The clinical phenomenon of glabrous skin with sweat glands (finger tips and soles of the feet) wrinkling or "pruning" in response to prolonged immersion in water has been observed for decades—with the first report as a potential test of autonomic function in 1977 (39). Recent studies in adults have demonstrated that this is a sympathetically mediated vasoconstrictive phenomenon (40,41). Other studies have replicated the same phenomenon by placing a topical anesthetic such as EMLA™ under an occlusive dressing (42,43). None of these methods have been studied systematically in children or adolescents.

OTHER CLINICAL APPLICATIONS

Identification of Risk Factors for Autonomic Dysregulation

Johansson et al. (44) documented increased sympathoadrenal activity in childhood (fractionated urinary catecholamines, higher baseline HR and greater increment in HR after mental arithmetic/stress test) in healthy children with a history of preterm or small-for-gestational-age (SGA) birth.

EARLY DETECTION AND MONITORING OF COMPLICATIONS OF SYSTEMIC DISEASE

Diabetes

Varechova and colleagues (45) demonstrated a decreased threshold to capsaicin-induced cough reflex in diabetic children with subclinical autonomic neuropathy and have suggested this as a screening test for autonomic neuropathy in diabetic children.

Cahill and colleagues (46) studied pupillography and response to pilocarpine (0.1%) and cocaine (4%) in 72 children with type I diabetes, 60 children with type II diabetes, and 120 age-matched controls. Smaller dark-adapted pupil size and denervation hypersensitivity to pilocarpine were noted in the diabetic patients even when VR testing of cardiovagal function was normal. This was recommended as an inexpensive way to detect early diabetic autonomic neuropathy (DAN).

Boysen et al. (47) tested 20 patients with diabetes I between 10 and 19 years of age and report that HRV measures and baroreflex sensitivity (BRS) were more sensitive at detecting abnormalities in diabetic patients than HR_{DB} or the 30:15 ratio. They speculated that incomplete cooperation or effort in some of the 136 control children studied may have led to the abnormalities noted with the later studies.

It remains to be seen whether early signs of autonomic dysregulation can be identified and used as a target for improved diabetic control in the pursuit of decreased long-term cardiac and renal complications of diabetes.

Screening for Other Systemic Illnesses

Trypanosomiasis

Bowman and colleagues (4) studied 38 children with confirmed but presymptomatic *Trypanosoma cruzi* infection in Peru and demonstrated blunted cardiovagal responses as compared to control children for the Valsalva maneuver (ratio of longest to shortest R-R interval), the cold pressor, and orthostatic tests. These simple, community-based tests requiring no expensive or high-technology equipment could serve well for screening programs.

Behcet's Disease

Borman et al. (48) documented abnormalities in HR variability and SSR in 70 Behcet's disease patients (primarily adults). While these abnormalities were primarily subclinical, there was a correlation between these changes and elevation of inflammatory markers, suggesting a relationship with disease activity.

Wilson's Disease

Soni et al. (49) studied 30 patients (mean age 19 years, range 11–47) with Wilson's disease and noted that 70% reported at least one autonomic symptom such as abnormal sweating, heat intolerance, early satiety, constipation, postural dizziness, bladder incontinence, palpitation, syncope, diarrhea, and dry mouth/dry skin. On testing, they noted increased HR at rest and decreased VRs and HR_{DB}. The SSR latency was significantly higher, and 10% of this cohort had absent SSR in at least one extremity. Parasympathetic and sympathetic deficits were both observed, with the former more prominent.

Asthma

Emin et al. (50) demonstrated a direct relationship between the severity of atopic asthma and the degree of abnormality in HRV and SSR in 77 children from 7 to 12 years old. Autonomic testing was suggested as a cost-effective manner to assess disease severity in cases of pediatric asthma.

High BP

Fitzgibbon et al. (51) studied 11- to 14-year-old children with high BP (HBP) (1) and normal BP (85) and calculated high-frequency (HF) and low-frequency (LF) power spectrum and BRS from 5 minutes of beat-to-beat BP and HR data. Children with HBP (> 95th percentile but not clinically hypertensive) demonstrated reduced autonomic regulation.

Obstructive Sleep Apnea

Montesano et al. (52) evaluated 18 children between 6 and 16 years of age who were undergoing evaluation for obstructive sleep apnea (OSA) and compared their autonomic test results (VR, HR_{DB}, HR 30:15, HUT BP response) with age-matched controls. The children with OSA demonstrated higher baseline BP and HR, greater increments in BP with HUT, and lower HR variability with deep breathing. These findings suggest an increase in sympathetic tone in children with OSA, and long-term implications need to be further evaluated.

IDENTIFYING UNDERLYING PATHOPHYSIOLOGY OF CLINICAL DISORDERS

Harlequin Syndrome/Flushing

Bremner and colleague (62) evaluated pupillary responses in 38 patients with Harlequin syndrome and noted Horner syndrome ipsilateral to the side with impaired facial sweating and flushing in two-thirds of the patients. Ten percent of the patients had a previously undetected mass lesion in the chest or neck presumably affecting the superior cervical ganglion or sympathetic chain.

Cyclic Vomiting Syndrome

Chelimsky et al. (53) studied six children between 6 and 16 years of age with classical cyclic vomiting syndrome and noted normal HR_{DB} and Valsalva maneuver. Sudomotor (QSART) testing was abnormal in all patients. Response to HUT demonstrated greater than 30 bpm increase in HR in all six children and a vasodepressor change in BP in three who developed dizziness. Autonomic testing therefore demonstrated sudomotor and sympathetic abnormalities, but not parasympathetic abnormalities, in a small cohort of children with cyclic vomiting syndrome.

Syncope/Orthostatic Intolerance

Martinon-Torres and colleagues (13) monitored end-tidal CO_2 during HUT in 34 children (mean age 10 yrs) referred for evaluation of syncope and noted that the time from onset of tilt and from onset of clinical symptoms to syncope were both significantly longer in children who were noted to hyperventilate. It was felt that this might identify a subgroup of children who would respond differently to preventive measures.

Singer et al. (11) performed an important study, which recruited 106 individuals under 20 years of age with good health and compared their HUT results (usually 5 minutes of tilt though a subset was tilted out to 10 minutes) with those of 654 patients of the same age who had been referred for testing due to clinical problems relating to orthostatic intolerance or lightheadedness. They observed that the HR increment in normal control children and adolescents was higher than previously estimated: The 95th percentile for the 5-minute orthostatic HR increment among normal controls was 43 bpm using HR averaged over 30 seconds. Further, an excessive orthostatic HR was considered to be 130 to 140 bpm in children 13 years of age or younger and greater than 120 bpm in adolescents 14 years and older. The authors suggested using the term "orthostatic symptoms without tachycardia" for symptomatic individuals who did not meet these criteria.

Antiel and colleagues (54) studied 31 patients between 12 and 17 years of age who presented with dyspepsia. A 10-minute HUT was performed as part of their clinical evaluation. Fifty percent of the 21 patients who demonstrated at least a 30-bpm increase in HR with HUT reported orthostatic dizziness as a daily complaint, while only 30% of the 10 patients with lower increases in HR with HUT reported orthostatic symptoms. The severity of the clinical GI symptoms and the results of gastric emptying did not relate to the amount of orthostatic tachycardia. While there is overlap between individuals with GI dysmotility and orthostatic intolerance, it is not universal and the magnitude of symptoms do not vary directly within an individual.

Longin et al. (55) studied 55 children with neurocardiogenic syncope and presyncope from 5 to 15 years of age and compared results of orthostatic testing in response to a 5-minute HUT and to 5 minutes of active standing with results from age-matched controls. HRV measures differed significantly from controls during tilt testing, with no overlap between LF power and total power calculated in control children and those with a history of neurocardiogenic syncope.

Characterization of Fiber-Type Involvement in Peripheral Neuropathies

Hilz (56) and colleagues demonstrated SSR changes in 13 patients with FD with different sensory stimuli used to evoke the responses. In patients with FD, preserved SSR in response to electrical stimuli with impaired or absent response to thermal stimuli confirmed small-fiber dysfunction.

Houlden et al. (57) studied 131 individuals with a wide spectrum of inherited peripheral neuropathies. Pupillary abnormalities were rare in hereditary neuropathy with liability to pressure palsy (HNPP) and Charcot-Marie-Tooth (CMT) I, but CMT II showed frequent and varied pupillary dysfunction. This was felt to be a differentiating finding between these two types of inherited neuropathy. Individuals with Refsum's disease and hereditary sensory and autonomic neuropathies also had abnormalities on pupillary testing.

Detecting Small-Fiber Dysfunction—Particularly as Cause of Pain Syndromes in Children and Adolescents

Oaklander and Klein (58) studied 41 consecutive children and adolescents with debilitating, unexplained widespread pain syndromes. A high fraction of autonomic tests were abnormal in this group (27% with decreased HR_{DB}, 42% with abnormal Valsalva maneuver, 75% with abnormal HUT, and 82% with abnormal QSART). Only two patients had a sural nerve biopsy; both (100%) were abnormal, and 11 of 37 (30%) who underwent skin biopsies for determination of nerve fiber density were abnormal. The noninvasiveness of the autonomic tests as well as the ability to repeat testing to assess treatment response strongly recommended consideration of autonomic testing for the evaluation of significant, unexplained widespread pain syndromes.

Abdominal Pain or GI Dysmotility

One recently described syndrome, the "4A" syndrome (adrenocortical insufficiency associated with achalasia, alacrima, and autonomic symptoms) can present with either abdominal pain/gastroesophageal motility problems or orthostatic intolerance (59). This can present from preschool years through adult life and has been associated with mutations in AAAS, a GTP-binding protein-linked hormone receptor. In addition to the symptomatic GI and orthostatic issues, patients have been demonstrated to lack normal HRV on HR_{DB} and VR testing and to have abnormalities of pupillary responsiveness.

Safder and colleagues (60) evaluated 76 children with functional abdominal pain on tilt table testing. They noted that the group of children whose symptoms were reproducible on HUT benefited more from treatment with fluids and fludrocortisone than those whose symptoms were not reproduced on the tilt test.

Safder et al. (61) recorded surface EMG over the gastric region (electrogastrography) in 49 adolescents undergoing HUT testing (25 meeting criteria for POTS and an age-matched group that did not meet POTS criteria). The two groups did not differ with respect to supine gastric activity. However, the adolescents meeting POTS criteria had significantly increased gastric activity in the upright HUT position. This data suggests an etiologic mechanism for the abdominal symptoms in children with POTS.

FUTURE DIRECTIONS

Using new technologies to develop faster, less intrusive methods of measuring autonomic function will be very useful in infants, children, and adolescents. This clearly has to be followed by collection of data from adequate cohorts of healthy children to allow precision in the interpretation of developmental changes over growth and aging.

SUMMARY

Many clinical disorders involve changes in the autonomic nervous system. It is important that pediatricians and pediatric specialists have the support available to evaluate, diagnose, and monitor autonomic involvement in the myriad of appropriate clinical problems that occur in children. While autonomic testing has an important role in detecting, diagnosing, and monitoring treatment, it is critical that it be performed using well-established protocols with adequate normative controls to facilitate interpretation.

REFERENCES

1. Low PA, Sleeten DM. Laboratory evaluation of autonomic failure. In: Low PA, Benarroch EE, eds. *Clinical Autonomic Disorders*. 3rd ed. Philadelphia, PA: Lippincott-Raven;2008:130–160.
2. Longin E, Dimitriadis C, Shazi S, et al. Autonomic nervous system function in infants and adolescents: impact of autonomic tests on heart rate variability. *Pediatr Cardiol*. 2009;30:311–324.
3. Staiano A, Santoro L, DeMarco R, et al. Autonomic dysfunction in children with Hirschsprung's disease. *Digestive Dis Sci*. 1999;44(5):960–965.
4. Bowman NM, Kawai V, Gilman RH, et al. Autonomic dysfunction and risk factors associated with Trpanosoma cruzi infection among children in Arequipa, Peru. *Am J Trop Med Hyg*. 2011;84(1):85–90.
5. Longin E, Schaible T, Lenz T, König S. Short term heart rate variability in healthy neonates: Normative data and physiologic observations. *Early Hum Dev*. 2005;81(8):663–671.
6. Marfella R, Giugliano D, diMaro G, et al. The squatting test. A useful tool to assess both parasympathetic and sympathetic involvement of the cardiovascular autonomic neuropathy in diabetes. *Diabetes*. 1994;43:607–612.
7. Nakagawa M, Shinohara T, Anan F, et al. New squatting test indices are useful for assessing baroreflex sensitivity in diabetes mellitus. *Diabet Med*. 2008;25(11):1309–1315.
8. Weiling W, Krediet CTP, van Dijk N, et al. Initial orthostatic hypotension: review of a forgotten condition. *Clin Sci(Lond)*. 2007;112:157–165.
9. Silvetti MS, Drago F, Ragonese P. Heart rate variability in healthy children and adolescents is partially related to age and gender. *Int J Cardiol*. 2001;81(2–3):169–174.
10. deJong-deVos van Steenwijk CC, Wieling W, Johannes HM, et al. Incidence and hemodynamic characteristics of near-fainting in healthy 6–16 year old subjects. *J Am Coll Cardiol*. 1995;25(7):1615–1621.
11. Singer W, Sletten DM, Opfer-Gehrking TL, et al. Postural tachycardia in children and adolescents—what is abnormal? *J Pediatr*. 2012;160(2):222–226.
12. Galland BC, Hayman RM, Taylor BJ, et al. Factors affecting heart rate variability and heart rate responses to tilting in infants aged 1 and 3 months. *Pediatr Res*. 2000;48(3):360–368.
13. Martinon-Torres F, Rodriguez-Nunez A, Fernandez-Cebrian S, et al. The relation between hyperventilation and pediatric syncope. *J Pediatr*. 2001;138(6):894–897.

14. Rao RP, Danduran MJ, Dixon JE, et al. Near intrared spectroscopy: guided tilt tzable testing for syncope. *Pediatgr Cardiol.* 2010;31:674–679.
15. Péréon Y, Laplaud D, Nguyen TT, Radafy E. A new application for the sympathetic skin response: the evaluation of auditory thresholds in cochlear implant patients. *Clin Neurophysiol.* 2001;112(2):314–318.
16. Jardim LB, Gomes I, Netto CB, et al. Improvement of sympathetic skin responses under enzyme replacement therapy in Fabry disease. *J Inherit Metab Dis.* 2006;29:653–659
17. Hilz MJ, Axelrod FB, Schweibold G, Kolodny EH. Sympathetic skin response following thermal, electrical, acoustic, and inspiratory gasp stimulation in familial dysautonomia patients and healthy persons. *Clin Auton Res.* 1999;9(4):165–177.
18. Vertugno, R, Liguori, R, Montagna, P, Cortelli, P. Sympathetic skin response: Basic mechanisms and clinical applications. *Clin Auton Res.* 2003;13:256–270.
19. Fealey RD. Thermorgulatory Sweat Test. In: Low PA, Benarroch EE, eds. *Clinical Autonomic Disorders.* 3rd ed. Philadelphia, PA: Lippincott-Raven;2008:245–257.
20. Kuntz NL, Fealey RE. Utility of diagnostic thermoregulatory sweat test in children. *Neurol.* 2010;76(9 Suppl 4):A 575.
21. Bremner F, Smith S. Pupil findings in a consecutive series of 150 patients with generalised autonomic neuropathy. *J Neurol Neurosurg Psychiatry.* 2006;77(10):1163–1168
22. Bremner F. Pupil evaluation as a test for autonomic disorders. *Clin Auton Res.* 2009;19(2):88–101.
23. Dundaroz R, Turkbay T, Erdem U, et al. Pupillometric assessment of autonomic nervous system in children with functional enuresis. *Int Urol Nephrol.* 2009;41(2):231–235.
24. Keivanidou A, Fotiou D, Arnaoutoglou C, et al. Evaluation of autonomic imbalance in patients with heart failure: a preliminary study of pupillomotor function. *Cardiol J.* 2010;17(1):65–72.
25. Maguire AM, Craig ME, Craighead A, et al. Autonomic nerve testing predicts development of complications; A 12 year followupstudy. *Diabetes Care.* 2007;30(11):77–82.
26. Karavanaki-Karanassiou K. Autonomic neuropathy in children and adolescents with Diabetes Mellitus. *J Pediatr Endocrinol Metab.* 2011;14 Suppl 5:1579–1586.
27. Dutsch M, Hilz MJ, Rauhut U, et al. Sympathetic and parasympathetic pupillary dysfunction in familial dysautonomia. *J Neurol Sci.* 2002;195(1):77–83.
28. Patwari PP, Stewart TM, Rand CM, et al. Pupillometry in Congenital Central Hypoventilation Syndrome (CCHS): Quantitative evidence of autonomic nervous system dysregulation. *Pediatr Res.* 2012;71(3):280–285.
29. Muppidi S, Adams-Hunt B, Tajzoy E, et al. Dynamic pupillometry as an autonomic testing tool. *Clin Auton Res.* 2013;23:297–303.
30. Boev A, Fountas K, Karampelas I, et al. Quantitative pupillometry: normative data in healthy pediatric volunteers. *J Neurosurg.* 2005;103(6 Suppl):496–500.
31. Muppidi S, Schribner M, Gibbons C, et al. A Unique manifestation of pupillary fatique in autoimmune autonomic ganglionopathy. *Arch Neurol.* 2012;69(5):644–648.
32. Rao SS, Camilleri M, Hasler WL, et al. Evaluation of gastrointestinal transit in clinical practice: position paper of the American and European Neurogastroenterology and Motility Societies. *Neurogastroenterol Motil.* 2011;23(1):8–23.
33. Weese-Mayer DE, Berry-Kravis EM, Ceccherini I, et al. An official ATS Clinical Policy Statement: Congenital central hypoventilation syndrome: Genetic basis, diagnosis, and management. *Am J Respir Crit Care Med.* 2010;181(6):626–644.
34. Casasnovas AB, Cives RV, Jeremias AV, et al. Measurement of colonic transit time in children. *J Pediatr Gastroenterol Nutr.* 1991;13(1):42–45.
35. Sutcliffe JR, King S, Hutson JM, Southwell B. What is new in radiology and pathology of motility disorders in children? *Semin Pediatr Surg.* 2010;19(2):81–85.
36. Wagener S, Shankar KR, Turnock RR, et al. Colonic transit time—what is normal? *J Pediatr Surg.* 2004;39(2):166–169.
37. Glassberg K, Combs AJ, Horowitz M. Non- neurogenic voiding disorders in children and adolescents: Clinical and Videourodynamic findings in 4 specific conditions. *J Urol.* 2010;184(5):2123–2127.
38. Van Batavia JP, Comb AJ, Hyun G, et al. Simplifying the Diagnosis of four common voiding conditions using uroflow/electromyography, electromyography lag time and voiding history. *J Urol.* 186(4 Suppl):1721–1726.

39. Bull C, Henry JA. Finger wrinkling as a test of autonomic function. *Br Med J*. 1997;1(6060):551–552.

40. Wilder-Smith EPV, Chow A. Water-immersion wrinkling is due to vasoconstriction. *Muscle Nerve*. 2003a;27:307–311.

41. Van Barneveld S, van der Palen J, van Putten MJ. Evaluation of the finger wrinkling test: a pilot study. *Clin Auton Res*. 2010;20(4):249–253.

42. Wilder-Smith E, Chow A. Water immersion and EMLA cause similar digit skin wrinkling and vasoconstriction. *J Microvasc Res*. 2003b;66:68–72.

43. Wilder-Smith EP, Guo Y, Chow A. Stimulated skin wrinkling for predicting intraepidermal nerve fibre density. *ClinNeurophysiol*. 2009;120(5):953–958.

44. Johansson S, Norman M, Legnevall L, et al. Increased catecholamines and heart rate in children with low birth weight: perinatal contributions to sympathoadrenal overactivity. *J Intern Med*. 2007;261(5):480–487.

45. Varechova S, Durdik P, Cervenkova V, et al. He influence of autonomic neuropathy on couge reflex sensitivity in children with diabetes mellitus type 1. *J Physiol and Pharmacol*. 2007;58 Suppl 5:705–715.

46. Cahill M, Eustace P, deJesus V. Pupillary autonomic denervation with increasing duration of diabetes mellitus. *Br J Ophthalmol*. 2001;85(10):1225–1230.

47. Boysen A, Lewin MA, Hecker W, et al. Autonomic function testing in children and adolescents with diabetes mellitus. *Pediatr Diabetes*. 2007;8(5):261–264.

48. Borman P, Tuncay F, Kocaoglu S, et al. The subclinic autonomic dysfunction in patients with Behcet disease: an electrophysiological study. *Clin Rheumatol*. 2012;31(1):41–47.

49. Soni D, Shukla G, Singh S, et al. Cardiovascular and sudomotor autonomic dysfunction in Wilson's disease—Limited correlation with clinical severity. *Auton Neurosci*. 2009;151:154–158.

50. Emin O, Esra G, Aysegul D, et al. Autonomic nervous system dysfunction and their relationship with disease severity in children with atopic asthma. *Respir Physiol Neurobiol*. 2012;183(3):206–210.

51. Fitzgibbon LK, Coverdale NSS, Phillips AA, et al. The association between baroreflex sensitivity and blood pressure in children. *Appl Physiol Nutr Metab*. 2012;37(2):301–307.

52. Montesano M, Siano S, chiari Paolino M, et al. Autonomic cardiovascular tests in children with obstructive sleep apnea syndrome. *Sleep*. 2010;33(10):1349–1355.

53. Chelimsky TC, Chelimsky GG. Autonomic abnormalities in cyclic vomiting syndrome. *J Pediatr Gastroenterol Nutr*. 2007;44(3):326–330.

54. Antiel RM, Risma JM, Grothe RM, et al. Orthostatic intolerance and gastrointestinal motility in adolescents with nausea and abdominal pain. *J Pediatr Gastroenterol Nutr*. 2008;46:285–288.

55. Longin E, Reinhard J, vonBuch D, et al. Autonomic function in children and adolescents with neurocardiogenic syncope. *Pediatr Cardiol*. 2008;29(4):763–770.

56. Hilz MJ. Assessment and evaluation of hereditary sensory and autonomic neuropathies with autonomic and neurophysiological examinations. *Clin Auton Res*. 2002;12 Suppl 1:133–143.

57. Houlden H, Reilly MM, Smith S. Pupil abnormalities in 131 cases of genetically defined inherited peripheral neuropathy. *Eye (Lond)*. 2009;23(4):966–974.

58. Oaklander Al, Klein MM. Evidence of small-fiber polyneuropathy in unexplained, juvenile-onset, widespread pain syndromes. *Pediatrics*. 2013;131(4):1091–1100.

59. Gazarian M, Cowell CT, Bonney M, Grigor WG. The "4A" syndrome: adrenocortical insufficiency associated with achalasia, alacrima, autonomic and other neurological abnormalities. *Eur J Pediatr*. 1995;154(1):18–23.

60. Safder S, Chelimsky TC, O'Riordan MA, Chelimsky G. Autonomic testing in functional gastrointestinal disorders: implications of reproducible gastrointestinal complaints during tilt table testing. *Gastroenterol Res Pract*. 2009;2009:1–6.

61. Safder S, Chelimsky TC, O'Riordan MA, Chelimsky G. Gastric electrical activity becomes abnormal in the upright position in patients with postural tachycardia syndrome. *J Pediatr Gastroenterol Nutr*. 2010;51(3):314–318.

62. Bremner F, Smith S. Pupillographic findings in 39 consecutive cases of harlequin syndrome. *J Neuroophthalmol*. 2008;28(3):171–177.

63. Daluwatte C, Miles JH, Christ SE, et al. Age-dependent pupillary light reflex parameters in children. *Conf Proc IEEE Eng Med Biol Soc*. 2012;2012:3776–3779.

64. Daluwatte C, Miles JH, Yao G. Simultaneously measured pupillary light reflex and heart rate variability in healthy children. *Physiol Meas.* 2012;33(6):1043–1052.
65. Grubb BP, Orecchio E, Kurcyzynski TW. Head-upright tilt table testing in evaluation of recurrent, unexplained syncope. *Pediatr Neurol.* 1992;8(6):423–427.

Clinical Neurophysiology: Future Role in Pediatric Neurologic Disorders

Aatif M. Husain, MD

Clinical neurophysiology (CNP) offers a unique method of analyzing the nervous system. Though the anatomy can be visualized in many different ways, the best and most common way of evaluating the function of the nervous system is with CNP. Most often, neurophysiologic procedures are used to help diagnose neurologic diseases. Though neurophysiologic abnormalities are often nonspecific, neurophysiologists are called upon to help confirm suspected diagnoses or suggest elusive ones. The field is growing rapidly, as evidenced by the increase in the number of publications each year (1).

The future role of CNP in pediatric (and adult) neurologic diseases will most certainly evolve from where it is today. Advances in neuroimaging and molecular and genetic testing have allowed much more specific diagnoses than allowed by CNP procedures. This coupled with advances in technology and the availability of new procedures is making the future of CNP more exciting than its past was. In this chapter, some ways in which CNP will evolve and the factors responsible for it are discussed. The discussion is not meant to be comprehensive, and many innovative CNP techniques are not reviewed due to space limitations. However, some of the more significant ways that CNP will be used in the future are noted.

HISTORICAL PERSPECTIVE

CNP has evolved much in the last 75 years. In the middle of the last century, though much had already been learned about electrical activity in the nervous system, clinical applications of neurophysiologic techniques were still in their infancy. Early neurophysiologists used machines and electrodes they made themselves (2,3). Oscilloscopes were used to display signals, and special paper was used to create hard copies (4). In the early and mid-20th century, the true utility of diagnostic CNP had yet to be realized. At the time, electroencephalography (EEG) and electromyography (EMG) were still research tools available only in large universities. That these tools could be used to diagnose many neurologic conditions had not yet been fully appreciated. Indeed, some of the initial diagnostic applications ended up not being as useful as originally thought; early investigators thought EEG would be helpful in determining the etiology of various psychopathologies (5).

In the latter part of the last century, CNP matured as a discipline and its value in the diagnosis of many neurologic conditions became well established. It was the primary method of objectively viewing the nervous system. The use of evoked potentials (EPs) allowed neurophysiologists the opportunity to analyze parts of the nervous system that were difficult to evaluate with other available methods, such as the spinal cord. Specialized training became necessary to properly interpret these tests so that accurate diagnostic information could be obtained from them. Certification examinations were created to test practitioners' proficiencies (6).

With maturity came the recognition that there were limits to the diagnostic utility of neurophysiologic testing. Despite their increasing popularity and utility, it was recognized that abnormalities detected by neurophysiologic tests were often nonspecific. This was particularly true for abnormalities detected with EPs (7). Moreover, in some situations, the sensitivity was limited as well. This was demonstrated by the relatively low sensitivity of a single EEG in diagnosing epilepsy (8). Another less well-recognized example is the low sensitivity and specificity of the multiple sleep latency test (MSLT) in the diagnosis of narcolepsy (9). These limitations were not unique to CNP; all tests used in medical diagnosis have limitations of sensitivity and specificity.

The improvements in electronics and integration of computers in medical testing allowed additional remarkable advances in CNP. Better amplifiers and commercially available equipment brought standardization to the field. Computers allowed the ability to digitize CNP data that were previously analog. Instead of paper, digital methods of displaying and storing data became available. Not only did this allow neurophysiologic tests to be done over longer periods of time, it reduced costs as well (10). The digitization of data also allowed better analysis and quantification.

Even as CNP matured and its vital place in neurologic diagnosis became established, there was evolution in its use. With the introduction and rapid development of neuroimaging, there became available another method of visualizing the nervous system. While neurophysiologic tests demonstrated physiologic injury, neuroimaging visualized anatomical changes. One example of now CNP was affected by neuroimaging was in the field of EPs. In the 1970s, EPs were the primary method of "visualizing" abnormalities in multiple sclerosis (MS) and detecting silent lesions (7). With the introduction of magnetic resonance imaging (MRI), the value of EPs diminished, and MRI along with cerebrospinal fluid analysis became the standard for investigating and diagnosing MS (11). Other advances have also had an impact on CNP. The development and availability of molecular and genetic testing has allowed many conditions to be precisely diagnosed. While CNP tests have proved to be sensitive, they are rarely specific for a particular condition. Many genetic and metabolic neurologic disorders could only be suggested by neurophysiologic tests, while molecular and genetic testing have made specific diagnoses possible. The utility of EEG and EMG in the diagnosis of these disorders has evolved (12,13).

Neuroimaging, molecular and genetic testing, and other advances have affected the use of all types of CNP procedures. In response, CNP has evolved and continues to evolve. Much like the pioneers of the early 20th century, the neurophysiologists of today are pushing the limits of neurophysiologic testing.

BETTER TECHNIQUE, BETTER ANALYSIS, BETTER INTERPRETATION

As the available equipment for performing neurophysiologic tests improves, the techniques for performing these tests have matured as well. Digital EEG acquisition techniques have allowed obtaining of data from many more electrodes in better detail. Better amplifiers have allowed improved sampling and signal resolution that was unheard of previously. Instead of 21 electrodes usually placed on the scalp, the dense array EEG uses 125 or more electrodes to generate data to help with the localization of seizure foci (source localization) (14,15). Further refinement of these techniques will lead to even better localization of ictal onset zones, which in turn will lead to better treatment for patients with epilepsy.

Concurrently, invasive EEG recordings have also improved. This type of EEG provides more than diagnosis—it aids in treatment as well. Rather than the conventional strip and grid electrodes, microelectrodes that are placed closer together are able to acquire data from much smaller areas of the cortex (16). Better electrode quality and recording characteristics also are allowing the detection of ultra-high and infra-slow frequency EEG activity. The correlation of these brain waves to pathology is being defined. Stereo-EEG is yet another advancement in invasive EEG recordings. Several stereotactically implanted depth electrodes can reach areas of the brain that are not accessible to subdural electrodes (17). These electrodes can localize epileptic zones more precisely. More widespread use of such techniques will lead to better treatment outcomes.

New methods are being used in EMG as well. Surface EMG was previously thought to add no additional value to needle analysis (18). However, with improved techniques and equipment, a more recent study found value in this technique, which offers a painless way of analysis of nerves and muscles (19). High-density surface EMG represents further enhancement of this technique. High-density analysis allows assessment of muscle fiber physiology that previously was not possible (20). While the diagnostic utility of this is not fully defined, continued research into noninvasive ways of neuromuscular assessment will lead to better diagnostic tools that will be more readily accepted by patients.

Many people believed that EPs had been supplanted by other imaging modalities. However, once again, with improved stimulation and recording techniques, EPs are now being applied for more refined assessment of the nervous system and are also finding utility in the diagnosis of nonneurologic conditions. Multifocal visual evoked potentials (mfVEPs) involve stimulation of small sectors of the visual field. This allows a more precise analysis of the optic nerve (21). Though still a research tool, mfVEP may prove to be a sensitive way to assess for optic neuritis in MS and various ophthalmologic disorders. Event-related potentials (ERPs) have long been thought of as useful in studying cognitive processing. Recent studies are showing utility of these diagnostic tests in neuropsychological disorders (21). More refinement of the various types of ERPs may lead to their adoption in diagnostic testing and monitoring therapeutic intervention in these conditions.

These are only a few ways in which currently established neurophysiologic tests may evolve in the future. There are many other examples in which technical advances and improved understanding of the procedures are pushing the boundaries of how these tests are currently used.

QUANTIFICATION OF DATA

The availability of digital acquisition of neurophysiologic data has allowed its quantification. Quantification involves processing the data through various algorithms to generate maps that reveal characteristics of the underlying data that are not evident on visual analyses of raw data. This has best been applied to EEG. Quantitative EEG has different meaning for different neurophysiologists. One way quantitative EEG has been used is to create "brain maps" of EEG data that has been processed. These brain maps change, based on various cognitive processes and can be measured when performing various tasks. In this way, it can also help monitor the effects of various therapeutic or other interventions (22). Brain maps will likely become a more valuable way of assessing higher cognitive functioning.

One of the most clinically useful applications of quantitative EEG has been in the analysis of long-term or continuous EEG (cEEG). Hours of data can be reviewed expeditiously by analyzing the quantitative EEG. This is particularly true of pediatric cEEG studies (23). Though many neurophysiologists continue to feel that review of the raw EEG is essential, the quantitative analysis certainly adds another dimension to interpretation. As the number of cEEG studies increases, algorithms for quantitative analysis improve, and the reviewers for raw EEG are limited, the need for and desirability of quantitative EEG will increase in the future.

Algorithms are also being used to quantify the number of functioning motor axons. This is process is known as motor unit number estimation (MUNE). Though MUNE has been done for many decades, recently, decomposition-enhanced spike-triggered averaging MUNE has been developed that uses computer algorithms. These quantitative assessments will prove to be valuable in studying disease evolution and response to treatment.

IMPROVED TEMPORAL RESOLUTION

Neurophysiologic studies traditionally have been done for short periods of time. Routine EEGs are typically 20 to 30 minutes, while neonatal EEGs are usually 60 minutes. EMGs provide neurophysiologic assessment of the peripheral nervous system at a finite time. Outside of video EEG (vEEG) monitoring, polysomnography (PSG) used to be the longest neurophysiologic test, lasting several hours. In the last 15 years, the utility of cEEG has become increasingly clear. Many more critically ill patients are found to be seizing when long-term EEG testing is performed as compared to 30- to 60-minute tracings (24–26). Investigations are suggesting that there may be features that are evident within the initial few minutes of the EEG that determine the likelihood of finding seizures later (27). cEEG tracings are often continued for 24 to 48 hours when a suspicion for seizures is present and longer if seizures are found. Pediatric and adult practitioners are realizing the need for cEEG monitoring, and it is rapidly becoming necessary for large hospitals to offer this type of monitoring. In addition to detecting more seizures, this improved temporal resolution is also revealing EEG patterns not appreciated before, such as stimulus-induced rhythmic, periodic, or ictal discharges (SIRPIDs) (28). The need for cEEG monitoring will continue to increase, and neurophysiologists will discover new patterns of EEG, the significance of which will have to be investigated.

The need for long-term analysis is also being realized in the assessment of sleep. While PSGs are multihour studies, they still only typically evaluate one night of sleep. Often a single night in a sleep laboratory does not reveal typical sleep. Long-term sleep-wake assessments in the form of actigraphy are becoming more popular. Not only can this test reveal abnormalities in circadian physiology, it can be useful to document hours of sleep over a multiweek period. This type of information may be necessary in various diagnostic evaluations, such as to determine the amount of sleep obtained before an MSLT (29). The need for assessing the sleep-wake schedule over several days to weeks is being recognized for various pediatric behavioral sleep disorders as well. The importance of sleep assessment can be realized by the popularity of commercially available devices that track exercise and sleep times (eg, FitBit®, others). The true sensitivity and utility of long-term sleep analysis will be further clarified in the future.

Other neurologic diseases with fluctuating signs and symptoms could also benefit from long-term neurophysiologic analysis. One such condition is myasthenia gravis. Though several neurophysiologic tests are available for diagnosis and determining the response to treatment, these tests are typically done at a given moment in time. Neurophysiologists may want to evaluate this and similar disorders over hours to days to get a better understanding of disease fluctuations that may not be evident clinically. Subtle subclinical changes may become evident that foretell clinical decompensation and allow early intervention.

EXPANDING THE SPHERE OF CLINICAL NEUROPHYSIOLOGY

The future of CNP will include an expanding sphere of how the nervous system is evaluated neurophysiologically. This will involve using traditional neurophysiological procedures and using them in new ways and using innovative techniques for evaluation. An example of an innovative use of a traditional neurophysiological test is the use of EPs in neurophysiologic intraoperative monitoring (NIOM). The application of EPs in NIOM enabled neurophysiologists to reduce the morbidity of many surgical procedures (30–32). NIOM continues to expand, and neurophysiologists are called upon to participate in many types of surgeries in which the nervous system is at risk. This field will continue to expand, limited only by the number of neurophysiologists wanting to pursue it (33).

Noninvasive brain stimulation is another exciting area of growth for neurophysiologists. Transcranial magnetic stimulation (TMS), a type of noninvasive brain stimulation, has evolved from being a research technique to being both a diagnostic and therapeutic tool. Moreover, it brings together and enhances collaboration between researchers from many different disciplines. TMS has allowed neurophysiologic assessment of pathways that were previously not possible in awake subjects (34). It has increased the pathophysiologic understanding of many neurologic disorders (35). Recalcitrant psychiatric disorders have also been treated with TMS (36). Moreover, it can also be used in the assessment of efficacy of drugs. This exciting neurophysiologic modality is just beginning to be integrated into clinical practice, and the future will see it increasing in popularity.

Magnetoencephalography (MEG) is another technique that has been available for decades, but more recently, its utility in evaluating patients for epilepsy surgery has become better defined. It serves as a useful complement to EEG in localizing neocortical epileptic zones (37). There are other uses for MEG as well. It has been used to study cognitive processes in fetuses and infants. Detection of problems can lead to earlier and more effective early intervention programs (38). The clinical availability of commercial MEG has certainly fueled its progress. Future neurophysiologists will be poised to further exploit this technology to help patients.

New techniques are also becoming available to investigate muscles and nerves. Electrical impedance myography (EIM) uses electricity to image muscles. Though currently still a research tool, EIM may lead to better diagnostic testing and longitudinal assessment of neuromuscular disorders (39). More research in the future will enable this technology to become integrated into clinical practice.

NEW DISEASES, BETTER ASSESSMENTS

The future of CNP will see neurophysiologists using their tools to assess conditions that have not traditionally been evaluated with neurophysiologic methods. TMS offers one of the best ways to study the pathophysiology of movement disorders like Parkinson's disease (PD) and dystonia (35). This technique has allowed investigators to study various symptoms of these conditions in detail, which hopefully will lead to better and more targeted therapies.

Various pain syndromes lend themselves well for analysis by neurophysiologic methods. Cortical hyperexcitability and hypoexcitability, also referred to as "dysexcitability," has been studied with EPs and TMS (40). Though conflicting results have been found, several theories about pathogenesis have emerged. Further investigations into this and other pain syndromes with newer techniques may bring these disease states into the clinical domain of the neurophysiologist.

Psychiatric conditions such as depression can be treated with TMS. Evaluation of some psychiatric conditions with TMS and other types of neurophysiologic tests may reveal clues to their pathophysiology. Conversion disorder and hysteria have been studied with a variety of neurophysiologic procedures, including cognitive EPs, EEGs, and MEGs. These studies have led to several theories that explain the cause of hysterical paralysis (41). More studies of this type will yield insights into the pathophysiology of not only neurologic but psychiatric conditions as well.

NEUROPHYSIOLOGY AS A BIOMARKER

Perhaps one of the most exciting advances in CNP has been the use of various neurophysiologic procedures as biomarkers of disease progression and severity. Though seemingly a natural fit, EEG has not been used much as a biomarker in treatment trials for seizures until recently. This is not surprising given the uncertain relationship between interictal abnormalities, epilepsy disease severity, and seizure control. With the availability of cEEG monitoring and the realization of frequent seizures in critically ill patients, the role of EEG as a biomarker has become possible. Recently a multicenter, randomized trial comparing the efficacy of antiepileptic drugs (AEDs) in the treatment of nonconvulsive seizures was completed (42). This was the first study to use EEG as a biomarker to evaluate the relative effectiveness of AEDs in critically ill patients. Other trials are already underway using EEG as a biomarker for treatment response of super refractory status epilepticus (SRSE) (43). SRSE is a diagnosis based on EEG, so it is certainly logical that treatment trials would use EEG as a measure of treatment success. The use of EEG is not without challenges, however. Interpretation of this test is still largely subjective; at times, consensus on what constitutes pathology (seizures) may be elusive. The use of EEG as a biomarker in epilepsy and status epilepticus studies has just started. The future hopefully will see many more similar clinical trials.

EPs have also found utility as biomarkers in clinical trials (44). MS/optic neuritis trials have used pattern reversal VEP to assess myelination of the optic nerve (45). Optic nerve conduction (VEP P100 latency) changes were used in a clinical trial as an objective way to compare the degree of remyelination with active drug versus placebo (46).

TMS has also been used as a biomarker. It has been combined with EMG and EEG to study the effect of drugs on muscles and the brain (47). TMS-EMG and TMS-EEG studies are also being used to predict which patients may respond to a particular therapy. This field is in its infancy, and in the future, it may enable physicians to better select medications for certain diseases.

The role of CNP in clinical trials is just being appreciated. Neurophysiologic tests offer an objective method of assessing symptoms that are currently assessed only subjectively. This may help remove a lot of noise from clinical trials and enable demonstration of therapeutic effect more clearly and with fewer subjects. Neurophysiologists will be well served in pursuing the use of neurophysiologic procedures as biomarkers in the assessment of therapy for neurologic and psychiatric disorders.

NONSCIENTIFIC INFLUENCES

Like any other medical discipline, nonscientific issues will also affect the future of CNP. Foremost among these influences are economic issues. Reimbursements for neurophysiologic procedures unfortunately affect how and how often they are performed. Favorable reimbursements may see an overuse of various procedures, while cuts may limit their availability. The last several years have seen government regulators reduce reimbursements for EMG/NCS (nerve conduction studies) and NIOM (48,49). How much this will affect patient care remains to be seen. It will undoubtedly have an immeasurable effect on students considering a career in CNP. These economic issues are most acute in the United States, but other practice settings are not immune to this either. Clearly, these issues will affect the future of CNP, but exactly how is unclear.

Naturally, clinical training in CNP will affect the future of the field as well. Though countries vary on how training is imparted, most developed countries have an organized process by which trainees can obtain specialization in this field. In the United States, formal fellowship programs provide the requisite training that is overseen by regulatory agencies. However, many training programs provide education in the more established disciplines in CNP, such as EEG and EMG. Few focus on fields such as NIOM or TMS (33). Professional trade organizations also provide education in CNP, and recently they have recognized the value in having programs in emerging CNP disciplines. More education in all areas of CNP and in research methods will be critical in ensuring further development of this field.

Education and training are important for not only physicians but also technologists. CNP technology has become too complex for the physicians to also serve as technologists, as was the case in the era of the pioneers of the field (50). Though board certification/registration examinations at basic and advanced levels are available for technologists, formal training programs are few and the number of graduates produced insufficient to maintain and grow CNP departments. Such is the situation in the United States; elsewhere in the world, the shortage of qualified technologists is even more acute. Training individuals on the job to perform these highly complex procedures often fills this void. While this helps ameliorate an acute shortage, it is not a viable long-term solution. Neurophysiologists will have to direct their attention to this problem urgently. Appropriate training programs, perhaps at a bachelor's or master's level, will be important to create and encourage a constant stream of qualified, professional technologists. Without this support staff, further progress in CNP will be greatly hampered.

CONCLUSIONS

The era of using CNP simply to diagnose neurologic disorders is coming to a close. No longer will neurophysiologists be content with providing a differential diagnosis for a condition or even diagnosing a disease; they will be using their procedures in many other ways. More traditional CNP tests will be used in novel ways to more accurately diagnose diseases. Long-term use of these tests will provide longitudinal data on disease progression. New neurophysiologic procedures are opening new chapters in diagnosis, management, and treatment of neurologic and psychiatric diseases that had not previously been evaluated with CNP. Abnormalities detected on neurophysiologic tests are being used as biomarkers of disease; these can be used in clinical trials and other ways to monitor the progression of a disease or response to treatment. Nonscientific influences will also affect CNP. The future of CNP is bright, and there remain many exciting opportunities for research, education, and teaching for young neurophysiologists.

REFERENCES

1. IFCN. Research & guidelines. http://www.ifcn.info/showcontent.aspx?MenuID=1137. Cited December 24, 2014.
2. Haas LF. Hans Berger (1873–1941), Richard Caton (1842–1926), and electroencephalography. *J Neurol Neurosurg Psychiatry.* 2003;74(1):9.
3. Kazamel M, Province P, Alsharabati M, Oh S. History of electromyography (EMG) and nerve conduction studies (NCS): a tribute to the founding fathers. *Neurology.* 2013;80(Meeting abstracts 1):P05.259.
4. Ladegaard J. Story of electromyography equipment. *Muscle Nerve Suppl.* 2002;11:S128–S133.
5. Schirmann F. "The wondrous eyes of a new technology"-a history of the early electroencephalography (EEG) of psychopathy, delinquency, and immorality. *Front Hum Neurosci.* 2014;8:232.
6. ABPN. Mission and history. http://www.abpn.com/mission_and_history.html. Cited December 26, 2014.
7. Aminoff MJ. The clinical role of somatosensory evoked potential studies: a critical appraisal. *Muscle Nerve.* 1984;7(5):345–354.
8. Hoefnagels WA, Padberg GW, Overweg J, et al. Syncope or seizure? The diagnostic value of the EEG and hyperventilation test in transient loss of consciousness. *J Neurol Neurosurg Psychiatry.* 1991;54(11):953–956.
9. Goldbart A, Peppard P, Finn L, et al. Narcolepsy and predictors of positive MSLTs in the Wisconsin Sleep Cohort. *Sleep.* 2014;37(6):1043–1051.
10. Husain AM, Hope VT, Mebust KA, et al. Cost analysis of analog versus digital electroencephalography. *Am J Electroneurodiagnostic Technol.* 1998;11:144–147.
11. McDonald WI, Compston A, Edan G, et al. Recommended diagnostic criteria for multiple sclerosis: guidelines from the International Panel on the diagnosis of multiple sclerosis. *Ann Neurol.* 2001;50(1):121–127.

12. Karakis I, Liew W, Darras DT, et al. Referral and diagnostic trends in pediatric electromyography in the molecular era. *Muscle Nerve.* 2014;50(2):244–249.
13. Swash M. What does the neurologist expect from clinical neurophysiology? *Muscle Nerve Suppl.* 2002;11:S134–S138.
14. Holmes MD, Tucker DM, Quiring JM, et al. Comparing noninvasive dense array and intracranial electroencephalography for localization of seizures. *Neurosurgery.* 2010;66(2):354–362.
15. Lantz G, Grave de Peralta R, Spinelli L, et al. Epileptic source localization with high density EEG: how many electrodes are needed? *Clin Neurophysiol.* 2003;114(1):63–69.
16. Schevon CA, Ng SK, Cappell J, et al. Microphysiology of epileptiform activity in human neocortex. *J Clin Neurophysiol.* 2008;25(6):321–330.
17. Panzica F, Varotto G, Rotondi F, et al. Identification of the Epileptogenic Zone from Stereo-EEG Signals: A Connectivity-Graph Theory Approach. *Front Neurol.* 2013;4:175.
18. Haig AJ, Gelblum JB, Rechtien JJ, Gitter AJ. Technology assessment: the use of surface EMG in the diagnosis and treatment of nerve and muscle disorders. *Muscle Nerve.* 1996;19(3):392–395.
19. Meekins GD, So Y, Quan D. American Association of Neuromuscular & Electrodiagnostic Medicine evidenced-based review: Use of surface electromyography in the diagnosis and study of neuromuscular disorders. *Muscle Nerve.* 2008;38(4):1219–1224.
20. Drost G, Stegeman DF, van Engelen BG, Zwarts MJ Clinical applications of high-density surface EMG: A systematic review. *J Electromyogr Kinesiol.* 2006;16(6):586–602.
21. Grover LK, Hood DC, Ghadiali Q, et al. A comparison of multifocal and conventional visual evoked potential techniques in patients with optic neuritis/multiple sclerosis. *Doc Ophthalmol.* 2008;117(2):121–128.
22. Michel CM, Murray MM. Towards the utilization of EEG as a brain imaging tool. *Neuroimage.* 2012;61(2):371–385.
23. Stewart CP, Otsubo H, Ochi A, et al. Seizure identification in the ICU using quantitative EEG displays. *Neurology.* 2010;75(17):1501–1508.
24. Jette N, Claassen J, Enerson RG, Hirsch LJ. Frequency and predictors of nonconvulsive seizures during continuous electroencephalographic monitoring in critically ill children. *Arch Neurol.* 2006;63(12):1750–1755.
25. Shafi MM, Westover MB, Cole AJ, et al. Absence of early epileptiform abnormalities predicts lack of seizures on continuous EEG. *Neurology.* 2012;79(17):1796–1801.
26. Claassen J, Mayer SA, Kowalski, et al. Detection of electrographic seizures with continuous EEG monitoring in critically ill patients. *Neurology.* 2004;62(10):1743–1748.
27. Swisher CB, Shah D, Sinha SR, Husain AM. Baseline EEG pattern on continuous ICU EEG monitoring and incidence of seizures. *J Clin Neurophysiol.* 2015;32(2):147–151.
28. Hirsch LJ, Claassen J, Mayer SA, Enmerson RG. Stimulus-induced rhythmic, periodic, or ictal discharges (SIRPIDs): a common EEG phenomenon in the critically ill. *Epilepsia.* 2004;45(2):109–123.
29. Baumann CR, Mignot E, Lammers GJ, et al. Challenges in diagnosing narcolepsy without cataplexy: a consensus statement. *Sleep.* 2014;37(6):1035–1042.
30. Nuwer MR, Dawson EG, Carlson LG, et al. Somatosensory evoked potential spinal cord monitoring reduces neurologic deficits after scoliosis surgery: results of a large multicenter survey. *Electroencephalogr Clin Neurophysiol.* 1995;96(1):6–11.
31. Radtke RA, Erwin CW, Wilkins RH. Intraoperative brainstem auditory evoked potentials: significant decrease in postoperative morbidity. *Neurology.* 1989;39(2 Pt 1):187–191.
32. Nuwer MR, Emerson RG, Galloway G, et al. Evidence-based guideline update: intraoperative spinal monitoring with somatosensory and transcranial electrical motor evoked potentials: report of the Therapeutics and Technology Assessment Subcommittee of the American Academy of Neurology and the American Clinical Neurophysiology Society. *Neurology.* 2012;78(8):585–589.
33. Husain AM, Emerson RG, Nuwer MN. Emerging subspecialties in neurology: neurophysiologic intraoperative monitoring. *Neurology.* 2011;76(15):e73–e75.
34. Galloway GM, Dias BR, Brown JL, et al. Transcranial magnetic stimulation--may be useful as a preoperative screen of motor tract function. *J Clin Neurophysiol.* 2013;30(4):386–389.
35. Hallett M, Rothwell J. Milestones in clinical neurophysiology. *Mov Disord.* 2011;26(6):958–967.
36. Slotema CW, Blom JD, Hoek HW, Sommer IE. Should we expand the toolbox of psychiatric treatment methods to include Repetitive Transcranial Magnetic Stimulation (rTMS)? A meta-analysis of the efficacy of rTMS in psychiatric disorders. *J Clin Psychiatry.* 2010;71(7):873–884.

37. Baumgartner C, Pataraia E. Revisiting the role of magnetoencephalography in epilepsy. *Curr Opin Neurol.* 2006;19(2):181–186.
38. Sheridan CJ, Matuz T, Draganova R, et al. Fetal Magnetoencephalography - Achievements and Challenges in the Study of Prenatal and Early Postnatal Brain Responses: A Review. *Infant Child Dev.* 2010;19(1):80–93.
39. Rutkove SB. Electrical impedance myography: Background, current state, and future directions. *Muscle Nerve.* 2009;40(6):936–946.
40. Cosentino G, Fierro B, Brighina F. From different neurophysiological methods to conflicting pathophysiological views in migraine: A critical review of literature. *Clin Neurophysiol.* 2014;125(9): 1721–1730.
41. Crommelinck M. Neurophysiology of conversion disorders: A historical perspective. *Neurophysiol Clin.* 2014;44(4):315–321.
42. Husain AM. Treatment of Recurrent Electrographic Nonconvulsive Seizures (TRENdS) study. *Epilepsia.* 2013;54 Suppl 6:84–88.
43. ClinicalTrials.gov. Study to evaluate SAGE-547 as adjunctive therapy for the treatment of super-refractory status epilepticus (SRSE). https://clinicaltrials.gov/ct2/show/NCT02052739?term=sage+547&rank=3. Cited December 26, 2014.
44. Kraft GH. Evoked potentials in multiple sclerosis. *Phys Med Rehabil Clin N Ame.* 2013;24(4):717–720.
45. Fernández O. Integrating the tools for an individualized prognosis in multiple sclerosis. *J Neurol Sci.* 2013;331(1–2):10–13.
46. ClinicalTrials.gov. 215ON201 BIB033 in acute optic neuritis (AON) (RENEW). https://clinicaltrials.gov/ct2/show/NCT01721161?term=lingo&rank=1. Cited December 26, 2014.
47. Ziemann U, Reis J, Schwenkreis P, et al. TMS and drugs revisited 2014. *Clin Neurophysiol.* 2014; pii: S1388-2457(14)00837-2.
48. Emerson RG, Husain AM. Blurring of local and remote practice models threatens IOM's future. *Neurology.* 2013;80(12):1076–1077.
49. Penz K. Medicare cuts impact access to care. http://www.aanem.org/About-Us/News/Reimbursement-Cuts-Impact-Access-to-Care.aspx. Cited December 26, 2014.
50. ASET. Competencies. http://www.aset.org/i4a/pages/index.cfm?pageid=3612. Cited December 26, 2014.

Index